Cancer Biomarkers and Targets in Digestive Organs

Cancer Biomarkers and Targets in Digestive Organs

Special Issue Editors

Nelson S. Yee
Nikki P. Lee

MDPI • Basel • Beijing • Wuhan • Barcelona • Belgrade

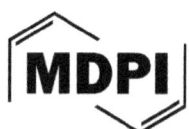

Special Issue Editors
Nelson S. Yee
Penn State Cancer Institute
USA

Nikki P. Lee
Department of Surgery,
The University of Hong Kong
China

Editorial Office
MDPI
St. Alban-Anlage 66
4052 Basel, Switzerland

This is a reprint of articles from the Special Issue published online in the open access journal *Biomedicines* (ISSN 2227-9059) from 2017 to 2019 (available at: https://www.mdpi.com/journal/biomedicines/special_issues/organs).

For citation purposes, cite each article independently as indicated on the article page online and as indicated below:

LastName, A.A.; LastName, B.B.; LastName, C.C. Article Title. *Journal Name* **Year**, *Article Number*, Page Range.

ISBN 978-3-03921-463-1 (Pbk)
ISBN 978-3-03921-464-8 (PDF)

© 2019 by the authors. Articles in this book are Open Access and distributed under the Creative Commons Attribution (CC BY) license, which allows users to download, copy and build upon published articles, as long as the author and publisher are properly credited, which ensures maximum dissemination and a wider impact of our publications.

The book as a whole is distributed by MDPI under the terms and conditions of the Creative Commons license CC BY-NC-ND.

Contents

About the Special Issue Editors vii

Nelson S. Yee and Nikki P. Lee
Special Issue: Cancer Biomarkers and Targets in Digestive Organs
Reprinted from: *Biomedicines* **2019**, 7, 3, doi:10.3390/biomedicines7010003 1

Yue Zhang, Kevin Zarrabi, Wei Hou, Stefan Madajewicz, Minsig Choi, Stanley Zucker and Wen-Tien Chen
Assessing Clinical Outcomes in Colorectal Cancer with Assays for Invasive Circulating Tumor Cells
Reprinted from: *Biomedicines* **2018**, 6, 69, doi:10.3390/biomedicines6020069 5

Nikki P. Lee, Haiyang Wu, Kevin T.P. Ng, Ruibang Luo, Tak-Wah Lam, Chung-Mau Lo and Kwan Man
Transcriptome Analysis of Acute Phase Liver Graft Injury in Liver Transplantation
Reprinted from: *Biomedicines* **2018**, 6, 41, doi:10.3390/biomedicines6020041 17

Jiajia Zhang, Shafat Quadri, Christopher L. Wolfgang and Lei Zheng
New Development of Biomarkers for Gastrointestinal Cancers: From Neoplastic Cells to Tumor Microenvironment
Reprinted from: *Biomedicines* **2018**, 6, 87, doi:10.3390/biomedicines6030087 26

Gail L. Matters and John F. Harms
Utilizing Peptide Ligand GPCRs to Image and Treat Pancreatic Cancer
Reprinted from: *Biomedicines* **2018**, 6, 65, doi:10.3390/biomedicines6020065 44

Lionel Kankeu Fonkoua and Nelson S. Yee
Molecular Characterization of Gastric Carcinoma: Therapeutic Implications for Biomarkers and Targets
Reprinted from: *Biomedicines* **2018**, 6, 32, doi:10.3390/biomedicines6010032 55

Leila Tchelebi, Nicholas Zaorsky and Heath Mackley
Stereotactic Body Radiation Therapy in the Management of Upper GI Malignancies
Reprinted from: *Biomedicines* **2018**, 6, 7, doi:10.3390/biomedicines6010007 69

Jeng-Wei Lu, Yi-Jung Ho, Shih-Ci Ciou and Zhiyuan Gong
Innovative Disease Model: Zebrafish as an In Vivo Platform for Intestinal Disorder and Tumors
Reprinted from: *Biomedicines* **2017**, 5, 58, doi:10.3390/biomedicines5040058 79

Nelson S. Yee, Eugene J. Lengerich, Kathryn H. Schmitz, Jennifer L. Maranki, Niraj J. Gusani, Leila Tchelebi, Heath B. Mackley, Karen L. Krok, Maria J. Baker, Claire de Boer and Julian D. Yee
Frontiers in Gastrointestinal Oncology: Advances in Multi-Disciplinary Patient Care
Reprinted from: *Biomedicines* **2018**, 6, 64, doi:10.3390/biomedicines6020064 96

Kristine Posadas, Anita Ankola, Zhaohai Yang and Nelson S. Yee
Tumor Molecular Profiling for an Individualized Approach to the Treatment of Hepatocellular Carcinoma: A Patient Case Study
Reprinted from: *Biomedicines* **2018**, 6, 46, doi:10.3390/biomedicines6020046 112

Nelson S. Yee
Update in Systemic and Targeted Therapies in Gastrointestinal Oncology
Reprinted from: *Biomedicines* **2019**, *6*, 34, doi:10.3390/biomedicines6010034 . . . . **123**

About the Special Issue Editors

Nelson S. Yee is the team leader of gastrointestinal oncology at Penn State Cancer Institute and Penn State Health Milton S. Hershey Medical Center and an associate professor of medicine at Penn State College of Medicine. As a board-certified medical oncologist, Dr. Yee specializes in diagnosing and treating patients with cancer in various digestive organs, including the pancreas, biliary tract, liver, and gastrointestinal tract and colon. As the principal investigator of clinical studies targeting malignant diseases of the digestive system, Dr. Yee develops new therapies, predictive biomarkers, and therapeutic targets. He has published numerous research articles, reviews, case reports, editorials, commentaries and book chapters and presented at research conferences in China, Hong Kong, Macao, Germany and the U.S. Additionally, he is an invited reviewer of grant applications for funding organizations around the globe. After completing dual Bachelor of Science degrees in pharmacy and chemistry at Massachusetts College of Pharmacy, Dr. Yee earned Doctor of Medicine and Doctor of Philosophy degrees at Weill Cornell Medical College and Memorial Sloan Kettering Cancer Center. At the Hospital of the University of Pennsylvania, he pursued clinical training in internal medicine, hematology and medical oncology. Before joining Penn State College of Medicine, Dr. Yee taught medicine at University of Pennsylvania and University of Iowa.

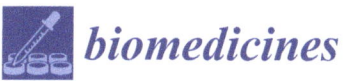

Editorial

Special Issue: Cancer Biomarkers and Targets in Digestive Organs

Nelson S. Yee [1],* and Nikki P. Lee [2]

1. Division of Hematology-Oncology, Department of Medicine, Penn State Health Milton S. Hershey Medical Center, Experimental Therapeutics Program, Penn State Cancer Institute, The Pennsylvania State University College of Medicine, Hershey, PA 17033, USA
2. Department of Surgery, The University of Hong Kong, Hong Kong, China; nikkilee@hku.hk
* Correspondence: nyee@pennstatehealth.psu.edu; Tel.: +1-717-531-0003

Received: 29 November 2018; Accepted: 27 December 2018; Published: 2 January 2019

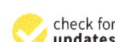

1. Introduction

The identification and development of cancer biomarkers and targets have greatly accelerated progress towards precision medicine in oncology. Studies of tumor biology have not only provided insights into the mechanisms underlying carcinogenesis, but have also led to discovery of molecules that have been developed into cancer biomarkers and targets. Multi-platforms for molecular characterization of tumors and blood-based biopsies have greatly expanded the portfolio of potential biomarkers and targets. These cancer biomarkers have been developed for diagnosis, early detection, prognosis, and prediction of treatment response. The molecular targets have been exploited for anti-cancer therapy with proven benefits in improving treatment response and survival. However, plenty of research opportunity exists for discovering, developing, and validating cancer biomarkers and targets for improving the clinical outcomes of patients with malignant diseases, particularly those in the digestive system.

2. Cancer Biomarkers and Targets in Digestive System

Pancreatic-hepato-biliary and gastrointestinal carcinoma are among the most lethal human malignant diseases [1]. With the advance in developing tumor biomarkers and targets, progress has been made to improve treatment response and survival for patients with cancer of the digestive system [2–7]. In clinical practice, a few biomarkers and targets have been utilized for patients with cancers of digestive organs. Serum levels of carcinoembryonic antigen (CEA), carbohydrate antigen 19-9 (CA 19-9), and alpha-fetoprotein (AFP) have been clinically used as tumor markers of gastrointestinal and hepato-pancreatic-biliary malignancies [8–10]. Yet the sensitivity and specificity of these biomarkers for disease diagnosis and prognosis are somewhat limited. However, there are several clinically developed predictive biomarkers of treatment response. For instance, the cell-surface human epidermal growth factor receptor 2 (HER2) when amplified or over-expressed, has been targeted for treatment using the anti-HER2 antibody, trastuzumab, with proven survival benefit in gastric carcinoma [11]. Expression of programmed death-ligand 1 (PD-L1) in gastric carcinoma predicts therapeutic responsiveness of the anti-PD-1 antibody, pembrolizumab [12]. Wild-type K-RAS in colorectal carcinoma predicts clinical benefits of the anti-epidermal growth factor receptor antibodies, cetuximab [13] or panitumumab [14]. Deficiency in mismatch repair protein, or a high level of microsatellite instability in colorectal carcinoma, suggest treatment response using anti-PD-1 antibody, pembrolizumab [15], or nivolumab [16]. In recent years, studies have been conducted to explore and develop molecular biomarkers and targets in gastrointestinal cancers. Intense research for clinical translation is ongoing, with the goal of attaining the goal of precision care for patients with cancers in digestive organs.

3. Recent Advances in Gastrointestinal Oncology

This Special Issue of *Biomedicines* comprises a variety of articles about recent advances in the discovery, characterization, translation, and clinical application of cancer biomarkers and targets in the digestive system. These articles include original research, reviews, case studies, and conference papers. At the Multi-Disciplinary Patient Care in Gastrointestinal Oncology conference in Hershey, Pennsylvania, the new frontiers in various aspects of digestive organ cancers were presented [17]. In this meeting report, Yee et al. provide updates and discuss advances in the epidemiology and genetics, diagnostic and screening evaluation, treatment modalities, and supportive care for patients with gastrointestinal cancers. In a critical review, Zhang et al. present new perspectives of the development of biomarkers for gastrointestinal cancers [18]. The biomarkers, including those derived from tumor genome, tumor-associated microenvironment, and liquid biopsies, are discussed. Complementary to the review on biomarkers, Yee presents an up-to-date report of the systemic treatment of gastrointestinal malignancies [19]. In this conference paper, results and implications of the recent clinical trials that investigated the efficacy of chemotherapy, targeted therapeutics, and immunotherapy in pancreatic, gastroesophageal, biliary tract, hepatocellular, and colorectal carcinoma are discussed. In addition to this, Tchelebi et al. provide an overview of the role of stereotactic body radiation therapy (SBRT) in the management of malignant diseases in the upper gastrointestinal tract [20]. Moreover, the emerging data on biomarkers of immunotherapy and SBRT are evaluated, with a focus on pancreatic and hepatocellular carcinoma.

4. Biomarkers and Targets in Cancer of Digestive Organs

A number of articles in this Special Issue examine the biomarkers and targets with a focus on cancer in individual organs, including liver. While liver transplantation is a potentially curative treatment of hepatocellular carcinoma, liver graft injury has been identified as an acute phase event that leads to post-transplant tumor recurrence. Lee et al. examined this acute phase event at the molecular level by transcriptomic analysis of liver grafts from recipients with or without tumor recurrence following liver transplantation [21]. This study reveals the altered genetic expression in liver grafts, and paves the way to identify key molecular pathways that may be involved in post-transplant tumor recurrence. On the other hand, Posadas et al. demonstrate the potential value of tumor molecular profiling for individualized therapy in hepatocellular carcinoma [22]. In this patient case study, the treatment response as determined by progression-free survival appears to correlate with the differential expression of biochemical markers and genetic mutations of the tumors.

Besides hepatocellular carcinoma, several articles focus on cancer biomarkers and targets in the gastrointestinal tract. Fonkoua and Yee present a critical review of the molecular characterization of gastric carcinoma by the Cancer Genome Atlas Research Network, the Asian Cancer Research Group, and tumor molecular profiling through expression analysis and genomic sequencing of tumor DNA [23]. These molecular analyses have generated a number of potential biomarkers and targets that may be translated into clinical use. Moreover, patient cases of gastroesophageal carcinoma are reported to demonstrate survival advantage of molecular profile-based treatment, suggesting the potential value of tumor molecular profiling in guiding selection of therapy tailored to the individual patient. For colorectal carcinoma, Zhang et al. evaluate circulating tumor cells and their expressed genes as biomarkers, along with assessment of the clinical outcomes [24]. Results of this study show that circulating tumor cells and their expression of both endothelial and tumor progenitor cell biomarkers are potential prognostic biomarkers in colorectal cancer. Complementary to clinical investigation in humans, Lu et al. described the zebrafish model to study human intestinal disorders and tumors [25]. In this review article, mutant and transgenic zebrafish as well as xenograft models as an in vivo platform for understanding the pathogenesis of gastrointestinal diseases and for evaluation of anti-cancer drugs are discussed.

Despite advances in developing clinically useful biomarkers and targets in gastrointestinal cancers, relatively little progress has been made for patients with pancreatic carcinoma. While early detection of pancreatic carcinoma is critical for improving patient survival, agents that selectively target pancreatic tumor are expected to enhance therapeutic efficacy. In this Special Issue, Matters and Harms present a detailed review of G protein-coupled receptors, which are key target proteins for drug discovery. They further discuss the potential of GPCRs as biomarkers for tumor imaging and targeted treatment of pancreatic carcinoma [26].

5. Conclusions and Future Perspectives

Research on discovery and development of cancer biomarkers and targets has been steadily progressing. Rigorous investigation for identification and validation of biomarkers and targets in both preclinical models and clinical studies are expected to generate new opportunities for making a positive impact on survival and quality of life in the patients. The articles in this Special Issue provide an update on the frontiers in gastrointestinal oncology, with a focus on biomarkers and targets in cancers of the digestive system. We hope this Special Issue will help stimulate research collaboration on developing strategies for prevention, early detection, diagnosis, and screening of cancers in digestive organs, as well as improving treatment outcomes and psychosocial support in patients with these malignant diseases. In particular, liquid biopsy for cancer biomarkers and targets has been a major focus of research with translation into clinical applications.

Recent advances in plasma-derived extracellular vesicles (EVs) have demonstrated the potential of making a clinically meaningful impact in the field of cancer biomarkers and targets. Analysis of EV-derived molecular markers is complementary to the conventional diagnostic modalities. By application of nano-, micro-, digital-, and microarray-based technologies, multiplex analysis of disease-specific markers is expected to improve the sensitivity and specificity of bodily fluid-based biopsies for diagnosis of cancer. These minimally invasive diagnostic tools that utilize ultra-low sample volume may prove to be economically cost effective for screening of cancer in the high-risk population and even in the general population. In addition to this, increasing evidence has indicated the potential value of blood-based biopsies in combination with tumor molecular profiling for developing predictive biomarkers of treatment response, as well as personalized targets of therapy. Further development, optimization, and clinical validation of these cancer biomarkers and targets will hopefully enable us to attain the goal of precision medicine in cancer of digestive organs.

Funding: This research received no external funding.

Conflicts of Interest: The authors declare no conflict of interest.

References

1. Siegel, R.L.; Miller, K.D.; Jemal, A. Cancer statistics, 2018. *CA Cancer J. Clin.* **2018**, *68*, 7–30. [CrossRef] [PubMed]
2. Yee, N.S. Toward the goal of personalized therapy in pancreatic cancer by targeting the molecular phenotype. *Adv. Exp. Med. Biol.* **2013**, *779*, 91–143. [PubMed]
3. Yee, N.S.; Kazi, A.A.; Yee, R.K. Current systemic treatment and emerging therapeutic strategies in pancreatic adenocarcinoma. *Curr. Clin. Pharmacol.* **2015**, *10*, 256–266. [CrossRef] [PubMed]
4. Marks, E.I.; Yee, N.S. Molecular genetics and targeted therapy in hepatocellular carcinoma. *Curr. Cancer Drug Targets* **2016**, *16*, 53–70. [CrossRef] [PubMed]
5. Ang, C.; Miura, J.T.; Gamblin, T.C.; He, R.; Xiu, J.; Millis, S.Z.; Gatalica, Z.; Reddy, S.K.; Yee, N.S.; Abou-Alfa, G.K. Comprehensive multiform biomarker analysis of 350 hepatocellular carcinomas identifies potential novel therapeutic options. *J. Surg. Oncol.* **2016**, *113*, 55–61. [CrossRef]
6. Marks, E.I.; Yee, N.S. Molecular genetics and targeted therapeutics in biliary tract carcinoma. *World J. Gastroenterol.* **2016**, *22*, 1335–1347. [CrossRef]
7. El-Deiry, W.S.; Vijayvergia, N.; Xiu, J.; Scicchitano, A.; Lim, B.; Yee, N.S.; Harvey, H.A.; Gatalica, Z.; Reddy, S. Molecular profiling of 6892 colorectal cancer samples suggests different possible treatment options specific to metastatic sites. *Cancer Biol. Ther.* **2015**, *16*, 1726–1737. [CrossRef]

8. Arnaud, J.P.; Koehl, C.; Adloff, M. Carcinoembryonic antigen (CEA) in diagnosis and prognosis of colorectal carcinoma. *Dis. Colon Rectum* **1980**, *23*, 141–144. [CrossRef]
9. Pleskow, D.K.; Berger, H.J.; Gyves, J.; Allen, E.; McLean, A.; Podolsky, D.K. Evaluation of a serologic marker, CA 19-9, in the diagnosis of pancreatic cancer. *Ann. Int. Med.* **1989**, *110*, 704–709. [CrossRef]
10. Johnson, P.J. The role of serum alpha-fetoprotein estimation in the diagnosis and management of hepatocellular carcinoma. *Clin. Liver Dis.* **2001**, *5*, 145–159. [CrossRef]
11. Bang, Y.J.; Van Cutsem, E.; Feyerislova, A.; Chung, H.C.; Shen, L.; Sawaki, A.; Lordick, F.; Ohtsu, A.; Omuro, Y.; Satoh, T.; et al. Trastuzumab in combination with chemotherapy versus chemotherapy alone for treatment of HER2-positive advanced gastric or gastro-oesophageal junction cancer (ToGA): A phase 3, open-label, randomised controlled trial. *Lancet* **2010**, *376*, 687–697. [CrossRef]
12. Fuchs, C.S.; Doi, T.; Jang, R.W.; Muro, K.; Satoh, T.; Machado, M.; Sun, W.; Jalal, S.I.; Shah, M.; Metges, J.-P.; et al. Safety and Efficacy of pembrolizumab monotherapy in patients with previously treated advanced gastric and gastroesophageal junction cancer. *JAMA Oncol.* **2018**, *4*, 3180013. [CrossRef] [PubMed]
13. Jonker, D.J.; O'Callaghan, C.J.; Karapetis, C.S.; Zalcberg, J.R.; Tu, D.; Au, H.-J.; Berry, S.R.; Krahn, M.; Price, T.; Simes, R.J.; et al. Cetuximab for the treatment of colorectal cancer. *N. Engl. J. Med.* **2007**, *357*, 2040–2048. [CrossRef] [PubMed]
14. Amado, R.G.; Wolf, M.; Peeters, M.; Van Cutsem, E.; Siena, S.; Freeman, D.J.; Juan, T.; Sikorski, R.; Suggs, S.; Radinsky, R.; et al. Wild-type KRAS is required for panitumumab efficacy in patients with metastatic colorectal cancer. *J. Clin. Oncol.* **2008**, *26*, 1626–1634. [CrossRef] [PubMed]
15. Le, D.T.; Uram, J.N.; Wang, T.; Bartlett, B.R.; Kemberling, H.; Eyring, A.D.; Skora, A.D.; Luber, B.S.; Azad, N.S.; Laheru, D.; et al. PD-1 blockade in tumors with mismatch-repair deficiency. *N. Engl. J. Med.* **2015**, *327*, 2509–2520. [CrossRef] [PubMed]
16. Overman, M.J.; McDermott, R.; Leach, J.L.; Lonardi, S.; Lenz, H.-J.; Morse, M.A.; Desai, J.; Hill, A.; Axelson, M.; Moss, R.A.; et al. Nivolumab in patients with metastatic DNA mismatch repair deficient/microsatellite instability-high colorectal cancer (Checkmate 142): Results of an open-label, multicenter, phase 2 study. *Lancet Oncol.* **2017**, *18*, 1182–1191. [CrossRef]
17. Yee, N.S.; Lengerich, E.J.; Schmitz, K.H.; Maranki, J.L.; Gusani, N.J.; Tchelebi, L.; Mackley, H.B.; Krok, K.L.; Baker, M.J.; de Boer, C.; et al. Frontiers in gastrointestinal oncology: Advances in multi-disciplinary patient care. *Biomedicines* **2018**, *6*, 64. [CrossRef]
18. Zhang, J.; Quadri, S.; Wolfgang, C.L.; Zheng, L. New development of biomarkers for gastrointestinal cancers: From neoplastic cells to tumor microenvironment. *Biomedicines* **2018**, *6*, 87. [CrossRef]
19. Yee, N.S. Update in systemic and targeted therapies in gastrointestinal oncology. *Biomedicines* **2018**, *6*, 34. [CrossRef]
20. Tchelebi, L.; Zaorsky, N.; Mackley, H. Stereotactic body radiation therapy in the management of upper GI malignancies. *Biomedicines* **2018**, *6*, 7. [CrossRef]
21. Lee, N.P.; Wu, H.; Ng, K.T.P.; Luo, R.; Lam, T.-W.; Lo, C.-M.; Man, K. Transcriptome analysis of acute phase liver graft injury in liver transplantation. *Biomedicines* **2018**, *6*, 41. [CrossRef] [PubMed]
22. Posadas, K.; Ankola, A.; Yang, Z.; Yee, N.S. Tumor molecular profiling for an individualized approach to the treatment of hepatocellular carcinoma: A patient case study. *Biomedicines* **2018**, *6*, 46. [CrossRef]
23. Fonkoua, L.K.; Yee, N.S. Molecular characterization of gastric carcinoma: Therapeutic implications for biomarkers and targets. *Biomedicines* **2018**, *6*, 32. [CrossRef]
24. Zhang, Y.; Zarrabi, K.; Hou, W.; Madajewicz, S.; Choi, M.; Zucker, S.; Chen, W.-T. Assessing clinical outcomes in colorectal cancer with assays for invasive circulating tumor cells. *Biomedicines* **2018**, *6*, 69. [CrossRef] [PubMed]
25. Lu, J.-W.; Ho, Y.-J.; Ciou, S.-C.; Gong, Z. Innovative disease model: Zebrafish as an in vivo platform for intestinal disorder and tumors. *Biomedicines* **2018**, *5*, 58. [CrossRef] [PubMed]
26. Matters, G.L.; Harms, J.F. Utilizing peptide ligand GPCRs to image and treat pancreatic cancer. *Biomedicines* **2018**, *6*, 65. [CrossRef] [PubMed]

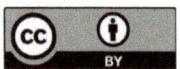

© 2019 by the authors. Licensee MDPI, Basel, Switzerland. This article is an open access article distributed under the terms and conditions of the Creative Commons Attribution (CC BY) license (http://creativecommons.org/licenses/by/4.0/).

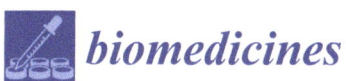

Article

Assessing Clinical Outcomes in Colorectal Cancer with Assays for Invasive Circulating Tumor Cells

Yue Zhang [1,2,*], Kevin Zarrabi [1], Wei Hou [1], Stefan Madajewicz [1,2], Minsig Choi [1,2], Stanley Zucker [1,2,3] and Wen-Tien Chen [1,4]

1. Stony Brook Medicine, Stony Brook, NY 11794, USA; kevin.zarrabi@stonybrookmedicine.edu (K.Z.); wei.hou@stonybrookmedicine.edu (W.H.); stefanmadajewicz@yahoo.com (S.M.); minsig.choi@stonybrookmedicine.edu (M.C.); s_zucker@yahoo.com (S.Z.); wentien@vitatex.com (W.-T.C.)
2. Division of Hematology/Oncology, Department of Medicine, Stony Brook University Hospital, Stony Brook, NY 11794, USA
3. Department of Medicine and Research, Veterans Affairs Medical Center, Northport, NY 11768, USA
4. Vitatex Inc., 25 Health Sciences Drive, Stony Brook, NY 11790, USA
* Correspondence: yue.zhang@stonybrookmedicine.edu

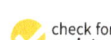

Received: 10 April 2018; Accepted: 1 June 2018; Published: 6 June 2018

Abstract: Colorectal carcinoma (CRC) is the second leading cause of cancer-related mortality. The goals of this study are to evaluate the association between levels of invasive circulating tumor cells (iCTCs) with CRC outcomes and to explore the molecular characteristics of iCTCs. Peripheral blood from 93 patients with Stage I–IV CRC was obtained and assessed for the detection and characterization of iCTCs using a functional collagen-based adhesion matrix (CAM) invasion assay. Patients were followed and assessed for overall survival. Tumor cells isolated by CAM were characterized using cell culture and microarray analyses. Of 93 patients, 88 (95%) had detectable iCTCs, ranging over 0–470 iCTCs/mL. Patients with Stage I–IV disease exhibited median counts of 0.0 iCTCs/mL ($n = 6$), 13.0 iCTCs/mL ($n = 12$), 41.0 iCTCs/mL ($n = 12$), and 133.0 iCTCs/mL ($n = 58$), respectively ($p < 0.001$). Kaplan–Meier curve analysis demonstrated a significant survival benefit in patients with low iCTC counts compared with in patients with high iCTC counts (log-rank $p < 0.001$). Multivariable Cox model analysis revealed that iCTC count was an independent prognostic factor of overall survival ($p = 0.009$). Disease stage ($p = 0.01$, hazard ratio 1.66; 95% confidence interval: 1.12–2.47) and surgical intervention ($p = 0.03$, HR 0.37; 95% CI: 0.15–0.92) were also independent prognostic factors. Gene expression analysis demonstrated the expression of both endothelial and tumor progenitor cell biomarkers in iCTCs. CAM-based invasion assay shows a high detection sensitivity of iCTCs that inversely correlated with overall survival in CRC patients. Functional and gene expression analyses showed the phenotypic mosaics of iCTCs, mimicking the survival capability of circulating endothelial cells in the blood stream.

Keywords: circulating tumor cells; colorectal carcinoma; CAM invasion assay; phenotypic mosaics; tumor progenitor

1. Introduction

Colorectal carcinoma (CRC) is the second leading cause of cancer-related mortality in the United States with an incidence rate of 135,430 new cases and an estimated 50,260 deaths in 2017 [1]. Patients with Stage IV disease have a 5-year survival rate under 10% [2]. Of patients with Stage II or III disease, 25–50% suffer from relapse, likely as a consequence of undetected spread of malignant cells, even after radical surgery and adjuvant therapy [3,4]. A prospective biomarker is needed to better predict disease recurrence, treatment response, and drug resistance, and to better understand the molecular mechanism of tumor cell invasion [5].

Circulating tumor cells (CTCs) have been isolated and have proven prognostic value in CRC patients [6–8]. We have developed a functional collagen-based adhesion matrix (CAM) enrichment assay for identifying CTCs that are positively expressing epithelial markers EpCAM and ESA/CD24 (Epi+), and for detecting the subpopulation that also expresses CAM uptake (CAM+) or invasion marker seprase and stem cell marker CD44, termed invasive CTCs (iCTCs) [9,10]. Detection, enrichment, and clinical utilities have been demonstrated in both metastatic and nonmetastatic cancers of the breast, ovary, and prostate [9–15]. Here, we utilized the CAM invasion assay to detect iCTCs from the blood of patients with colorectal carcinoma. Patients with biopsy-proven colorectal carcinoma were recruited. Peripheral blood samples (2 mL each assay) were collected from patients with Stage I–IV disease and were applied to the CAM system. iCTCs were quantified and the patients were followed with routine clinic exams. Herein, we have shown that iCTCs have prognosticative value in patients with CRC. Specifically, we assess the association between overall survival and the level of iCTCs. This study supports the paradigm that assessment for iCTCs may be utilized by clinicians in identifying individuals with CRC who are at high risk for aggressive disease [16]. Furthermore, we evaluated the clinical significance of iCTCs in patients receiving surgery, chemotherapy, and radiation. Microarray and cell culture analyses further demonstrated the possibility for iCTCs to be potentially used as a prognostic biomarker in CRC patients.

2. Materials and Methods

2.1. Patient and Clinical Samples

This study was performed through Stony Brook University Medical Center and the Department of Veterans Affairs Medical Center, Northport, NY, USA. The study was performed with the approval of the Institutional Review Board and the Committee on Research in Human Subjects (ID code 100593, renewed 7 November 2016). Specimens were collected from 19 October 1999 to 24 November 2015. Patients were followed and monitored for disease recurrence and mortality. The patients were staged according to the American Joint Committee on Cancer TNM system. Samples were obtained via three to twenty milliliter (mL) collections of peripheral blood ($n = 93$). Blood was collected in Vacutainer™ tubes (Becton Dickinson, Franklin Lakes, NJ, USA; green top, lithium heparin as anticoagulant) and processed within four hours of collection. Two milliliter aliquots of blood were employed for quantification of iCTCs. Blood was collected in the clinic and processed in the laboratory according to the workflow below; detailed steps were described in a previous paper [14].

2.2. Clinical Data Collection

All clinical data and end points were collected and documented in a de-identified fashion. All data was entered and stored in a Microsoft Excel worksheet. Data was extracted from the electronic medical record of the patient's medical charts and collected through 1 November 2016. Overall survival length was calculated from the date of blood sample collection to the date of death or most recent documented contact.

2.3. Cell Culture, Identification of CTCs and iCTCs, and Functional Proliferation/Invasion Assays

Cell culture, identification of CTCs and iCTCs, and proliferation/invasion assays using the functional CAM enrichment platform have been described previously [9,14]. Briefly, nuclear cells from 2 mL whole blood aliquots were seeded onto one well of a CAM-coated 6-well plate (Vita-Assay™, Vitatex Inc., Stony Brook, NY, USA) with the complete cell culture (CCC) medium and incubated in a CO_2 incubator for 12–18 h for capture of CTCs, iCTCs, and approximately 0.1% leukocytes, collectively called CAM-avid cells. Using the experimental tumor-cell-spiked-in blood, the Vita-Assay™ enrichment platform functionally captured and enriched (up to one-million-fold) 98% of tumor cells spiked in blood—CTCs—with 0.01–1.0% purity (most co-isolating cells were leukocytes). Furthermore, the platform exhibited the unique advantage that CAM-avid cells could be identified as iCTCs after subsequent ingestion of fluorescent CAM (CAM+). Since the functional proclivities to degrade and ingest the extracellular matrix are major acquired capabilities of invasive and metastatic cells, CAM+ cells represent a unique way to identify iCTCs.

To culture iCTCs ex vivo, old media and nonadherent cells in the same plate were removed and replaced with fresh media every three days for continued culture. Proliferative and differentiative activities of iCTCs were determined by their capability to duplicate and form stem-cell-like colonies and epithelial morphology.

To identify CTCs and iCTCs, cells adhered on CAM-coated plates were collected, fixed, and stained for microscopy using anti-hematopoietic lineage (HL) antibody against CD45 (clone T29/33, DakoCytomation, Carpinteria, CA, USA); anti-epithelial pan-cytokeratins 4, 5, 6, 8, 10, 13, and 18 (CK) (clone C11, Sigma, St. Louis, MO, USA); or anti-endothelial CD31 (Clone JC/70A, NeoMarkers, Fremont, CA, USA); this was followed by red or blue color alkaline-phosphatase-anti-alkaline-phosphatase (APAAP) secondary antibodies (DakoCytomation), then by staining with fluorescein isothiocyanate (FITC)- or tetramethylrhodamine (TRITC)-conjugated anti-tumor progenitor (TP) antibodies (anti-CD44 and anti-seprase, Vitatex) or anti-epithelia (EPI) antibodies (ESA clone B29.1, Biomeda; EPCAM clone Ber-Ep4). Stained cells in suspension were mounted using a Cytospin device (StatSpin cytofuge and Filter Concentrators). Microscopic analyses were performed on a Nikon Eclipse E400 inverted fluorescence microscope equipped with a Microfire digital camera system and Image Pro Plus software. EPI + CD45- cells were identified as CTCs; EPI + CD45-CAM+ or TP+ cells were iCTCs. Microscopic counting of cells was performed by trained personnel and confirmed by a second observer.

The invasive activity of iCTCs was determined by the CAM uptake assay using fluorescently labeled CAM-coated 6-well plates, as described [14]. Cells exhibiting CAM uptake (CAM+) were identified as a functional label for iCTCs. To demonstrate the acquired endothelial function by iCTCs, CAM-adherent cells were incubated with fluorescein-acetylated low-density lipoprotein (acLDL, Invitrogen, Carlsbad, CA, USA) at 37 °C in a CO_2 incubator for three hours. Cells exhibiting acLDL uptake were identified as either circulating endothelial cells or iCTCs in CRC blood (Figure 1).

2.4. Microarray Data Analysis

CAM-adherent cells that were directly isolated from 1 mL of whole blood using a CAM-coated tube (Vita-Cap™, Vitatex Inc., Stony Brook, NY, USA) were used in DNA microarray analysis, as described [9]. Briefly, generation of cRNA, labeling, hybridization, and scanning of the Affymetrix high-density oligonucleotide microarray HG_U133_Plus_2 chip (containing 54,675 gene probes) were performed according to the manufacturer's specifications (Affymetrix, Santa Clara, CA, USA). Analysis of each chip was performed using the Affymetrix Microarray Suite 5.1 Software to generate raw expression data. GeneSpring 7.2 software (Silicon Genetics, Redwood City, CA, USA) was used to assist in the statistical analysis and the selection of genes specific for CAM-enriched circulating cells.

2.5. Statistical Analysis

Patient data was stratified as continuous or categorical variables. Continuous variables, such as patient age and iCTC counts, were analyzed by way of medians, means, and standard errors. Due to the fact the data distribution was not normal, nonparametric statistics (Kruskal–Wallis test for multiple groups and Mann–Whitney U test for two groups) were employed. Categorical variables, such as patient gender, race, disease stage, and history of chemotherapy/radiation therapy/surgery were listed as frequencies and percentages. Categorical data was analyzed with chi-square tests.

Effects of iCTC counts on overall survival were evaluated using the Cox proportional hazards models. For multivariable analyses, iCTC and other characteristics (e.g., gender, race, chemotherapy, stage, surgery, and radiation) and their interactions were all included in the Cox model. For univariable analyses, iCTC counts were included as a sole predictor in the Cox model. To determine an optimal cutoff point of iCTCs, which can best differentiate the survival curve by high- and low-iCTC groups, the Cox model was fitted iteratively using all possible cutoff points. The cutoff point with the best model fitting index akaike information criterion (AIC) (lowest value) was selected as the optimal point. The patients were categorized into the high- and low-iCTC groups using the optimal cutoff point. The survival curve for each group was estimated using the Kaplan–Meier method. Log-rank tests were used to assess survival differences between patients who had high iCTC counts versus low iCTC counts. iCTC detection was defined as the presence of at least one detectable iCTC. Results with two-tailed p-values less than 0.05 were considered statistically significant. All analyses were performed using SAS v9.4 (the SAS Institute, Cary, NC, USA).

3. Results

3.1. Patient Characteristics

Ninety-three patients (M/F: 63/30; median age: 62.0 years, range: 35–82 years) with colon and rectal cancers had samples collected and were analyzed in this study. Of the 93 total patients, 88 patients (95%) had detectable iCTCs and iCTC positives correlated with disease status: Stage I, 6 patients (7%); Stage II, 12 patients (14%); Stage III, 12 patients (14%); and Stage IV, 58 patients (65%) (Table 1). A total of 64 (69%) patients were undergoing treatment for tumors in the colon and 29 (31%) for tumors in the rectum. Patients received various treatments: chemotherapy, 71 (81%); surgical resection, 74 (84%); and radiation therapy, 30 (34%). There was no significant correlation between iCTCs and patient gender, race, disease stage, or age.

Table 1. Characteristics by cancer type.

		Total (n = 88 *)
Male		63 (72%)
Race	Caucasian	70 (80%)
	African American	5 (6%)
	Asian	2 (2%)
	Hispanic	3 (3%)
	Unknown	8 (9%)
Stage	1	6 (7%)
	2	12 (14%)
	3	12 (14%)
	4	58 (65%)
Chemotherapy		71 (81%)
Surgery		74 (84%)
Radiation		30 (34%)

Patient baseline clinical–pathological characteristics. * Of 93 total patients, 88 patients had detectable iCTCs.

3.2. Clinical Characteristics of iCTCs: Stage and Survival

A baseline of 5.0 iCTCs/mL was used as a predetermined cutoff for iCTC positivity with readings below 5.0 iCTCs/mL considered undetectable levels (Table 2). Data comparing iCTCs and CTCs were available for 31 patients, in which 38% to 72% of CTCs overlapped with iCTCs. However, CTCs as identified using Epi+ markers were high in patients with benign disease (85%, n = 30), suggesting low specificity. Analyses were performed to establish a correlation between iCTC measurements and clinical staging. Overall, 95% (n = 88) of patients had detectable iCTCs at the time of evaluation. There is a significant correlation between disease stage and iCTCs: 92% (n = 12) of patients with Stage III disease and 97% (n = 58) of patients with Stage IV disease had detectable iCTCs. This is opposed to only 17% (n = 6) and 50% (n = 12) of patients with Stages I and II disease, respectively (Figure 2, p-value < 0.001). Analysis of the median iCTC count as a function of disease stage demonstrated significance (Figure 3; Table 3). Median iCTC counts of 0.0 iCTCs/mL (n = 6), 13.0 iCTCs/mL (n = 12), 41.0 iCTCs/mL (n = 12), and 133.0 iCTCs/mL (n = 58) were observed for Stages I, II, III, and IV disease, respectively (Figure 3; p-value < 0.001); mean iCTC counts of 8.3 iCTCs/mL (n = 6), 35.8 iCTCs/mL (n = 12), 65.9 iCTCs/mL (n = 12), and 144.8 iCTCs/mL (n = 58) were observed for Stages I, II, III, and IV disease, respectively.

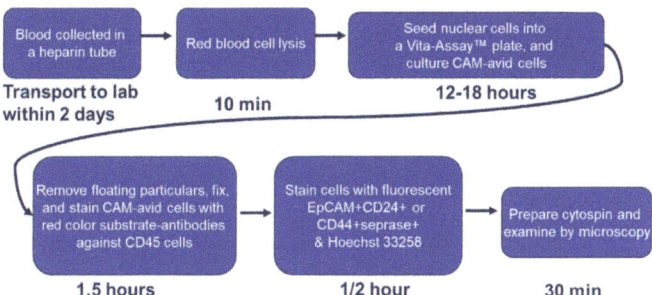

Figure 1. Flow chart representing the procedural steps of invasive circulating tumor cell (iCTC) isolation and quantification.: CAM indicates collagen-based adhesion matrix.

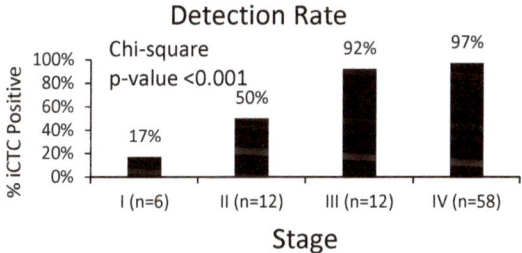

Figure 2. iCTC detection rate by disease stage. Percentage of patients within each stage group and their detectable iCTC rates. iCTC detection varied considerably between Stage III/IV disease and Stage I/II disease (p-value < 0.001).

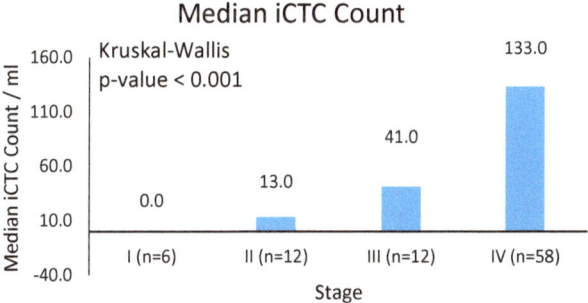

Figure 3. Mean iCTC counts. Median iCTCs by stage with SD. Median iCTC counts differ significantly between Stage IV disease and Stage I–III disease (p-value < 0.001).

Table 2. CTC detectability by stage.

Stage	CTC < 5	CTC ≥ 5	CTC ≥ 5%
I (n = 6)	5	1	17%
II (n = 12)	6	6	50%
III (n = 12)	1	11	92%
IV (n = 58)	2	56	97%

Distribution of iCTC counts over different stage groups.

Table 3. iCTC median, mean and SD.

Stage	iCTC Median	iCTC Mean	iCTC Standard Error
I ($n = 6$)	0.0	8.3	8.3
II ($n = 12$)	13.0	35.8	13.5
III ($n = 12$)	41.0	65.9	23.1
IV ($n = 58$)	133.0	144.8	13.8

Patients were followed to assess the correlation of iCTC counts and patient survival. Mean follow-up time was 71.7 months (range 1.0–143.2 months). At the conclusion of the study, 28% ($n = 26$) of patients were living and 72% of patients ($n = 67$) were deceased. Patients were stratified by an arbitrary cutoff of 30 iCTCs/mL for survival analysis and survival times were compared between patients with high iCTC counts (>30 iCTCs/mL) and low iCTC counts (≤30 iCTCs/mL; lowest AIC = 506.8). A significant decrease in survival time was observed in patients who had iCTC counts greater than 30 iCTCs/mL (Figure 4; log-rank p-value < 0.001). The hazard ratio of survival increases by 5% for every 10 iCTCs/mL (hazard ratio 1.05, 95% CI: 1.03–1.07, $p < 0.001$). When evaluated by cancer type, iCTC counts correlate significantly with survival in colon cancer (hazard ratio: 1.06, 95% CI: 1.03–1.09, $p < 0.0001$) but with a trend toward significance in rectal cancer (hazard ratio: 1.03, 96% CI: 1.00–1.07, $p = 0.06$).

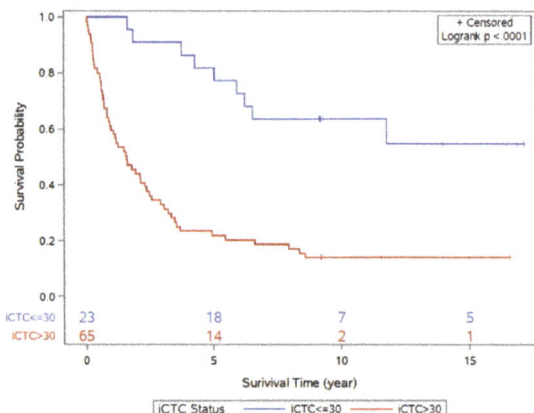

Figure 4. Kaplan–Meier curve analysis for disease outcome according to high-iCTC-count groups and low-iCTC-count groups using optimal iCTC cutoff point (≤30 iCTCs/mL vs. >30 iCTCs/mL). The two survival curves are significantly different (log-rank p-value < 0.001). The red line indicates the high iCTC count group; blue line indicates the low iCTC count group.

A multivariable analysis of the survival data from this patient cohort was performed to establish correlations between iCTC counts and patient characteristics (e.g., cancer type, stage, gender, chemotherapy, surgery, radiation, and age); iCTC counts, stage, and surgical treatment remained significant with adjustments for other covariates (Table 4). These results indicate that iCTC count is an independent prognostic factor for distant metastases (hazard ratio = 1.66, 95% CI: 1.12–2.47, $p = 0.01$). As expected, surgical intervention as assessed by iCTC count was associated with improved outcome (hazard ratio = 0.37, 95% CI: 0.15–0.92, $p = 0.03$). As iCTC counts increase by 10 units, the hazard ratio increases by 4% (Table 4; 95% CI 1.12–2.47, $p = 0.01$). If the disease status increases by one stage, the hazard ratio increases by 66% (95% CI: 1.12–2.47, $p = 0.01$). For patients who had undergone surgery, the hazard ratio is reduced by 63% ($p = 0.03$).

Table 4. Hazard ratio (HR) for stage and surgery.

Factor	Univariable Model		Multivariable Model	
	Hazard Ratio (95% CI)	*p* Value	Hazard Ratio (95% CI)	*p* Value
iCTCs	1.05 (1.03–1.07)	<0.0001	1.04 (1.01–1.06)	0.009
Stage	1.89 (1.37–2.61)	0.0001	1.66 (1.12–2.47)	0.01
Surgery	0.17 (0.08–0.36)	<0.0001	0.37 (0.15–0.92)	0.03

Cox regression multivariate analysis of prognostic factors for colorectal carcinoma.

3.3. Molecular and Functional Phenotyping of iCTCs in CRC Patients

iCTCs represent a subpopulation of CTCs that exhibit the phenotype of a metastasis-initiating cell in blood [17], including proliferation and tumor differentiation, invasion, progenitor cell potency, and survival capability in the blood stream.

To determine the proliferative and functional activities of iCTCs, we captured iCTCs in CRC blood using Vita-Assay™ plates and cultured the cells on the same CAM substrata. We successfully cultured iCTCs for up to four weeks in blood of 56 out of 61 CRC patients (92%), a result similar to those in both metastatic and nonmetastatic cancers of the breast, ovary, and prostate [9–15]. The number and size of cells increased over time in culture, resulting in sizeable colonies within 10 days (Figure 5a) and large-spread cells with epithelial morphology after 20 days (Figure 5a), whereas co-purified hematopoietic cells were observed in reduced number over time (Figure 5a). The growth rate of iCTCs was estimated by counting numbers of cells in colonies formed in Day 5 cultures, which were composed of 16–32 iCTCs, suggesting a doubling time of about 34–42 h for iCTCs. These ex vivo results indicate that the iCTC phenotype includes the ability to propagate and progress to tumor cell morphology.

To examine whether iCTCs surviving in the blood stream acquire the phenotype of circulating endothelial cells, cells captured in the CAM-coated wells were immuno-stained with antibodies against epithelial CK and endothelial CD31, and underwent functional analyses using CAM uptake for invasive tumor cells as described [14] and acLDL uptake for circulating endothelial cells as described [18]. iCTCs showed tumor-cell-like morphology, were CK+ and CD31+, and showed both acLDL and CAM uptakes (Figure 5b). This finding shows that iCTCs acquire the phenotypic characteristics of circulating endothelial cells, such as the expression of the endothelial lineage marker and the endothelial function to adopt for their survival in the blood stream and extravasation.

Based on the assumption that subsets of endothelial cell genes are upregulated in iCTCs, global gene expression profiling of cells isolated by CAM from the blood of healthy subjects and of CRC and breast cancer patients were conducted using Affymetrix HG_U133_Plus_2 chips containing 54,675 gene probes (Figure 6). Genes related to multiple cell lineage–progenitor potency (*DTR, SOX1, FGFR2, NOTCH1, FOLH1, NEUROG2, FLT3LG, TEKT3, CDH5, FLT4, TEK*) and tumor immune response (*DPP4/CD26*) were upregulated in 9 CRC samples and 20 breast cancer samples, but other endothelial genes (*FGF4, SOX2, NRG1, FLT1, CDC2, MCAM, EGFR, FGFR1, BMP1, PECAM1, FGF6, FGF5, VWF*) were not (Figure 5). In addition, four cytokeratin genes (*KRT8, KRT16, KRT17,* and *KRT19*) and eight tumor-associated genes (*TERT, MUC16/M17S2/CA125, CD44, TWIST1, TACSTD1/EpCAM/CD326/ESA/HEA125/GA733, DPP4/CD26, ESR1,* and *PGR*), were upregulated in CRC and breast cancer samples, as described previously [9]. The expression data strongly suggest that iCTCs express a subset of endothelial markers, in addition to their own tumor progenitor markers.

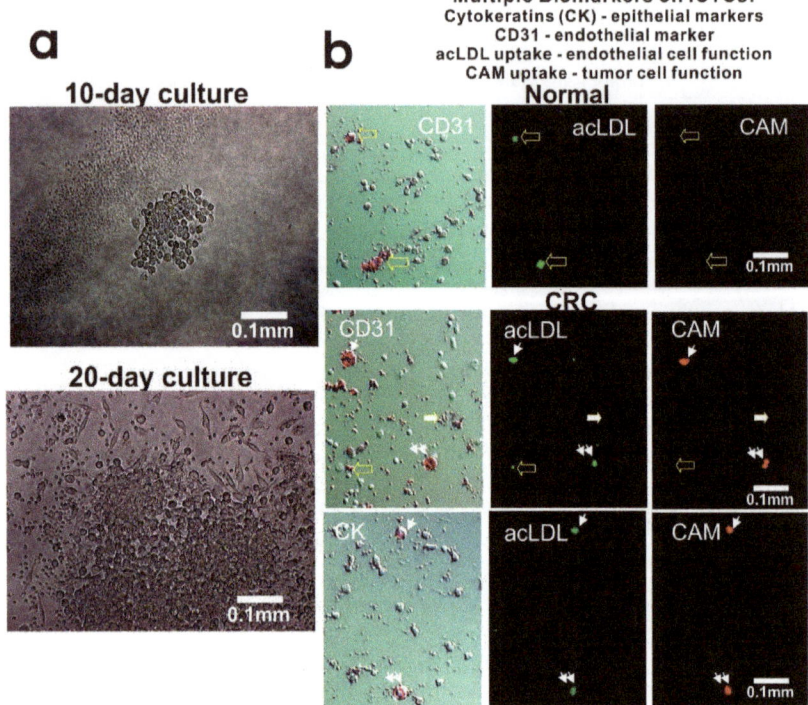

Figure 5. Proliferative and invasive activities and expression of multiple cell lineage markers of iCTCs in blood of CRC patients. (**a**) Proliferation and differentiation of iCTCs into epithelial colonies ex vivo. CAM-enriched cells were cultured on the CAM scaffold for ten days and twenty days. Live cells were photographed under phase contrast microscopy. Tumor cells grew in clusters with large epithelioid cells but hematologic cells (solitary small cells and platelet-like cell fragments seen in the lower image) decreased in number and became not evident; (**b**) iCTCs express epithelial and endothelial biomarkers as well as display epithelial and endothelial functions. Cell multipotency of iCTCs was verified in single cells using expression of epithelial cytokeratins (CK) and endothelial CD31, acLDL uptake of endothelial function, and CAM uptake of tumor progenitor cell function. Background cells that were not labeled with antibody staining were leukocytes and platelets co-isolated with iCTCs. (**Upper**) panel: circulating endothelial cells in normal blood were seen to be CD31+ acLDL uptake+ but CAM uptake−. (**Middle**) panel: iCTCs in blood of a Stage IV CRC patient were seen to show CD31+ acLDL uptake+ CAM uptake+ (indicated by small arrows and double small arrows). However, circulating endothelial cells and platelets were seen to be CD31+ acLDL uptake± CAM uptake− (indicated by large solid and open arrows). (**Lower**) panel: iCTCs in blood of a Stage IV CRC patient were seen to show CK+ acLDL uptake+ CAM uptake+ (indicated by small arrows and double small arrows).

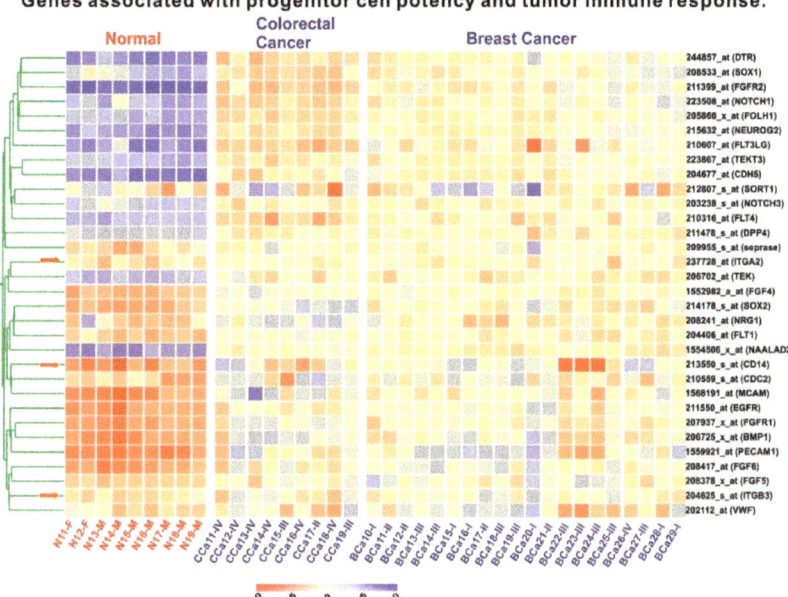

Figure 6. Expression of tumor-progenitor-associated genes in iCTCs isolated by CAM from blood of patients with CRC and breast cancer. Global gene expression profiling of circulating cells isolated by Vita-Cap™ from 9 healthy subjects, 9 CRC patients, and 20 patients with breast cancer. Columns represent catalogues of cell samples analyzed: circulating Normal (N) cells isolated from healthy donors with suffix M for Male and F for Female; CCa are circulating Colorectal Cancer (CCa) cells and BCa are circulating Breast Cancer (BCa) cells with suffixes I–IV being stages of the disease. Colorgram depicts high (red) and low (blue) relative levels of gene expression. Red arrows indicate the three internal control genes that exhibited no difference between normal and cancer cell samples.

4. Discussion

CTCs have been demonstrated to have potential clinical validity in a variety of different cancers [19]. CTC enumeration is a potential method for early detection, treatment monitoring, and response assessment in colorectal cancer patients [20,21]. Unfortunately, the relationship between CTC counts and clinicopathological parameters remains unknown [22]. There is a paucity of data regarding CTC counts and clinical outcomes. It has not been used in clinical practice to date [23].

In this study, we utilized an iCTC detection system, which assesses for CAM adhesive and invasive properties in conjunction with tumor progenitor marker expression in patients with colorectal cancer. We showed that microscopic examination of CAM-avid cells detected iCTCs with a high sensitivity, i.e., 88 of 93 patients (95%) had detectable iCTCs, ranging over 0–470 iCTCs/mL. In addition, we found that patients with Stages I, II, III, and IV disease exhibited median iCTC counts of 0.0 iCTCs/mL, 13.0 iCTCs/mL, 41.0 iCTCs/mL, and 133.0 iCTCs/mL, respectively (p-value < 0.001), suggesting that our iCTC detection method may have the highest sensitivity compared with previous methods [20–23], which detected 1 CTC/7.5 mL blood from fractions of patients with Stage IV disease. A possible explanation for the more than 10-fold detection sensitivity and specific detection in early stages of disease from our method is that CAM is an artificial extracellular matrix mimic that exerts powerful attractive force for solid-tissue-derived cells themselves including CTCs and iCTCs circulating in blood. Other methods rely on devices with specific filtration, microfluidic dynamics, or antibody-coated microcarriers to extract CTCs from whole blood. Other methods, therefore, might miss a portion of CTCs that are small in size, lack specified physical properties, or are low in expression of needed cell surface antigens.

Our data supports the paradigm whereby iCTC count is a promising biomarker with diagnostic and prognostic value. In our cohort of 93 patients, those with advanced disease harbored significantly higher iCTCs. We found that surgical intervention affected iCTCs in colorectal cancer (HR 0.37), in contrast to previous studies that focused on CTC count correlation with chemotherapy [24]. Analysis of our patients revealed a significant survival benefit in those with low iCTC counts. iCTC counts were not significantly associated with gender, age, or race. Due to limitations in sample size, data was not stratified to account for differences in patients with colon or rectal cancers.

CTCs provide a unique source of tumor-derived material for molecular analysis [24]. The majority of the genes identified were involved in cell motility, cell adhesion, chemokine activity, signal transduction, and cell proliferation in a previous study using cDNA from CTCs [25]. We performed global gene expression profiling from the isolated iCTCs and found upregulation of multiple cell lineage–progenitor potency (*DTR, SOX1, FGFR2, NOTCH1, FOLH1, NEUROG2, FLT3LG, TEKT3, CDH5, FLT4, TEK*), tumor immune response (*DPP4/CD26*), cytokeratin genes (*KRT8, KRT16, KRT17,* and *KRT19*), and tumor-associated genes (*TERT, MUC16/M17S2/CA125, CD44, TWIST1, TACSTD1/EpCAM/CD326/ESA/HEA125/GA733, DPP4/CD26, ESR1,* and *PGR*). In this study, gene expression profiling supports the hypothesis that iCTCs are a subpopulation of CTCs that exhibit the phenotype of a metastasis-initiating cell in blood [17], including proliferation and tumor differentiation, invasion, progenitor cell potency, and tumor immune response. This pattern is consistent with a previous report of cDNA from CTCs in CRC using microarray analysis [25].

In this study, the detected iCTC counts correlated with tumor burden and disease staging, suggesting that iCTCs have the potential to be a monitoring and prognostic biomarker in CRC. Also, we have validated use of the CAM method in detection of iCTCs in patients with CRC and provided groundwork for future prospective studies. For example, treatment monitoring for early recurrence of disease has yet to be evaluated using iCTCs in the CRC patient cohort. Pearl et al. has reported that increases in iCTCs predated relapse of epithelial ovarian cancer earlier than cancer antigen 125 (CA-125) monitoring [12]. Wang et al. demonstrated that postoperative detection of CTCs detects disease relapse early while carcinoembryonic antigen (CEA) levels are within normal limits. CTC levels were found to have a six-month lead time over CEA levels with relation to disease recurrence [26]. These studies exemplify the promising role of CTCs as a surrogate tumor marker. However, while the small sample size of 93 patients only in this study allowed for proof-of-principle demonstrations and hypothesis generation of iCTCs in colorectal cancer, a larger cohort study is warranted to determine the prognostic relevance of iCTCs in CRC patients. Moreover, that there are no studies to date investigating a head-to-head comparison between CAM assay and the traditional anti-EpCAM approach, although such studies may be technically challenging [27].

In summary, we provide data on iCTCs enriched through a functional CAM assay in the CRC patient cohort. iCTCs are readily enriched and detectable with the approach. We found that iCTC levels correlate clinically with disease stage and tumor burden, providing promising evidence for the prognosticative value of iCTCs. iCTCs may serve as a surrogate biomarker for colorectal tumors. Further studies are warranted to determine if iCTCs may have a role in early detection of disease recurrence, drug response testing, and genomic studies. Our findings highlight the clinical significance of iCTCs in CRC and suggest a role for iCTC quantification in disease diagnosis, treatment monitoring, and post-treatment surveillance.

Author Contributions: Y.Z., K.Z., S.M., M.C., S.Z. and W.-T.C., had the initial idea of this manuscript, wrote the manuscript, and conceived the project and supervised all research. W.H. performed the statistical analysis and prepared data presentations. Y.Z., S.M. and S.Z. provided and analyzed clinical data.

Acknowledgments: We thank the patients and clinical research nurses at Stony Brook Medicine and Veterans Affairs Medical Center for participation in this research. We are grateful for the technical assistance of Wei Zheng, Huan Dong, and Qiang Zhao of Vitatex Inc. We are most grateful to Mohammad Hossein Zarrabi who participated in the beginning of this study. This study was supported by SBIR grant R44CA140047 and Contract HHSN261201500011C from the NCI awarded to Vitatex Inc. that holds a subcontract with Stony Brook Medicine.

Conflicts of Interest: According to the policy, the five authors (Y.Z., K.Z., W.H., S.M. and S.Z.) do not have any relevant financial relationship with a commercial interest. The reported study was performed at Stony Brook Medicine, as NCI-funded, SBIR collaborative projects between Vitatex Inc. and SUNY Stony Brook. W.-T.C. has significant equity holdings or similar interests in the licensee Vitatex Inc. from SUNY Stony Brook for technology described in this presentation. W.-T.C. is the inventor of patents for the Cell Adhesion Matrix (CAM) technology used in this study.

Abbreviations

Progression-free survival	PFS
Overall survival	OS
Colorectal carcinoma	CRC
Circulating tumor cells	CTCs
Epithelial cell adhesion molecule	EpCAM
Collagen adhesion matrix	CAM
Epithelial markers	Epi+
Hazard ratio	HR
Confidence interval	CI
Akaike information criterion	AIC
Invasive CTCs	iCTCs
Carcinoembryonic antigen	CEA

References

1. American Cancer Society. *Cancer Facts & Figures*; The Society: Atlanta, GA, USA, 2017.
2. Brenner, H.; Kloor, M.; Pox, C.P. Colorectal cancer. *Lancet* **2014**, *383*, 1490–1502. [CrossRef]
3. Torino, F.; Bonmassar, E.; Bonmassar, L.; De Vecchis, L.; Barnabei, A.; Zuppi, C.; Capoluongo, E.; Aquino, A. Circulating tumor cells in colorectal cancer patients. *Cancer Treat Rev.* **2013**, *39*, 759–772. [CrossRef] [PubMed]
4. Hayashi, M.; Inoue, Y.; Komeda, K.; Shimizu, T.; Asakuma, M.; Hirokawa, F.; Miyamoto, Y.; Okuda, J.; Takeshita, A.; Shibayama, Y.; et al. Clinicopathological analysis of recurrence patterns and prognostic factors for survival after hepatectomy for colorectal liver metastasis. *BMC Surg.* **2010**, *10*, 27. [CrossRef] [PubMed]
5. Fakih, M.G. Metastatic colorectal cancer: Current state and future directions. *J. Clin. Oncol.* **2015**, *33*, 1809–1824. [CrossRef] [PubMed]
6. Hou, J.M.; Krebs, M.; Ward, T.; Sloane, R.; Priest, L.; Hughes, A.; Clack, G.; Ranson, M.; Blackhall, F.; Dive, C. Circulating tumor cells as a window on metastasis biology in lung cancer. *Am. J. Pathol.* **2011**, *178*, 989–996. [CrossRef] [PubMed]
7. Huang, M.Y.; Tsai, H.L.; Huang, J.J.; Wang, J.Y. Clinical Implications and Future Perspectives of Circulating Tumor Cells and Biomarkers in Clinical Outcomes of Colorectal Cancer. *Transl. Oncol.* **2016**, *9*, 340–347. [CrossRef] [PubMed]
8. Sequist, L.V.; Nagrath, S.; Toner, M.; Haber, D.A.; Lynch, T.J. The CTC-chip: An exciting new tool to detect circulating tumor cells in lung cancer patients. *J. Thorac. Oncol.* **2009**, *4*, 281–283. [CrossRef] [PubMed]
9. Lu, J.; Fan, T.; Zhao, Q.; Zeng, W.; Zaslavsky, E.; Chen, J.J.; Frohman, M.A.; Golightly, M.G.; Madajewicz, S.; Chen, W.T. Isolation of circulating epithelial and tumor progenitor cells with an invasive phenotype from breast cancer patients. *Int. J. Cancer* **2010**, *126*, 669–683. [CrossRef] [PubMed]
10. Pearl, M.L.; Zhao, Q.; Yang, J.; Dong, H.; Tulley, S.; Zhang, Q.; Golightly, M.; Zucker, S.; Chen, W.T. Prognostic analysis of invasive circulating tumor cells (iCTCs) in epithelial ovarian cancer. *Gynecol. Oncol.* **2014**, *134*, 581–590. [CrossRef] [PubMed]

11. Fan, T.; Zhao, Q.; Chen, J.J.; Chen, W.T.; Pearl, M.L. Clinical significance of circulating tumor cells detected by an invasion assay in peripheral blood of patients with ovarian cancer. *Gynecol. Oncol.* **2009**, *112*, 185–191. [CrossRef]
12. Pearl, M.L.; Dong, H.; Tulley, S.; Zhao, Q.; Golightly, M.; Zucker, S.; Chen, W.T. Treatment monitoring of patients with epithelial ovarian cancer using invasive circulating tumor cells (iCTCs). *Gynecol. Oncol.* **2015**, *137*, 229–238. [CrossRef] [PubMed]
13. Paris, P.L.; Kobayashi, Y.; Zhao, Q.; Zeng, W.; Sridharan, S.; Fan, T.; Adler, H.L.; Yera, E.R.; Zarrabi, M.H.; Zucker, S.; et al. Functional phenotyping and genotyping of circulating tumor cells from patients with castration resistant prostate cancer. *Cancer Lett.* **2009**, *277*, 164–173. [CrossRef] [PubMed]
14. Tulley, S.; Zhao, Q.; Dong, H.; Pearl, M.L.; Chen, W.T. Vita-Assay (TM) Method of Enrichment and Identification of Circulating Cancer Cells/Circulating Tumor Cells (CTCs). *Methods Mol. Biol.* **2016**, *1406*, 107–119. [PubMed]
15. Friedlander, T.W.; Ngo, V.T.; Dong, H.; Premasekharan, G.; Weinberg, V.; Doty, S.; Zhao, Q.; Gilbert, E.G.; Ryan, C.J.; Chen, W.T.; et al. Detection and characterization of invasive circulating tumor cells derived from men with metastatic castration-resistant prostate cancer. *Int. J. Cancer* **2014**, *134*, 2284–2293. [CrossRef] [PubMed]
16. Tsai, W.S.; Chen, J.S.; Shao, H.J.; Wu, J.C.; Lai, J.M.; Lu, S.H.; Hung, T.F.; Chiu, Y.C.; You, J.F.; Hsieh, P.S.; et al. Circulating Tumor Cell Count Correlates with Colorectal Neoplasm Progression and Is a Prognostic Marker for Distant Metastasis in Non-Metastatic Patients. *Sci. Rep.* **2016**, *6*, 24517. [CrossRef] [PubMed]
17. Alix-Panabieres, C.; Bartkowiak, K.; Pantel, K. Functional studies on circulating and disseminated tumor cells in carcinoma patients. *Mol. Oncol.* **2016**, *10*, 443–449. [CrossRef] [PubMed]
18. Asahara, T.; Murohara, T.; Sullivan, A.; Silver, M.; van der Zee, R.; Li, T.; Witzenbichler, B.; Schatteman, G.; Isner, J.M. Isolation of putative progenitor endothelial cells for angiogenesis. *Science* **1997**, *275*, 964–967. [CrossRef] [PubMed]
19. Micalizzi, D.S.; Haber, D.A.; Maheswaran, S. Cancer metastasis through the prism of epithelial to mesenchymal transition in circulating tumor cells. *Mol. Oncol.* **2017**, *11*, 770–780. [CrossRef] [PubMed]
20. Cohen, S.J.; Punt, C.J.; Iannotti, N.; Saidman, B.H.; Sabbath, K.D.; Gabrail, N.Y.; Picus, J.; Morse, M.; Mitchell, E.; Miller, M.C.; et al. Relationship of circulating tumor cells to tumor response, progression-free survival, and overall survival in patients with metastatic colorectal cancer. *J. Clin. Oncol.* **2008**, *26*, 3213–3221. [CrossRef] [PubMed]
21. Tol, J.; Koopman, M.; Miller, M.C.; Tibbe, A.; Cats, A.; Creemers, G.J.; Vos, A.H.; Nagtegaal, I.D.; Terstappen, L.W.; Punt, C.J. Circulating tumour cells early predict progression-free and overall survival in advanced colorectal cancer patients treated with chemotherapy and targeted agents. *Ann. Oncol.* **2010**, *21*, 1006–1012. [CrossRef] [PubMed]
22. Wu, W.; Zhang, Z.; Gao, X.H.; Shen, Z.; Jing, Y.; Lu, H.; Li, H.; Yang, X.; Cui, X.; Li, Y.; et al. Clinical significance of detecting circulating tumor cells in colorectal cancer using subtraction enrichment and immunostaining-fluorescence in situ hybridization (SE-iFISH). *Oncotarget* **2017**, *8*, 21639–21649. [CrossRef] [PubMed]
23. Cabel, L.; Proudhon, C.; Gortais, H.; Loirat, D.; Coussy, F.; Pierga, J.Y.; Bidard, F.C. Circulating tumor cells: Clinical validity and utility. *Int. J. Clin. Oncol.* **2017**. *22*, 421–430. [CrossRef]
24. León-Mateos, L.; Casas, H.; Abalo, A.; Vieito, M.; Abreu, M.; Anido, U.; Gómez-Tato, A.; López, R.; Abal, M.; Muinelo-Romay, L. Improving circulating tumor cells enumeration and characterization to predict outcome in first line chemotherapy mCRPC patients. *Oncotarget* **2017**, *8*, 54708–54721. [CrossRef] [PubMed]
25. Wang, J.Y.; Yeh, C.S.; Tzou, W.S.; Hsieh, J.S.; Chen, F.M.; Lu, C.Y.; Yu, F.J.; Cheng, T.L.; Huang, T.J.; Lin, S.R. Analysis of progressively overexpressed genes in tumorigenesis of colorectal cancers using cDNA microarray. *Oncol. Rep.* **2005**, *14*, 65–72. [PubMed]
26. Wang, J.Y.; Lin, S.R.; Wu, D.C.; Lu, C.Y.; Yu, F.J.; Hsieh, J.S.; Cheng, T.L.; Koay, L.B.; Uen, Y.H. Multiple molecular markers as predictors of colorectal cancer in patients with normal perioperative serum carcinoembryonic antigen levels. *Clin. Cancer Res.* **2007**, *13*, 2406–2413. [CrossRef] [PubMed]
27. Paterlini-Brechot, P.; Benali, N.L. Circulating tumor cells (CTC) detection: Clinical impact and future directions. *Cancer Lett.* **2007**, *253*, 180–204. [CrossRef] [PubMed]

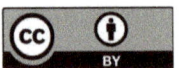 © 2018 by the authors. Licensee MDPI, Basel, Switzerland. This article is an open access article distributed under the terms and conditions of the Creative Commons Attribution (CC BY) license (http://creativecommons.org/licenses/by/4.0/).

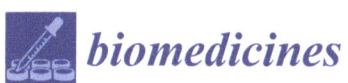

Article

Transcriptome Analysis of Acute Phase Liver Graft Injury in Liver Transplantation

Nikki P. Lee [1,2,*], Haiyang Wu [3], Kevin T.P. Ng [1], Ruibang Luo [3], Tak-Wah Lam [3], Chung-Mau Lo [1,2] and Kwan Man [1,2]

1. Department of Surgery, The University of Hong Kong, Hong Kong, China; ledodes@hku.hk (K.T.P.N.); chungmlo@hkucc.hku.hk (C.-M.L.); kwanman@hku.hk (K.M.)
2. Collaborative Innovation Center for Diagnosis and Treatment of Infectious Diseases, Zhejiang University, Hangzhou 310003, China
3. Department of Computer Science, The University of Hong Kong, Hong Kong, China; repurpledeep@gmail.com (H.W.); rbluo2@hku.hk (R.L.); twlam@cs.hku.hk (T.-W.L.)
* Correspondence: nikkilee@hku.hk; Tel: +852-3917-9652; Fax: +852-3917-9634

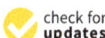

Received: 22 December 2017; Accepted: 5 April 2018; Published: 6 April 2018

Abstract: Background: Liver transplantation remains the treatment of choice for a selected group of hepatocellular carcinoma (HCC) patients. However, the long-term benefit is greatly hampered by post-transplant HCC recurrence. Our previous studies have identified liver graft injury as an acute phase event leading to post-transplant tumor recurrence. Methods: To re-examine this acute phase event at the molecular level and in an unbiased way, RNA sequencing (RNA-Seq) was performed on liver graft biopsies obtained from the transplant recipients two hours after portal vein reperfusion with an aim to capture frequently altered pathways that account for post-transplant tumor recurrence. Liver grafts from recurrent recipients (n = 6) were sequenced and compared with those from recipients without recurrence (n = 5). Results: RNA expression profiles comparison pointed to several frequently altered pathways, among which pathways related to cell adhesion molecules were the most involved. Subsequent validation using quantitative polymerase chain reaction confirmed the differential involvement of two cell adhesion molecules *HFE* (hemochromatosis) and *CD274* and their related molecules in the acute phase event. Conclusion: This whole transcriptome strategy unravels the molecular landscape of liver graft gene expression alterations, which can identify key pathways and genes that are involved in acute phase liver graft injury that may lead to post-transplant tumor recurrence.

Keywords: Liver transplantation; liver graft injury; intragraft gene expression profiles; cell adhesion molecules; *CD274*; *HFE*

---

1. Introduction

Hepatocellular carcinoma (HCC) is a clinically challenging liver malignancy with a nearly equal worldwide incidence and death. Among various treatments, liver transplant results in a favorable survival in a well selected patient subgroup [1]. However, this treatment unavoidably accompanies ischemia and reperfusion injury that can trigger acute phase graft injury, or even rejection [2]. Acute phase liver graft injury is a hallmark event leading to late phase HCC recurrence in liver transplantation. Our previous studies using a liver transplant animal model have revealed a deregulation of signaling pathways related to inflammation, invasion and migration in the acute phase event and their associations with late phase tumor recurrence [3,4]. Besides, various molecules, e.g., CXCL10 (C-X-C motif chemokine ligand 10), and certain cells, e.g., endothelial progenitor cells, were found capable of promoting tumor recurrence after liver transplantation in studies using relevant animal models and clinical specimens [5,6].

These studies have unequivocally demonstrated that acute phase liver graft injury is an early event leading to post-transplant tumor recurrence. A better understanding of the acute phase event is important for developing new or prophylactic treatments for post-transplant tumor recurrence.

Despite the efforts that have been devoted to the study of acute phase liver graft injury and late phase HCC recurrence in liver transplantation, the molecular mechanisms underlying these events were not fully uncovered. Here, we revisited this theme by using RNA sequencing to capture intragraft gene expression changes in acute phase liver graft injury that account for post-transplant tumor recurrence, for which some of them are known for their effects on recipient outcomes. In a liver transplant animal study, cDNA microarray results revealed a number of genes, especially those inflammatory genes, were up-regulated in liver grafts that are more prone to develop tumors [4]. On the other hand, certain genes, such as *GPx3* (glutathione peroxidase 3), experienced down-regulation [7]. Apart from the above effects, intragraft gene expression changes can also influence other post-transplant outcomes, such as graft rejection. A preferential expression of genes related to signal transduction, inflammation, and immune response was detected in liver grafts undergoing acute cellular rejection, which is a common situation leading to graft loss in a specific recipient group [8]. Overall, these prior studies have put forth the importance of studying intragraft gene expression patterns in acute phase liver graft injury and their correlation with post-transplant outcomes. The derived results can enhance the understanding of acute phase liver graft injury, for which the knowledge can improve patient management in terms of risk stratification, prophylaxis and treatment of post-transplant tumor recurrence. Our long-term goal is to improve the recipient outcomes after liver transplantation.

2. Experimental Section

2.1. Clinical specimens

HCC patients that were included in this study received their liver transplant in Queen Mary Hospital, Pokfulam, Hong Kong (March 2004 to April 2010). Written patient consents were obtained. The last follow-up date was September 2013. The clinicopathological information between HCC patients with and without HCC recurrence after liver transplantation including sex, age, type of liver transplant, Milan criteria, vascular permeation, HBsAg before liver transplantation, new TNM stage, AST level (24 h after liver transplantation), and ALT level (24 h after liver transplantation) were listed in Supplementary Table S1. Among them, both the AST and ALT level in recurrence group were significantly higher than the non-recurrence group (Supplementary Table S1). The recurrence period and recurrence sites are listed in Supplementary Table S2. Liver graft biopsies collected 2 h after portal vein reperfusion during liver transplantation were frozen immediately and stored at −80 °C. The use of clinical specimens for research was approved by the Institutional Review Board of The University of Hong Kong/Hospital Authority Hong Kong West Cluster (HKU/HA HKW IRB).

2.2. RNA sequencing (RNA-Seq) and data processing

RNA-Seq was performed on liver grafts from recipients with (n = 6) or without (n = 5) post-transplant HCC recurrence. The 5 patients without post-transplant HCC recurrence are patients treated with deceased donor liver transplant (DDLT). Total RNA was extracted from liver grafts using TRIzol reagent (Life Technologies, Waltham, MA, USA) as before [9,10]. RNA quality was analyzed in an Agilent 2100 Bioanalyzer (Agilent Technologies, Santa Clara, CA, USA). RNA sequencing was performed in a HiSeq 2500 System sequencer (Illumina, San Diego, CA, USA) in BGI, Hong Kong. A total of eight billion bases of sequencing data (quality control passed) was produced. The data were preprocessed using cutadapt version 1.1 to remove sequencing adapters. Then the data were mapped to the human reference genome GRCh37 (hg19) using aligner BWA version 0.6.2 with default options and then converted into BAM file format using SAMtools version 0.1.19. The gene expression level of each sample was calculated using the method introduced by Mortazavi et al. [11]. More specifically, the gene expression level difference between any given two samples was gauged by the number of sequencing data mapped to the gene, RPKM (reads per kilobase per million mapped reads). Each recurrence sample was compared to each non-recurrence sample to identify the up-regulated and down-regulated genes (Figure 1), together with their expression ratios. Using this method, a total of 30 differentially expressed gene lists were generated, which were then merged. Genes with inconsistent expression changes were removed. An average expression difference for each gene was calculated.

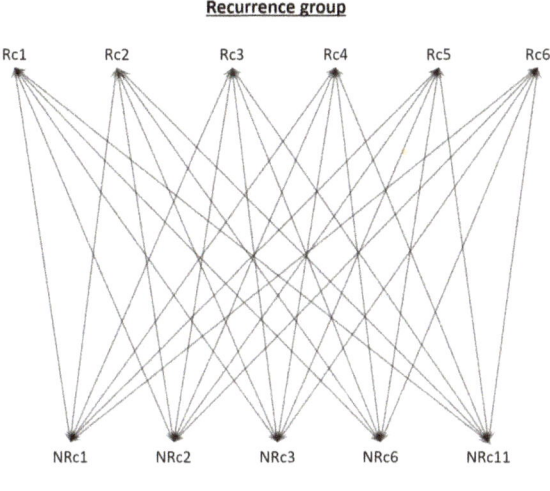

Figure 1. RNA-Seq data comparison method. RNA-Seq data of liver grafts from recipients with (n = 6) or without (n = 5) post-transplant hepatocellular carcinoma (HCC) recurrence was individually compared to identify differentially expressed genes, for which this result was used to map the frequently altered pathways. Rc, recurrence; NRc, non-recurrence.

2.3. Bioinformatics analyses

Pathway enrichment analyses were performed using Kyoto Encyclopedia of Genes and Genomes (KEGG) and Gene Ontology (GO). STRING database (http://string-db.org, version 9) was used to find related molecules for the candidate genes [12]. High confidence level at 0.700 was used.

2.4. Reverse transcription-quantitative polymerase chain reaction (RT-qPCR)

RT-qPCR was performed, as described [9,10]. Total RNA from liver graft biopsies were extracted as above. Reverse transcription was performed using High-Capacity cDNA Reverse Transcription kit (Applied Biosystems, Foster City, CA, USA). qPCR was performed using Power SYBR Green PCR Master Mix (Applied Biosystems) and gene-specific primers (Supplementary Table S3). *β-Actin* expression was used as an internal normalization control. The relative expression level of each gene in each sample was normalized with the average expression level in healthy donor livers using $2^{-\Delta\Delta Ct}$ method [13].

2.5. Statistical analyses

Continuous variables were compared by *t*-test or Mann-Whitney *U* test. The categorical variables were compared by chi-square Fisher's test. Gene expression level correlation was analyzed by Pearson correlation analysis. $p < 0.05$ was considered statistically significant.

3. Results

3.1. Cell adhesion molecules-related pathways in acute phase liver graft injury

Eleven sets of RNA-Seq data of liver grafts from recipients with (n = 6) or without (n = 5) post-transplant HCC recurrence were subjected to pathway enrichment analyses based on the use of differentially expressed genes between these two recipient groups. The top five pathways frequently altered in our studied condition are those related to steroid hormone biosynthesis, retinol metabolism, metabolism of xenobiotics by cytochrome P450, drug metabolism by cytochrome P450, and finally, cell adhesion molecules (Supplementary Table S4). Among these pathways, we focused on pathways related to cell adhesion molecules for further study, not only because of their diversified roles in liver tumorigenesis, but also because of their expression in immune cells important for post-transplant tumor recurrence [14–16].

3.2. HFE and CD274 are two cell adhesion molecules with differential involvement in acute phase liver graft injury

Cell adhesion molecules represent a broad class of membrane-associated molecules with diversified functions in pathophysiological processes, ranging from cell adhesion, inflammation, tissue injury, to tumorigenesis. In this category, seventy-five genes were differentially expressed in liver grafts in the recurrence group compared to the non-recurrence group (Supplementary Table S5), implicating their involvement in post-transplant HCC recurrence. Six genes with more than two-fold expression level difference between these two groups, i.e., *ITGA8, SELE, HFE, CDH26, HLA-DQA2*, and *CD274* (Figure 2 and highlighted in Supplementary Table S5), were subjected to RT-qPCR validation in a sample set of seven recurrences and seven non-recurrences. Among the four genes down-regulated in recurrence samples (*ITGA8, SELE, HFE,* and *CDH26*), only *HFE* maintained its down-regulation (Figure 3). The *CDH26* validation result was not shown due to its nearly undetectable expression level in our current experimental setting. For the two genes up-regulated in recurrence samples (*HLA-DQA2* and *CD274*), an up-regulation of *CD274* was maintained (Figure 4). No validation experiment was performed on *HLA-DQA2* due to its ubiquitous nature.

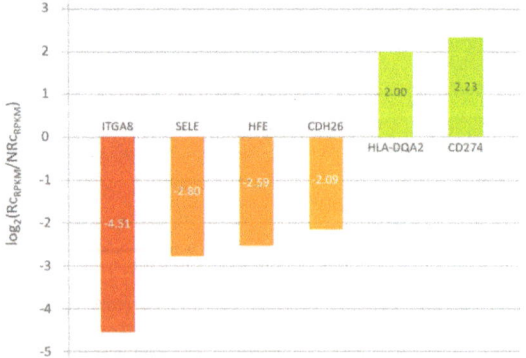

Figure 2. RNA-Seq result shows cell adhesion molecules that had more than two-fold gene expression level difference between recurrence and non-recurrence samples in acutely injured liver grafts. Six cell adhesion molecules with intragraft gene expression level difference of more than two-fold when recurrence samples were compared to non-recurrence ones. Four molecules (*ITGA8, SELE, HFE,* and *CDH26*) have been down-regulated in recurrence samples, whereas two molecules (*HLA-DQA2* and *CD274*) were found to have been up-regulated.

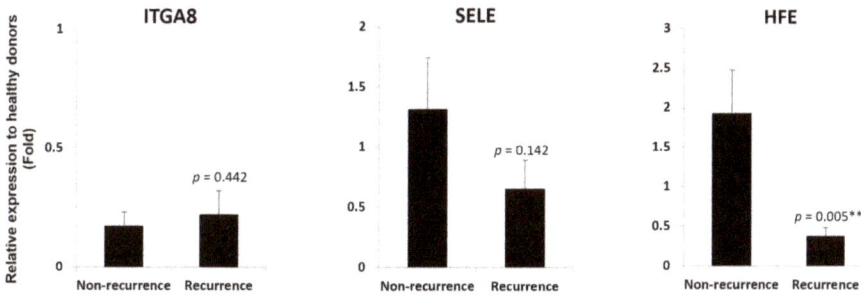

Figure 3. *HFE* down-regulation in liver grafts from recipients with post-transplant HCC recurrence. RT-qPCR result demonstrated a down-regulation of *HFE*, but not *ITGA8* and *SELE*, in liver grafts from recipients with post-transplant HCC recurrence. ** $p < 0.01$.

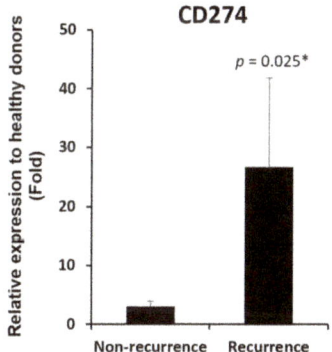

Figure 4. *CD274* up-regulation in liver grafts from recipients with post-transplant HCC recurrence. RT-qPCR result demonstrated an up-regulation of *CD274* in liver grafts from recipients with post-transplant HCC recurrence. * $p < 0.05$.

3.3. HFE- and CD274-related molecules in acutely injured liver grafts

STRING database result revealed four *HFE*-related molecules (*B2M*, *TF*, *TFR2*, and *TFRC*) (Figure 5A and Supplementary Table S6) and two *CD274*-related molecules (*CD80* and *PDCD1*) (Figure 6A and Supplementary Table S6). Their gene expression level correlation with HFE and CD274 was performed in liver grafts from 43 transplant recipients (6 recurrence and 37 non-recurrence) using RT-qPCR. Among the *HFE*-related molecules, *B2M*, *TF*, and *TFR2*, but not *TFRC*, demonstrated positive gene expression level correlation with *HFE* (Figure 5B). Among the *CD274*-related molecules, *CD80*, but not *PDCD1*, exhibited positive gene expression level correlation with *CD274* (Figure 6B). Collectively, our results revealed that the involvement of *HFE* and *CD274* and their related molecules in acute phase liver graft injury and their concurrent involvement in post-transplant tumor recurrence.

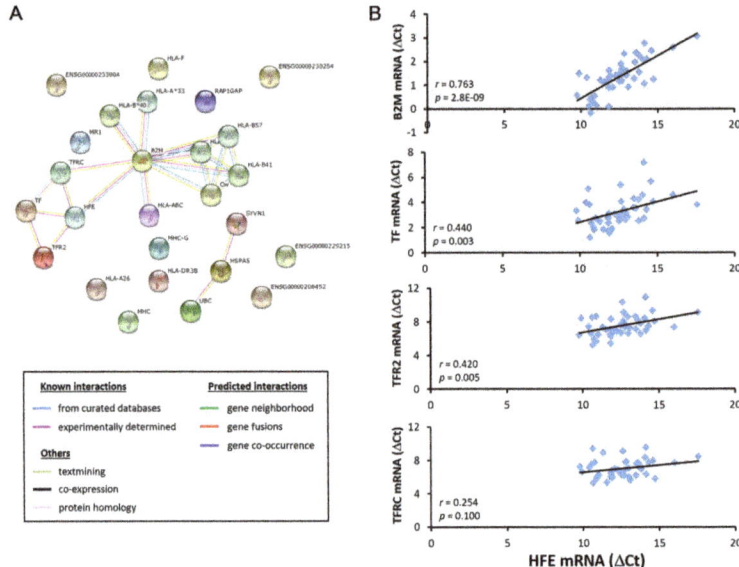

Figure 5. Correlation analysis of *HFE* and its related molecules in liver grafts from transplant recipients. (**A**) Bioinformatics analysis revealed *B2M*, *TF*, *TFR2* and *TFRC* as *HFE*-related molecules; (**B**) Among these molecules, *B2M*, *TF* and *TFR2*, but not *TFRC*, demonstrated a positive gene expression correlation with *HFE* in liver grafts from 43 transplant recipients using RT-qPCR.

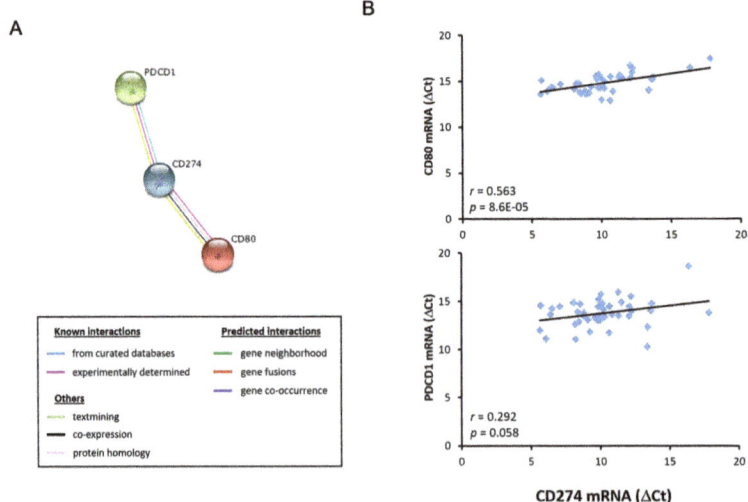

Figure 6. Correlation analysis of *CD274* and its related molecules in liver grafts from transplant recipients. (**A**) Bioinformatics analysis revealed that *CD80* and *PDCD1* were *CD274*-related molecules; (**B**) *CD80*, but not *PDCD1*, demonstrated a positive gene expression correlation with *CD274* in liver grafts from 43 transplant recipients using RT-qPCR.

4. Discussion

Our previous studies have identified that the acute phase liver graft injury is a key event leading to post-transplant HCC recurrence. In this study, we adopted a more comprehensive and unbiased approach using RNA sequencing to analyze differentially expressed genes in this acute phase event, with an aim to identify key players. The sequencing data revealed a subset of cell adhesion molecules differentially expressed in liver grafts from recipients with or without post-transplant tumor recurrence. Cell adhesion molecules belong to a class of cell surface molecules with diversified functions from adhesion, migration, to inflammation [16]. In liver transplantation, inflammation is initiated in the hallmark event of ischemia and reperfusion injury resulting from hepatic surgery. Massive recruitment of immune cells, which express various cell adhesion molecules, takes place during acute phase liver graft injury that can eventually lead to post-transplant tumor recurrence [17]. Certain cell adhesion molecules, e.g., MHC molecules [18], are involved in ischemia and reperfusion liver injury. In addition, our previous studies have demonstrated that certain molecules, e.g., aldose reductase and repressor and activator protein, are capable of regulating hepatic ischemia and reperfusion injury through their effects on inflammation [19,20]. Collectively, our and other findings have exemplified the key roles of cell adhesion molecules in inflammation, ischemia, and reperfusion liver graft injury, as well as post-transplant tumor recurrence. However, due to the small sample size that was used, findings that were derived from this study should be further validated in a separate cohort of large sample size. To minimize variations between patients, we tried to analyze specimens from patients that were selected based on the Milan criteria.

HFE (hemochromatosis) is a cell adhesion molecule that was identified in this study to have down-regulated gene expression level in liver grafts from recipients with post-transplant HCC recurrence. It is an atypical MHC class I molecule with diversified cellular functions, such as iron homeostasis maintenance and immune function regulation [21,22]. Mutation of this gene can lead to iron overload, which is a predisposing factor for HCC [21,23]. Besides, two studies have reported the close link between hepatic iron overload and poor survival of liver transplant recipients [24,25]. In this study, we have also established a positive correlation in the intragraft gene expression of *HFE* and its related molecules (*B2M*/β2-microglobulin, *TF*/transferrin, and *TFR2*/transferrin receptor 2) in liver transplant recipients, for which these molecules are known iron metabolism regulators with close interaction with *HFE* [21,26]. Taken together, it is convincing to believe that *HFE* down-regulation in liver grafts, as observed in this study, can lead to iron overload and eventually post-transplant tumor recurrence.

In contrary to *HFE*, we have demonstrated a high intragraft gene expression level of *CD274* from recipients with post-transplant tumor recurrence. *CD274*, also known as PD-L1, is expressed on immune cells, as well as non-hemopoietic cells [27]. In addition to its general immunoregulatory functions, *CD274* is also involved in tumorigenesis, as reflected by its high expression level in tumor tissues rather than in adjacent non-tumor tissues of various cancers [27,28]. The tumor-related function of *CD274* can also help to explain for its high intragraft gene expression level in transplant recipients with tumor recurrence as observed in this study. The tumor-inducing effect of *CD274* may also involve other immunoregulatory molecules, such as *CD80*, whose intragraft gene expression level correlated positively with *CD274* in transplant recipients as reported here. Like *CD274*, *CD80* is also found on immune cells and is involved in an array of immune pathways [29]. Indeed, both molecules are known to participate in transplantation immunity [30]. In view of these interesting observations from this and other studies, it is plausible that *CD274* may work with its related molecule, e.g., *CD80*, in triggering acute phase liver graft injury and post-transplant tumor recurrence.

Taken together, we have successfully used RNA sequencing to unravel the molecular landscape of acute phase liver graft injury that accounts for post-transplant tumor recurrence. Certain cell adhesion molecules, e.g., *HFE* and *CD274*, were found to have differential roles in our studied condition. These molecules have potential function as a prognostic marker for risk assessment to identify transplant recipients more prone to tumor recurrence and to guide them for prophylactic treatment for prevention. Apart from the preventive measure, the identified molecules can also form a basis for research on new treatment targets.

Supplementary Materials: The following are available online at http://www.mdpi.com/2227-9059/6/2/41/s1.

Author Contributions: Nikki P. Lee, Kevin T.P. Ng, Ruibang Luo, Tak-Wah Lam, Chung-Mau Lo, Kwan Man conceived and designed the experiments; Haiyang Wu, Kevin T.P Ng, Ruibang Luo performed the experiments; Haiyang Wu, Kevin T.P. Ng, Ruibang Luo analyzed the data; Tak-Wah Lam, Chung-Mau Lo, Kwan Man contributed reagents/materials/analysis tools; Nikki P. Lee, Kevin T.P. Ng, Ruibang Luo wrote the paper.

Conflicts of Interest: The authors declare no conflict of interest.

References

1. Lo, C.M. Liver transplantation in 2012: Transplantation for liver cancer—More with better results. *Nat. Rev. Gastroenterol. Hepatol.* **2013**, *10*, 74–76. [CrossRef] [PubMed]
2. Zhai, Y.; Busuttil, R.W.; Kupiec-Weglinski, J.W. Liver ischemia and reperfusion injury: New insights into mechanisms of innate-adaptive immune-mediated tissue inflammation. *Am. J. Transplant.* **2011**, *11*, 1563–1569. [CrossRef] [PubMed]
3. Man, K.; Lo, C.M.; Xiao, J.W.; Ng, K.T.; Sun, B.S.; Ng, I.O.; Cheng, Q.; Sun, C.K.; Fan, S.T. The significance of acute phase small-for-size graft injury on tumor growth and invasiveness after liver transplantation. *Ann. Surg.* **2008**, *247*, 1049–1057. [CrossRef] [PubMed]
4. Man, K.; Shih, K.C.; Ng, K.T.; Xiao, J.W.; Guo, D.Y.; Sun, C.K.; Lim, Z.X.; Cheng, Q.; Liu, Y.; Fan, S.T.; et al. Molecular signature linked to acute phase injury and tumor invasiveness in small-for-size liver grafts. *Ann. Surg.* **2010**, *251*, 1154–1161. [CrossRef] [PubMed]
5. Ling, C.C.; Ng, K.T.; Shao, Y.; Geng, W.; Xiao, J.W.; Liu, H.; Li, C.X.; Liu, X.B.; Ma, Y.Y.; Yeung, W.H.; et al. Post-transplant endothelial progenitor cell mobilization via CXCL10/CXCR3 signaling promotes liver tumor growth. *J. Hepatol.* **2014**, *60*, 103–109. [CrossRef] [PubMed]
6. Li, C.X.; Ling, C.C.; Shao, Y.; Xu, A.; Li, X.C.; Ng, K.T.; Liu, X.B.; Ma, Y.Y.; Qi, X.; Liu, H.; et al. CXCL10/CXCR3 signaling mobilized-regulatory T cells promote liver tumor recurrence after transplantation. *J. Hepatol.* **2016**, *65*, 944–952. [CrossRef] [PubMed]
7. Qi, X.; Ng, K.T.; Shao, Y.; Li, C.X.; Geng, W.; Ling, C.C.; Ma, Y.Y.; Liu, X.B.; Liu, H.; Liu, J.; et al. The Clinical Significance and Potential Therapeutic Role of GPx3 in Tumor Recurrence after Liver Transplantation. *Theranostics* **2016**, *6*, 1934–1946. [CrossRef] [PubMed]
8. Asaoka, T.; Kato, T.; Marubashi, S.; Dono, K.; Hama, N.; Takahashi, H.; Kobayashi, S.; Takeda, Y.; Takemasa, I.; Nagano, H.; et al. Differential transcriptome patterns for acute cellular rejection in recipients with recurrent hepatitis C after liver transplantation. *Liver Transplant.* **2009**, *15*, 1738–1749. [CrossRef] [PubMed]
9. Ng, K.T.; Xu, A.; Cheng, Q.; Guo, D.Y.; Lim, Z.X.; Sun, C.K.; Fung, J.H.; Poon, R.T.; Fan, S.T.; Lo, C.M.; et al. Clinical relevance and therapeutic potential of angiopoietin-like protein 4 in hepatocellular carcinoma. *Mol. Cancer* **2014**, *13*, 196. [CrossRef] [PubMed]
10. Ng, K.T.; Lo, C.M.; Guo, D.Y.; Qi, X.; Li, C.X.; Geng, W.; Liu, X.B.; Ling, C.C.; Ma, Y.Y.; Yeung, W.H.; et al. Identification of transmembrane protein 98 as a novel chemoresistance-conferring gene in hepatocellular carcinoma. *Mol. Cancer Ther.* **2014**, *13*, 1285–1297. [CrossRef] [PubMed]
11. Mortazavi, A.; Williams, B.A.; McCue, K.; Schaeffer, L.; Wold, B. Mapping and quantifying mammalian transcriptomes by RNA-Seq. *Nat. Methods* **2008**, *5*, 621–628. [CrossRef] [PubMed]
12. Szklarczyk, D.; Franceschini, A.; Wyder, S.; Forslund, K.; Heller, D.; Huerta-Cepas, J.; Simonovic, M.; Roth, A.; Santos, A.; Tsafou, K.P.; et al. STRING v10: Protein-protein interaction networks, integrated over the tree of life. *Nucleic Acids Res.* **2015**, *43*, D447–D452. [CrossRef] [PubMed]
13. Livak, K.J.; Schmittgen, T.D. Analysis of relative gene expression data using real-time quantitative PCR and the 2(-Delta Delta C(T)) method. *Methods* **2001**, *25*, 402–408. [CrossRef] [PubMed]
14. Cescon, M.; Bertuzzo, V.R.; Ercolani, G.; Ravaioli, M.; Odaldi, F.; Pinna, A.D. Liver transplantation for hepatocellular carcinoma: Role of inflammatory and immunological state on recurrence and prognosis. *World J. Gastroenterol.* **2013**, *19*, 9174–9182. [CrossRef] [PubMed]
15. Li, C.X.; Man, K.; Lo, C.M. The impact of liver graft injury on cancer recurrence posttransplantation. *Transplantation* **2017**, *101*, 2665–2670. [CrossRef] [PubMed]

16. Jaeschke, H. Cellular adhesion molecules: Regulation and functional significance in the pathogenesis of liver diseases. *Am. J. Physiol.* **1997**, *273*, G602–G611. [CrossRef] [PubMed]
17. Martinez-Mier, G.; Toledo-Pereyra, L.H.; Ward, P.A. Adhesion molecules in liver ischemia and reperfusion. *J. Surg. Res.* **2000**, *94*, 185–194. [CrossRef] [PubMed]
18. Viebahn, R.; Thoma, M.; Kinder, O.; Schenk, M.; Lauchart, W.; Becker, H.D. Analysis of intragraft adhesion molecules and their release in clinical liver transplantation: Impact of reperfusion injury. *Transplant. Proc.* **1998**, *30*, 4257–4259. [CrossRef]
19. Li, C.X.; Ng, K.T.; Shao, Y.; Liu, X.B.; Ling, C.C.; Ma, Y.Y.; Geng, W.; Qi, X.; Cheng, Q.; Chung, S.K.; et al. The inhibition of aldose reductase attenuates hepatic ischemia-reperfusion injury through reducing inflammatory response. *Ann. Surg.* **2014**, *260*, 317–328. [CrossRef] [PubMed]
20. Li, C.X.; Lo, C.M.; Lian, Q.; Ng, K.T.; Liu, X.B.; Ma, Y.Y.; Qi, X.; Yeung, O.W.; Tergaonkar, V.; Yang, X.X.; et al. Repressor and activator protein accelerates hepatic ischemia reperfusion injury by promoting neutrophil inflammatory response. *Oncotarget* **2016**, *7*, 27711–27723. [CrossRef] [PubMed]
21. Weston, C.; Connor, J. Evidence for the influence of the iron regulatory MHC class I molecule HFE on tumor progression in experimental models and clinical populations. *Transl. Oncog.* **2014**, *6*, 1–12.
22. Brissot, P.; Bardou-Jacquet, E.; Jouanolle, A.M.; Loreal, O. Iron disorders of genetic origin: A changing world. *Trends. Mol. Med.* **2011**, *17*, 707–713. [CrossRef] [PubMed]
23. Kew, M.C. Hepatic iron overload and hepatocellular carcinoma. *Liver Cancer* **2014**, *3*, 31–40. [CrossRef] [PubMed]
24. Kowdley, K.V.; Brandhagen, D.J.; Gish, R.G.; Bass, N.M.; Weinstein, J.; Schilsky, M.L.; Fontana, R.J.; McCashland, T.; Cotler, S.J.; Bacon, B.R.; et al. National Hemochromatosis Transplant Registry. Survival after liver transplantation in patients with hepatic iron overload: The national hemochromatosis transplant registry. *Gastroenterology* **2005**, *129*, 494–503. [CrossRef] [PubMed]
25. Brandhagen, D.J.; Alvarez, W.; Therneau, T.M.; Kruckeberg, K.E.; Thibodeau, S.N.; Ludwig, J.; Porayko, M.K. Iron overload in cirrhosis-HFE genotypes and outcome after liver transplantation. *Hepatology* **2000**, *31*, 456–460. [CrossRef] [PubMed]
26. Barton, J.C.; Edwards, C.Q.; Acton, R.T. HFE gene: Structure, function, mutations, and associated iron abnormalities. *Gene* **2015**, *574*, 179–192. [CrossRef] [PubMed]
27. Gianchecchi, E.; Delfino, D.V.; Fierabracci, A. Recent insights into the role of the PD-1/PD-L1 pathway in immunological tolerance and autoimmunity. *Autoimmun. Rev.* **2013**, *12*, 1091–1100. [CrossRef] [PubMed]
28. Keir, M.E.; Butte, M.J.; Freeman, G.J.; Sharpe, A.H. PD-1 and its ligands in tolerance and immunity. *Annu. Rev. Immunol.* **2008**, *26*, 677–704. [CrossRef] [PubMed]
29. Carreno, B.M.; Collins, M. The B7 family of ligands and its receptors: New pathways for costimulation and inhibition of immune responses. *Annu. Rev. Immunol.* **2002**, *20*, 29–53. [CrossRef] [PubMed]
30. Del Rio, M.L.; Buhler, L.; Gibbons, C.; Tian, J.; Rodriguez-Barbosa, J.I. PD-1/PD-L1, PD-1/PD-L2, and other co-inhibitory signaling pathways in transplantation. *Transpl. Int.* **2008**, *21*, 1015–1028. [CrossRef] [PubMed]

© 2018 by the authors. Licensee MDPI, Basel, Switzerland. This article is an open access article distributed under the terms and conditions of the Creative Commons Attribution (CC BY) license (http://creativecommons.org/licenses/by/4.0/).

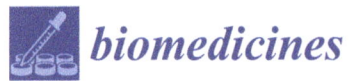

Review

New Development of Biomarkers for Gastrointestinal Cancers: From Neoplastic Cells to Tumor Microenvironment

Jiajia Zhang [1], Shafat Quadri [2], Christopher L. Wolfgang [1] and Lei Zheng [1,*]

1. Departments of Oncology and Surgery, the Sidney Kimmel Comprehensive Cancer Center, the Bloomberg-Kimmel Institute for Cancer Immunotherapy, the Pancreatic Cancer Precision Medicine Center of Excellence Program, the Johns Hopkins University School of Medicine, Baltimore, MD 21287, USA; zhangjiajia@jhmi.edu (J.Z.); cwolfga2@jhmi.edu (C.L.W.)
2. Merck Research Laboratory, Merck & Co., Kenilworth, NJ 07033, USA; shafat.quadri@merck.com
* Correspondence: lzheng6@jhmi.edu; Tel.: +1-410-502-6241; Fax: +1-410-614-8216

Received: 5 June 2018; Accepted: 10 August 2018; Published: 13 August 2018

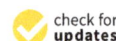

Abstract: Biomarkers refer to a plethora of biological characteristics that can be quantified to facilitate cancer diagnosis, forecast the prognosis of disease, and predict a response to treatment. The identification of objective biomarkers is among the most crucial steps in the realization of individualized cancer care. Several tumor biomarkers for gastrointestinal malignancies have been applied in the clinical setting to help differentiate between cancer and other conditions, facilitate patient selection for targeted therapies, and to monitor treatment response and recurrence. With the coming of the immunotherapy age, the need for a new development of biomarkers that are indicative of the immune response to tumors are unprecedentedly urgent. Biomarkers from the tumor microenvironment, tumor genome, and signatures from liquid biopsies have been explored, but the majority have shown a limited prognostic or predictive value as single biomarkers. Nevertheless, use of multiplex biomarkers has the potential to provide a significantly increased diagnostic accuracy compared to traditional single biomarker. A comprehensive analysis of immune-biomarkers is needed to reveal the dynamic and multifaceted anti-tumor immunity and thus imply for the rational design of assays and combinational strategies.

Keywords: biomarker; gastrointestinal malignancies; immunotherapy

1. Introduction

Biomarkers are defined as objective, quantifiable biological indicators of a normal or abnormal process, a condition or disease, or a response to treatment [1]. Prognostic biomarkers allow a selection of patients with a high risk for disease recurrence or rapid progression and help regarding decision making for a treatment regimen. Predictive biomarkers represent an array of indicators that project the patient's response to the treatment. Currently, biomarkers are genetic, epigenetic, proteinic, or cellular alterations that are inherent to cancer cells, and have been an integral part of individualized cancer care.Glycoproteins, such as carcinoembryonic antigen (CEA) and cancer antigen 19-9 (CA19-9), are classical proteinic biomarkers for disease monitoring [2–4]. Biomarkers at the genome level, which are often driver mutations such as *KRAS* and epidermal growth factor receptor (EGFR), have been widely used as a guide for a selection of patients that might benefit from targeted therapies [4–7]. More recent literature has highlighted *BRCA*, a tumor suppressor gene involved in the repair of double-stranded DNA breaks, as a viable predictive biomarker for response to platinum agents and poly(ADP-ribose) polymerase (PARP) inhibitors [8]. Immunotherapy has revolutionized human cancer treatment by unleashing the potential of the antitumor immune response;

however, only 15–20% of patients respond to immunotherapy [9,10]. This underpins the importance of identifying novel biomarkers that can select the patients for immunotherapy. Programmed death ligand 1 (PD-L1) positivity, T cell-inflamed phenotype, and high tumor mutational burden have been reported to enrich the patient populations that benefit from the treatment of immune checkpoint inhibitors (ICIs) [11–15]; however, these makers alone are insufficiently accurate for patient selection across different cancer types. Microsatellite instability (MSI), a pan-cancer biomarker, predicts the response of solid tumors to anti-PD-1/PD-L1 (Programmed death-1/Programmed death ligand 1) blockade, is only found in 1–2% of most of malignancies [12,16]. Preliminary clinical findings showed that the signatures that reflect the composition and metabolites of the gut microbiota would impact the antitumor immune response in patients receiving ICIs, including anti-cytotoxic T-lymphocyte antigen 4 [CTLA-4] and anti-PD-1/PD-L1 antibodies, and have the potential to predict durable clinical responses in non-small cell lung cancer (NSCLC), renal cell carcinoma (RCC), and melanoma; however, the role of the microbiome in predicting the benefits from the ICIs remains unclear for gastrointestinal (GI) cancer [17–21]. A few studies have also suggested the association of members of the gut microbiome with ICI toxicities, but evidence is lacking in the GI setting [21,22]. In addition, biomarkers that can guide the choice of combination immunotherapy are scarce [23]. Quantitative multiplexed approaches, which exert unique advantages in revealing the tumor-immune complexity, may represent a new avenue for biomarker discovery in the tumor microenvironment, especially for combinational therapies targeting the suppressive myeloid/stromal compartment [24,25]. This review summarizes the advances of biomarkers in gastrointestinal malignancies, with a focus on the development of new biomarkers that are of predictive and/or prognostic values in cancer therapies.

2. Current Clinical Application of Biomarkers in Gastrointestinal Malignancies

2.1. Tumor Markers

The tumor markers currently being used in the clinic are all surrogate markers of malignant diseases (Table 1). CEA is one of the most commonly used tumor markers for gastrointestinal malignancies and a member of the immunoglobulin superfamily [26]. It acts as a mediator for cell adhesion on cancer cells. The overexpression of CEA occurs in >90% of colorectal cancers (CRC) and 60% of other types of cancer, including gastric, lung, and pancreatic cancers [27]; thus, it has been widely used as a serum tumor marker. Its sensitivity and specificity are not high, particularly for the early stages of the disease [28]; therefore, it cannot be used as a biomarker for screening gastrointestinal cancers. However, in the patients with an established disease, the absolute level of the serum CEA correlates with the disease burden and has a prognostic value [29]. In CRC, CEA is the only laboratory test routinely recommended for surveillance. High levels of CEA after surgical resection imply the presence of a persistent disease and the need for further evaluation [30]. The serial measurement of the CEA levels after surgery in patients with colorectal cancer can detect recurrences earlier; nevertheless, this information does not lead to an improved treatment outcome [28]. Currently, the American Society of Clinical Oncology (ASCO) guidelines recommend that the serum CEA levels be obtained in most patients with CRC, so as to aid surgical treatment planning, posttreatment follow-up, and the assessment of prognosis [31]. Another common glycoprotein biomarker is CA19-9, which is used primarily to assess the disease response to therapy or to detect cancer recurrence in patients with gastric cancer, pancreatic cancer, gallbladder cancer, cholangiocarcinoma, or adenocarcinoma of the ampulla of Vater. It is the most useful tumor marker for pancreatic cancer, with sensitivity and specificity rates of 70–92% and 68–92%, respectively [32–34]. In addition, an elevated preoperative CA19-9 level is strongly associated with the presence of subradiographic unresectable diseases, and can be used for a selection of patients for staging the laparoscopy [35]. The lack of tumor specificity is the limitation of the currently used tumor markers. Tumor specific markers, particularly those reflecting the tumor biology, are highly demanded.

Table 1. Major molecular markers in clinical application.

Molecule	Tumor Type	Implication
Tumor markers		
CEA	Colorectal, gastric, and pancreatic cancers	Indicating residual disease, progressive, or recurrent disease
		Measuring treatment response
CA19-9	Pancreatic cancer	Indicating residual disease, progressive, or recurrent disease
		Measuring treatment response
Targets of matched therapies		
HER2	Gastric or esophagogastric-junction cancers	Selecting for targeted therapy
KRAS	Colorectal, gastric, and pancreatic cancers	Predicting for treatment unresponsiveness
Mismatch repair Genes		
MMR	Solid tumors	Predicting for treatment responsiveness
Biomarkers in tumor microenvironment		
PD-L1 expression	Gastric cancer	Enriching patient population responding to anti-PD-1/PD-L1 therapies

CEA—carcinoembryonic antigen; MMR—mismatch repair; PD-L1—programmed death ligand 1; PD-1—programmed death-1.

2.2. Targets of Matched Therapies

HER2, a tyrosine kinase receptor belonging to the epidermal growth factor receptor (EGFR) family, is an established prognostic factor and a therapeutic target for gastroesophageal adenocarcinoma [36–39]. Through the activation of downstream signaling pathways, including RAS/RAF/mitogen-activated protein kinase (RAS/RAF/MAPK) and phosphatidylinositol-3 kinase/protein kinase-B/mammalian target of rapamycin (PI3K/AKT/mTOR), aberrant HER2 amplification or overexpression can lead to uncontrolled cell-cycle progression, cell division, motility, survival, invasion, and adhesion [7]. Approximately 7–38% of gastroesophageal adenocarcinomas have an amplification and/or overexpression of HER2, with a slightly higher positivity in gastroesophageal junction (GEJ), intestinal-type, and well-moderately differentiated tumors [6,7,40,41]. The inhibition of HER2 with the monoclonal antibody trastuzumab in patients with HER2-amplified/overexpressed advanced-stage gastric or esophagogastric-junction adenocarcinomas, confers an improved response rate, progression-free survival, and overall survival when trastuzumab is combined with cisplatin and fluoropyrimidine [5]. Based on the above evidence from the phase III ToGA trial, the current guideline suggests that patients with advanced gastric cancer who are potential candidates for trastuzumab should be screened to determine their HER2 status.

Another biomarker for therapeutic target is c-MET, of which the aberrant expression has been reported in 18–100% of gastrointestinal tumors [42,43]. Activated c-MET signaling results in enhanced cancer cell proliferation, survival, and invasion, and is an independent prognostic factor for inferior survival [44–46]. Several monoclonal antibodies and small-molecule inhibitors of c-MET have been evaluated in clinical trials, however, most of the phase III trials of MET inhibitors showed negative results for gastric cancer. In hepatocellular carcinoma, although encouraging results were reported in phase II studies [47–49], the phase III trial failed to show an improvement in the overall survival compared with the placebo in patients with c-MET-positive advanced hepatocellular cancer (HCC), casting doubt on the role of MET inhibition as a viable therapeutic strategy [50,51]. Therefore, the development of biomarkers for therapeutic target is still a challenge.

In metastatic CRC, the *KRAS* mutation status has been widely reported as a prognostic and predictive biomarker [52]. *KRAS* mutations can be identified in 12–75% of colon cancers and are independently associated with a worse prognosis in the majority of the studies, albeit not all of the studies [53,54]. As the *RAS* oncogene is located at the downstream of the EGFR signaling pathway, the *RAS* mutations can lead to an activation of the pathway, even if the EGFR is blocked [55]. Thus, the *KRAS* mutation status is a biomarker for unresponsiveness to anti-EGFR therapy. Interestingly, there is a bias toward the right-sided CRC for the *KRAS* mutation, this may partially explain an inferior survival and poor response to targeted therapy with EGFR inhibitors for the right proximal CRC compared to the left colon CRC [56]. The characteristics of the HER2, c-MET, and KRAS expression in GI cancers are summarized in Table 2.

Table 2. Characteristics of HER2, c-Met, and KRAS expression in gastrointestinal (GI) cancers.

Molecule	Genomic Alterations	Pathways Involved	Cancer types	Treatment
HER2	Amplification/ overexpression	Activation of the MAPK and the PI3K/AKT axis	Gastric or esophagogastric-junction cancers	Monoclonal antibodies (e.g., cetuximab and trastuzumab)
c-MET	Amplification/ overexpression	Activation of GRB2-SOS-RAS-MAPK, the PI3K/AKT axis, and STAT3 pathway	Colorectal cancer, gastric cancer, pancreatic cancers and hepatocellular carcinoma	Monoclonal antibodies (e.g., rilotumumab, ficlatuzumab, and TAK-701); Tyrosine kinase inhibitors (e.g., tivantinib, cabozantinib, and crizotinib)
KRAS	Activating mutation within catalytic RAS domain	RAS–RAF–MEK	Colorectal cancer	Downstream pathway inhibitors (e.g., *MEK* inhibitors selumetinib and trametinib)

MAPK—mitogen-activated protein kinase; GRB2—growth factor receptor-bound protein 2; STAT—signal transducer and activator of transcription; PI3K—the p85 subunit of phosphatidylinositol 3-kinase; SOS—son of sevenless homologue 1.

2.3. Mismatch Repair Genes

Mismatch repair (MMR) gene products function to repair the nucleotide base mispairings and small insertions or deletions that occur during DNA replication [57,58]. Thus, the MMR-deficient tumors could accumulate hundreds to thousands of somatic mutations, regardless of their cell of origin. It has been implicated in the pathogenesis of the hereditary nonpolyposis colorectal cancer syndromes, as well as a variety of different sporadic cancers. MMR-deficiency is present in 15–20% of all colorectal cancers (CRCs), 8.5–20% of gastric cancers, 3–7% in esophageal/GEJ adenocarcinomas, and 2–3% of pancreatic cancers [12,16,59,60]. MMR-deficiency has been shown to be positively prognostic for survival in patients with colon, gastric, and pancreatic cancers [57,60,61]. It could also serve as a potential predictive marker for a lack of efficacy of fluoropyrimidine based adjuvant chemotherapy in gastric cancer and colon cancer [62–64]. Importantly, MMR deficiency is a pan-cancer predictor for response to anti-PD-1/PD-L1 blockade therapies [65]. It is hypothesized that tumors with an MMR deficiency are enriched with missense mutations that are presented as neoepitopes to T cells, which are subsequently targets of anti-PD-1/PD-L1 therapies. Le et al. reported a phase II clinical trial of progressive metastatic carcinoma with or without MMR deficiency, and revealed significantly increased somatic mutations per tumor in the MMR–deficient tumors compared with the MMR-proficient tumors (mean, 1782 vs. 73). The MMR deficient patients had a remarkably increased immune-related objective response rate (40% vs. 0%) and prolonged immune-related progression-free survival rate (78% vs. 11%), compared to their counterparts [16]. In an expanded cohort of 86 patients with MMR-deficient tumors, the objective radiographic responses were noted in 53% of the patients (46 of 86 patients; 95% CI, 42–64%), with 21% ($n = 18$) achieving a complete radiographic response. Disease control (measured as partial response + complete response + stable disease) was achieved in 66 (77%) of the 86 patients (95% CI, 66–85%) [12]. This led to the approval from the Food and Drug Administration (FDA) for testing MMR-deficiency in order to identify the candidate patients who may benefit from a second-line PD-1 pathway blockade, regardless of the tumor types [66]. Of note, this is the first and only FDA approved pan-cancer biomarker for immune checkpoints blockade.

Clinical trials investigating its role as predictive biomarkers in the first-line and (neo)adjuvant settings are ongoing [67,68].

3. New Development of Biomarkers

3.1. Biomarkers in Tumor Microenvironment

3.1.1. PD-L1 Expression

As above described, PD-1, which is expressed on activated lymphocytes, including T cells, B cells, and natural killer cells, limits the T cell effector functions within tissues. By upregulating the ligands for PD-1 (PD-L1), tumor cells induce the apoptosis of the effector T cells [69,70]. The reported incidence of PD-L1 expression ranges differently in the different tumor types (14–100%), whether or not these tumors respond to anti PD-1/PD-L1 treatment [71–76]. Early studies have suggested that PD-L1 positivity enriches the patient populations that can benefit from PD-1/PD-L1 axis inhibition [77,78], with the hypothesis that pre-existing immunity suppressed by PD-1/PD-L1 could be re-invigorated on antibody treatment with checkpoint blockade. However, more studies questioned the accuracy of PD-L1 as an effective predictive biomarker. In the recent phase III trials testing the adjuvant anti-PD-1 in resected stage III melanoma, the first-line anti-PD-1 antibody in combination with chemotherapy in metastatic NSCLC, and the combination of anti-PD-1 and anti-CTLA4 antibodies in NSCLC with a high mutational burden, the benefit of immunotherapy did not correlate with the PD-L1 expression level [79–81]. In the Keynote 059 trial, objective responses and complete responses (CRs) were observed in both the PD-L1-positive and negative gastric and gastroesophageal adenocarcinoma patients who had previously received at least two lines of treatment [82]. The PD-L1-positivity was defined as a combined positive score (CPS) $\geq$1%, where CPS is the number of PD-L1 staining tumor cells, lymphocytes, and macrophages divided by the total number of viable tumor cells multiplied by 100, using PD-L1 Immunohistochemistry (IHC) 22C3 pharmDx immunohistochemistry. Although the objective response rate (ORR) seemed higher in the patients with PD-L1–positive compared with the PD-L1–negative tumors (23 of 148 [15.5%] vs. 7 of 109 [6.4%], respectively), the patients with PD-L1–negative tumors also experienced objective responses, including CR in three patients (2.8%) [82]. Nevertheless, this study has gained the FDA approval of using PD-L1 positivity (Table 1) at the 1% cutoff as a biomarker to select patients with metastatic gastric and gastroesophageal adenocarcinoma for the treatment of pembrolizumab [83]. In the Asian population, Nivolulab was approved for the treatment of the unresectable, advanced, or recurrent gastric cancer that has progressed after using conventional chemotherapy, based on the results from the phase III ATTRACTION-2 trial, regardless of PD-L1 status. In hepatocellular cancer (HCC), the report from the phase I/II trial suggests that ICIs elicited a promising response rate of 16–19% (49/255) in advanced HCC, but the response rate to the ICIs did not differ according to the PD-L1 expression status [82–85]. In PDACs, reports of the PD-L1 expression vary from 12–90%, however, single agent anti-PD1 treatment has shown no efficacy, except for MMR deficient patients, regardless of PD-L1 status [86].

Therefore, evolving evidence suggests that PD-L1 testing alone is insufficiently accurate to predict patient response to immunotherapy, although it may be used in some GI cancers to enrich the patients that may more likely benefit from anti-PD-1/PD-L1 antibodies (Table 3). Several factors may explain the heterogeneity of the predictive values for the PD-L1 expression, including differences in the PD-L1 IHC assay platforms and detection antibodies, differing IHC cutoffs, tissue preparation, processing variability, primary versus metastatic lesions, oncogenic versus induced PD-L1 expression, and the staining of tumor versus immune cells [42,47,75,87,88]. It should be noted that the PD-L1 expression measured in the clinical assays may only represent a snapshot of the dynamic and multifaceted immune cells and their complex interaction with neoplastic cells. A comprehensive characterization of the tumor microenvironment is necessary to adequately assess the strength of PD-L1 in predicting the immune response to anti-PD-L1/PD-1 therapies.

Table 3. New development of biomarkers.

Molecule	Tumor Type	Implication
Biomarkers in tumor microenvironment		
PD-L1 expression	Other cancer types, except gastric cancer	Enriching patient population responding to anti-PD-1/PD-L1 therapies
Tumor infiltrating lymphocyte	Colon and gastric cancers	Indicating good prognosis
Immunosuppressive myeloid cells	Pancreatic, hepatocellular, and gastric cancers	Indicating poor prognosis
Intratumoral stroma	Gastric, pancreatic, esophageal, and colon cancers	Indicating poor prognosis
Biomarkers in tumor genomics		
Targeted gene panels	Pan-cancer	Selecting patients for targeted therapies
Mutational burden	Pan-cancer	Enriching patient population responding to anti-PD-1/PD-L1 therapies
Biomarkers in liquid biopsies		
ctDNA/CTC/Exosomes	Pan-cancer	Indicating residual disease, progressive, or recurrent disease Measuring treatment response

CTC—circulating tumor cells.

3.1.2. Tumor Infiltrating Lymphocyte

Tumor infiltrating lymphocytes (TILs) represent a potent machinery of the adaptive immunity that has the antitumor potential. TILs have been shown to be associated with improved prognoses and response to immunotherapy in various cancer type (Table 3) [24,44–46,89–91]. In colorectal cancers, the type, density, and location of the immune cells, specifically the cytotoxic and memory T cells, has been reported to be a better predictor of survival than (Union for International Cancer Control) UICC-TNM staging 89]. Among the tumors with similar degrees of T cell infiltration, those with the greatest proportion of CD103+ memory T cells have the best prognosis [92]. To standardize the method of evaluating TILs in CRC, a new method that measures the area occupied by mononuclear cells over the stromal area on hematoxylin and eosin (H-E)-stained sections was proposed. The results from such a method confirmed the density of TILs as a useful prognostic factor in CRC [93]. In Epstein–Barr virus (EBV)-associated gastric cancer an association between a high percentage of TILs, low intratumoral PD-L1 expression, and longer disease-free survival (DFS) was demonstrated [94]. A meta-analysis on 23 relevant studies of 3173 hepatocellular carcinoma (HCC) patients showed that high levels of CD8+ and CD3+ TILs had a better prognostic value on the overall survival (OS), yet high levels of FoxP3+ TILs had a worse prognostic value on OS and DFS/Relapse-free survival (RFS), implicating that TILs may serve as a prognostic biomarker in HCC [95]. A TIL density of ≥5% was reported to be associated with a better objective response as well as the progression free survival (PFS) in NSCLC patients treated with Nivolumab [96]. Recently, a T cell inflamed expression score utilizing 18 gene signatures was shown to be significantly associated with a Pembrolizumab response in gastric/GEJ cancer [97,98]. A significant but nonlinear association was found between the T cell-inflamed gene expression score and PD-L1 expression. These results suggest the potential for a T cell-inflamed gene expression profiling score in association with the PD-L1 expression as biomarkers for treatment selection in gastric/GEJ cancers. In pancreatic cancer, variable frequencies of endogenous CD8+ T cells, CD4+Foxp3− T cells, and CD4+Foxp3+ regulatory T cells (Treg) were reported. Notably, these T cells were enriched within CD20+ lymphoid aggregates, with a trend toward longer survival in those patients with tumoral Tertiary lymphoid structures [99]. In our cohort of 24 pancreatic ductal adenocarcinomas receiving neoadjuvant GVAX® vaccination, which is a tumor vaccine composed of autologous tumor cells genetically modified to secrete granulocyte–macrophage colony-stimulating factor (GM-CSF), the ratios of CD8+ T cell to CD68+ T cell are favorable predictors of survival, as reported in other malignancies [100,101]. Nevertheless, the above results need to be confirmed in future trials and more studies on whether and how TILs or effector T cells can be used to predict the response to immunotherapy in gastrointestinal malignancies are warranted.

3.1.3. Immunosuppressive Myeloid Cells

Tumor-associated myeloid cells not only create a suppressive or anergic environment by blocking T cell functions and proliferation, but also accelerate tumor growth by promoting cancer stemness, angiogenesis, stroma deposition, epithelial-to-mesenchymal transition, and metastasis [102]. The accumulation of the intratumoral and circulating myeloid derived suppressive cells (MDSCs) has been shown to be associated with disease progressiveness and prognosis in pancreatic adenocarcinoma, hepatocellular carcinoma, and gastric cancer (Table 3) [102–106]. In our study evaluating 24 pancreatic ductal adenocarcinomas from patients who received neoadjuvant GVAX vaccination, although, essentially all of the tumors have induction of TILs and PD-L1 expression, the survival of patients is correlated with the infiltration of myeloid cells [76]. Nevertheless, myeloid cells are also critical for an innate immune response. It is unlikely that a single myeloid marker would be able to predict the immune response. Multiplex biomarker assays will need to be developed for characterizing immunosuppressive myeloid cells before a clinical assay can be used for predicting their response to immunotherapy.

3.1.4. Intratumoral Stroma

The intratumoral stromal (ITS) proportion, composition, and activation status represent another array of biomarkers for the disease prognosis. Stromal proportion, quantified by histopathological microscopy analysis of the conventional hematoxylin and eosinstained slides, has been reported to be independently associated with poor prognosis in several types of cancers, including gastric cancer, esophageal, and colon cancers (Table 3) [107–111]. Wu et al. showed that the stromal gene expression signature as well as the ITS proportion quantified by morphometry in tissue sections of patient samples, correlated with the survival of gastric cancer patients in multiple independent cohorts. Measuring the relative amount of ITS may enable the identification of subgroups of gastric cancer patients that benefit from stroma-directed therapies [112]. More recently, transforming growth factor beta (TGFβ) activated stroma was found to represent a primary mechanism of immune evasion that engenders T cell exclusion and primary resistance to anti-PD-1–PD-L1 therapy in microsatellite-stable (MSS) CRC. In murine models, the authors showed that the inhibition of TGFβ signaling in the stroma with a TGF-β receptor 1 (TGF-βR1) specific inhibitor could lead to a potent anti-tumour cytotoxic T cell response and prevent metastasis [113]. Admittedly, there are promising applications in immunotherapies targeting intratumoral stroma and in combination with immune checkpoint inhibitors, however, the identification of accompanying predictive features from intratumoral stroma to enrich for populations that can benefit from combinational therapies are crucial. A summary of biomarkers in the tumor microenvironment is depicted in Figure 1.

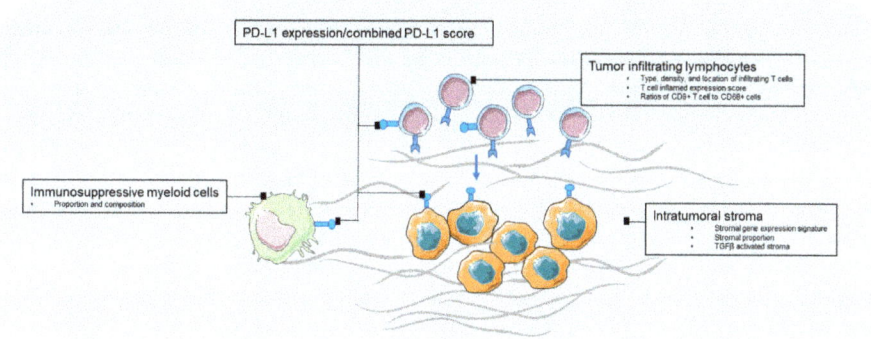

Figure 1. Biomarkers in tumor microenvironment. PD-L1—programmed death-1 ligand-1.

3.2. Biomarkers in Tumor Genomics

3.2.1. Targeted Gene Panels

Targeted gene sequencing is an emerging approach for identifying potentially targetable genomic biomarkers and matching them for treatments. However, a number of challenges remain. For example, the Memorial Sloan Kettering Cancer Center has developed an (IMPAC) targeted gene sequencing panel, which included 341 genes initially, and has expanded to 410 cancer-associated genes [114]. As reported, 10,945 tumors from 10,366 patients with advanced cancer were sequenced. Eleven percent of the patients were enrolled in a genomically matched clinical trial. Among the 10,366 patients, 338 patients had pancreatic cancer. Five of these pancreatic cancer patients died before the results were finalized. Potentially actionable findings were noted in 26% of these pancreatic cancer patients. Nevertheless, only three of the 225 patients (1%) who would need treatments received matched therapy based on the sequencing results [115]. Two had no benefit and one had an unknown response. Therefore, the practical application of molecular results to guide individual patient treatment is currently limited in patients with pancreatic adenocarcinoma.

3.2.2. Mutational Burden

The tumor mutational burden (TMB) has been shown to be significantly associated with a clinical benefit to immune checkpoint blockade in various cancer types [6,11,13–15,35,116]. However, most of the GI cancers have low mutation burdens [5], except those with MMR-deficiency. In a cohort of 1375 patients across various GI tumors, colon cancer was reported to have the highest TMB (mean: 11.6 and 9.9 mutations [mut]/megabase [MB]), whereas biliary cancers and pancreatic adenocarcinomas had the lowest TMB (mean: 5.7 and 4.9 mut/MB) [117]. Using a cut-off of 17 mut/MB to define high vs. low TMB, the high TMB was seen most frequently in right sided colon cancer (12%), gastric cancer (11%), and anal cancer (8%), and least frequently in pancreatic cancer (1.3%) and esophageal squamous cell carcinoma (0%). In addition, primary tumors, MSI-H and/or MSS with *POLE* mutations were observed to have a higher TMB. Those with a higher frequency of somatic mutations and tumor-specific neoantigens were found to have more abundant infiltration of CD8+ T lymphocytes and a higher expression of regulatory molecules (CTLA-4, PD-1, Lymphocyte-activation gene 3[LAG-3] and indolamine 2,3-dioxygenase 1 [IDO1]) [118].

3.3. Biomarkers in Liquid Biopsies

A tumor tissue biopsy would be necessary to establish the diagnosis; however, it would not be feasible for monitoring the treatment response [119]. The analysis of biomarkers from peripheral blood, including the circulating tumor DNA (ctDNA), circulating tumor cells (CTC), and exosomes, using a noninvasive approach known as liquid biopsy, has emerged as a way to overcome the restrictions of tumor tissue biopsies and has exhibited a great potential of being used to detect the recurrence and measure the treatment response [120].

3.3.1. ctDNA

ctDNAs are predominantly released as a result of the apoptosis or necrosis of actively growing cancer cell, but can also be secreted directly from the circulating tumor cells [121]. Notably, ctDNA can maintain tumor-specific genomic aberrations, including point mutations in tumor suppressors and oncogenes, copy number variants, DNA methylation patterns, and chromosomal rearrangements, providing a comprehensive genomic profiling for tumor evolution and dynamics disease monitoring [119]. In CRC, ctDNA has been shown to successfully gather the real-time molecular evolution in patients treated with EGFR targeted therapy [122,123]. The ctDNA analyses can not only identify genetic alterations that are likely to be responsible for resistance to EGFR blockade, but also can guide the selection of rare populations of patients who are likely to respond to targeted agents [124]. Changes of circulating tumor DNA (ctDNA) levels during therapy might also be an indicator of clinical efficacy with ICIs. In a small prospective pilot study ($n = 15$), the ctDNA levels at week eight showed synchronous changes with tumor size and as well as an association with PFS in various cancer types [125]. In the chemotherapy setting, the RAS/BRAF mutations detected in ctDNA correlated with a worse PFS in the metastatic CRC patients ($n = 27$) treated with first-line chemotherapy [126]. However, the role of ctDNA in predicting the response to treatment needs to be validated in a larger population.

3.3.2. CTC

CTCs are surrogates of tumor cells in the bloodstream. CTC prevalence differs with cancer type and stage. In patients with metastatic GI malignancies, CTC could be detected in 30–66% of patients [127], and its presence has been shown to correlate with decreased OS or decreased PFS [128]. The value of CTCs as a therapeutic target to monitor the treatment response and detect relapse has also been reported [129]. Nevertheless, the prognostic and predictive role of CTC is not established in a non-metastatic setting, given the scarcity of CTC in this patient population [130,131]. On the other hand, CTC recently demonstrated its value in monitoring the response to immunotherapy. In a prospective cohort of 49 metastatic melanoma patients treated with ICI, a decrease in an RNA signature score of CTC within seven weeks of therapy correlated with a marked improvement in PFS (hazard ratio [HR], 0.17; $p = 0.008$) and overall survival (OS) (HR, 0.12; $p = 0.04$) [132]. The promising results support the rationale to apply CTCs in monitoring the tumor burden in other cancer types such as GI cancers.

Thus far, despite the interesting and promising results from small cohorts of studies on liquid biopsy approaches as predictive or prognostic biomarkers, there is insufficient evidence of clinical utility of the majority of ctDNA/CTC assays in either advanced cancer or early-stage cancer [133]. Discordance exists between the results of different platforms [134]. Prospective trials in large populations will be required to establish the clinical utility of ctDNA and CTC.

3.3.3. Exosomes

Exosomes are endosome derived extracellular vesicles (EVs) ranging in 30–120 nm [135]. They carry a cargo of proteins, metabolites, RNAs (mRNA, miRNA, long non coding RNA), DNAs (mtDNA, ssDNA, and dsDNA), and lipids [136], and represent an important source as a biomarker from liquid biopsies. In pancreatic cancer, the glypican-1 (GPC1)+ endosomes were reported as a diagnostic biomarker to distinguish healthy subjects and patients with a benign pancreatic disease from patients with early- and late-stage pancreatic cancer, with absolute specificity and sensitivity. The levels of the GPC1(+) endosomes correlated with the tumor burden and the survival of pre- and post-surgical patients [137]. A rapid, highly sensitive, and widely usable detection method based on the amplified luminescent proximity homogeneous assay, using photosensitizer-beads for cancer cell-derived EVs was proposed, with the utilization of monitoring the circulating EVs with the antigen CD147 for the detection of colorectal cancer [138]. Although endosomes held great promise for non-invasive early detection and target for potential therapeutics, it has several limitations. One of the biggest challenges in exosome biology is how to accurately measure the quantity and purity of the exosomes. Only a small subset of EVs carry the relevant communication content, thus its actual efficiency may be difficult to detect. In addition, more knowledge of the specific markers of the EV subtypes and fundamental roles of each type of EV is required to better inform their utilization in various disease settings. The advantages and limitations of various liquid biopsy approaches are summarized in Table 4.

Table 4. Advantages, disadvantages of ctDNA, CTC, and exosome as biomarkers.

Approaches	Advantages	Disadvantages	References
ctDNA	Higher sensitivity; quick renew/short half-life; maintain tumor-specific genomic aberrations	Not suitable for functional assay, noises from normal cell-free DNA, challenges in methods' standardization	[134,138,139]
CTC	Allow morphological/molecular/functional study; potentials for therapeutic targets	Low specificity, particularly in early stage setting; challenges in methods' standardization limited capture techniques	[121,127,128,134,140]
Exosomes	Higher sensitivity; higher serum concentration; diverse EV contents; Potential for therapeutic targets	Isolation and purification of exosomes; specific exosome marker to identify subset of EVs; not suitable for functional assay; challenges in methods' standardization	[135–137]

EV—extracellular vesicles.

4. Prospective

There are only a handful of biomarkers used in clinics for the management of GI malignancies. Although many new biomarkers have been identified for GI malignancies, their clinical assays have not been validated. On the other hand, biomarker assays are highly demanded by a selection of patients for appropriate treatment. Nevertheless, such a biomarker is often not conceived until a clinical trial of experimental therapeutics fails to meet its endpoint because of a lack of patient selection. The development of experimental therapeutics will not be advanced until an adequate biomarker assay is established. Therefore, in the future, biomarker development should be done in parallel with drug development. Whenever a potential therapeutic target is identified, a companion biomarker assay should be developed. For immunotherapy, a single biomarker is often not sufficient in predicting the treatment response. A comprehensive analysis of immune-biomarkers can not only provide the rational design of combination immunotherapy, but can also identify multiple immune-biomarkers, and subsequently develop a multiplex assay to co-evaluate multiple immune-biomarkers. In addition, recent research on ion channels and aquaporins have suggested their function as possible modulators of important processes in gastrointestinal carcinogenesis, including colorectal, pancreatic, gastric, and esophageal cancers, as well as their potential as new cancer biomarkers once appropriately validated [141–143].

Acknowledgments: This study is partially funded by NIH grants R01 CA169702 (L.Z.); R01 CA197296 (L.Z.); NIH grant K23 CA148964 (L.Z.); the Commonwealth Foundation (L.Z.), the Bloomberg-Kimmel Institute for Cancer Immunotherapy(L.Z., J.Z.), the Viragh Foundation and the Skip Viragh Pancreatic Cancer Center at Johns Hopkins (L.Z.); the Sol Goldman Pancreatic Cancer Research Center (L.Z.); the Zhang Family Gift Fund (L.Z.); National Cancer Institute Specialized Programs of Research Excellence in Gastrointestinal Cancers grant P50 CA062924 (L.Z.); Sidney Kimmel Comprehensive Cancer Center grant P30CA006973 (L.Z., C.L.W.).

Conflicts of Interest: S.Q. is an employee of Merck and Co. L.Z. receives grant supports from Bristol-Meyer Squibb, Merck, iTeos, Amgen, Gradalis, and Halozyme. L.Z.'s laboratory receives the royalty for licensing GVAX to Aduro Biotech. L.Z. received the consultant fee from Biosynergies, NovaRock, Merck, and Astrozeneca.

References

1. Institute National Cancer Biomarkers. Available online: https://www.cancer.gov/publications/dictionaries/cancer-terms/def/biomarker (accessed on 27 July 2018).
2. Badreddine, R.; Wang, K.K. Biomarkers in gastrointestinal cancers. *Am. J. Gastroenterol.* **2008**, *103*, 2106–2110. [CrossRef] [PubMed]
3. Papadopoulou, E.; Metaxa-Mariatou, V.; Tsaousis, G.; Tsoulos, N.; Tsirigoti, A.; Efstathiadou, C.; Apessos, A.; Agiannitopoulos, K.; Pepe, G.; Bourkoula, E.; et al. Molecular predictive markers in tumors of the gastrointestinal tract. *World J. Gastrointest. Oncol.* **2016**, *8*, 772–785. [CrossRef] [PubMed]
4. Deschoolmeester, V.; Lardon, F.; Pauwels, P.; Peeters, M. *Biomarkers in Gastrointestinal Cancer: Focus on Colon, Pancreas and Gastric Cancer*; InTech: London, UK, 2012.
5. Bang, Y.J.; Van Cutsem, E.; Feyereislova, A.; Chung, H.C.; Shen, L.; Sawaki, A.; Lordick, F.; Ohtsu, A.; Omuro, Y.; Satoh, T.; et al. Trastuzumab in combination with chemotherapy versus chemotherapy alone for treatment of HER2-positive advanced gastric or gastro-oesophageal junction cancer (toga): A phase 3, open-label, randomised controlled trial. *Lancet* **2010**, *376*, 687–697. [CrossRef]
6. Van Cutsem, E.; Bang, Y.J.; Feng-Yi, F.; Xu, J.M.; Lee, K.W.; Jiao, S.C.; Chong, J.L.; Lopez-Sanchez, R.I.; Price, T.; Gladkov, O.; et al. HER2 screening data from toga: Targeting HER2 in gastric and gastroesophageal junction cancer. *Gastric Cancer* **2015**, *18*, 476–484. [CrossRef] [PubMed]
7. Okines, A.; Cunningham, D.; Chau, I. Targeting the human EGFR family in esophagogastric cancer. *Nat. Rev. Clin. Oncol.* **2011**, *8*, 492–503. [CrossRef] [PubMed]
8. Yu, I.S.; Cheung, W.Y. A contemporary review of the treatment landscape and the role of predictive and prognostic biomarkers in pancreatic adenocarcinoma. *Can. J. Gastroenterol. Hepatol.* **2018**, *2018*, 10. [CrossRef] [PubMed]
9. Murala, S.; Alli, V.; Kreisel, D.; Gelman, A.E.; Krupnick, A.S. Current status of immunotherapy for the treatment of lung cancer. *J. Thorac. Dis.* **2010**, *2*, 237–244. [PubMed]
10. Topalian, S.L.; Drake, C.G.; Pardoll, D.M. Immune checkpoint blockade: A common denominator approach to cancer therapy. *Cancer Cell* **2015**, *27*, 450–461. [CrossRef] [PubMed]
11. Rizvi, N.A.; Hellmann, M.D.; Snyder, A.; Kvistborg, P.; Makarov, V.; Havel, J.J.; Lee, W.; Yuan, J.; Wong, P.; Ho, T.S.; et al. Cancer immunology. Mutational landscape determines sensitivity to PD-1 blockade in non-small cell lung cancer. *Science* **2015**, *348*, 124–128. [CrossRef] [PubMed]
12. Le, D.T.; Durham, J.N.; Smith, K.N.; Wang, H.; Bartlett, B.R.; Aulakh, L.K.; Lu, S.; Kemberling, H.; Wilt, C.; Luber, B.S.; et al. Mismatch repair deficiency predicts response of solid tumors to PD-1 blockade. *Science* **2017**, *357*, 409–413. [CrossRef] [PubMed]
13. Chan, T.A.; Wolchok, J.D.; Snyder, A. Genetic basis for clinical response to CTLA-4 blockade in melanoma. *N. Engl. J. Med.* **2015**, *373*, 1984. [CrossRef] [PubMed]
14. Van Allen, E.M.; Miao, D.; Schilling, B.; Shukla, S.A.; Blank, C.; Zimmer, L.; Sucker, A.; Hillen, U.; Foppen, M.H.G.; Goldinger, S.M.; et al. Genomic correlates of response to CTLA-4 blockade in metastatic melanoma. *Science* **2015**, *350*, 207–211. [CrossRef] [PubMed]
15. Hugo, W.; Zaretsky, J.M.; Sun, L.; Song, C.; Moreno, B.H.; Hu-Lieskovan, S.; Berent-Maoz, B.; Pang, J.; Chmielowski, B.; Cherry, G.; et al. Genomic and transcriptomic features of response to anti-PD-1 therapy in metastatic melanoma. *Cell* **2016**, *165*, 35–44. [CrossRef] [PubMed]
16. Le, D.T.; Uram, J.N.; Wang, H.; Bartlett, B.R.; Kemberling, H.; Eyring, A.D.; Skora, A.D.; Luber, B.S.; Azad, N.S.; Laheru, D.; et al. PD-1 blockade in tumors with mismatch-repair deficiency. *N. Engl. J. Med.* **2015**, *372*, 2509–2520. [CrossRef] [PubMed]
17. Matson, V.; Fessler, J.; Bao, R.; Chongsuwat, T.; Zha, Y.; Alegre, M.-L.; Luke, J.J.; Gajewski, T.F. The commensal microbiome is associated with anti–PD-1 efficacy in metastatic melanoma patients. *Science* **2018**, *359*, 104–108. [CrossRef] [PubMed]
18. Routy, B.; Le Chatelier, E.; Derosa, L.; Duong, C.P.M.; Alou, M.T.; Daillère, R.; Fluckiger, A.; Messaoudene, M.; Rauber, C.; Roberti, M.P.; et al. Gut microbiome influences efficacy of PD-1–based immunotherapy against epithelial tumors. *Science* **2018**, *359*, 91–97. [CrossRef] [PubMed]
19. Gopalakrishnan, V.; Spencer, C.N.; Nezi, L.; Reuben, A.; Andrews, M.C.; Karpinets, T.V.; Prieto, P.A.; Vicente, D.; Hoffman, K.; Wei, S.C.; et al. Gut microbiome modulates response to anti–pd-1 immunotherapy in melanoma patients. *Science* **2018**, *359*, 97–103. [CrossRef] [PubMed]

20. Zitvogel, L.; Ma, Y.; Raoult, D.; Kroemer, G.; Gajewski, T.F. The microbiome in cancer immunotherapy: Diagnostic tools and therapeutic strategies. *Science* **2018**, *359*, 1366–1370. [CrossRef] [PubMed]
21. Chaput, N.; Lepage, P.; Coutzac, C.; Soularue, E.; Le Roux, K.; Monot, C.; Boselli, L.; Routier, E.; Cassard, L.; Collins, M.; et al. Baseline gut microbiota predicts clinical response and colitis in metastatic melanoma patients treated with ipilimumab. *Ann. Oncol.* **2017**, *28*, 1368–1379. [CrossRef] [PubMed]
22. Dubin, K.; Callahan, M.K.; Ren, B.; Khanin, R.; Viale, A.; Ling, L.; No, D.; Gobourne, A.; Littmann, E.; Huttenhower, C. Intestinal microbiome analyses identify melanoma patients at risk for checkpoint-blockade-induced colitis. *Nat. Commun.* **2016**, *7*, 10391. [CrossRef] [PubMed]
23. Hazama, S.; Tamada, K.; Yamaguchi, Y.; Kawakami, Y.; Nagano, H. Current status of immunotherapy against gastrointestinal cancers and its biomarkers: Perspective for precision immunotherapy. *Ann. Gastroenterol. Surg.* **2018**, *2*, 289–303. [CrossRef] [PubMed]
24. Tsujikawa, T.; Kumar, S.; Borkar, R.N.; Azimi, V.; Thibault, G.; Chang, Y.H.; Balter, A.; Kawashima, R.; Choe, G.; Sauer, D.; et al. Quantitative multiplex immunohistochemistry reveals myeloid-inflamed tumor-immune complexity associated with poor prognosis. *Cell Rep.* **2017**, *19*, 203–217. [CrossRef] [PubMed]
25. Gorris, M.A.J.; Halilovic, A.; Rabold, K.; van Duffelen, A.; Wickramasinghe, I.N.; Verweij, D.; Wortel, I.M.N.; Textor, J.C.; de Vries, I.J.M.; Figdor, C.G. Eight-color multiplex immunohistochemistry for simultaneous detection of multiple immune checkpoint molecules within the tumor microenvironment. *J. Immunol.* **2018**, *200*, 347–354. [CrossRef] [PubMed]
26. Hatakeyama, K.; Wakabayashi-Nakao, K.; Ohshima, K.; Sakura, N.; Yamaguchi, K.; Mochizuki, T. Novel protein isoforms of carcinoembryonic antigen are secreted from pancreatic, gastric and colorectal cancer cells. *BMC Res. Notes* **2013**, *6*, 381. [CrossRef] [PubMed]
27. Kuppusamy, P.; Govindan, N.; Yusoff, M.M.; Ichwan, S.J.A. Proteins are potent biomarkers to detect colon cancer progression. *Saudi J. Biol. Sci.* **2017**, *24*, 1212–1221. [CrossRef] [PubMed]
28. Fletcher, R.H. Carcinoembryonic antigen. *Ann. Intern. Med.* **1986**, *104*, 66–73. [CrossRef] [PubMed]
29. Arnaud, J.P.; Koehl, C.; Adloff, M. Carcinoembryonic antigen (cea) in diagosis and prognosis of colorectal carcinoma. *Dis. Colon Rectum* **1980**, *23*, 141–144. [CrossRef] [PubMed]
30. Goldstein, M.J.; Mitchell, E.P. Carcinoembryonic antigen in the staging and follow-up of patients with colorectal cancer. *Cancer Investig.* **2005**, *23*, 338–351. [CrossRef]
31. Meyerhardt, J.A.; Mangu, P.B.; Flynn, P.J.; Korde, L.; Loprinzi, C.L.; Minsky, B.D.; Petrelli, N.J.; Ryan, K.; Schrag, D.H.; Wong, S.L.; et al. Follow-up care, surveillance protocol, and secondary prevention measures for survivors of colorectal cancer: American society of clinical oncology clinical practice guideline endorsement. *J. Clin. Oncol.* **2013**, *31*, 4465–4470. [CrossRef] [PubMed]
32. Pleskow, D.K.; Berger, H.J.; Gyves, J.; Allen, E.; McLean, A.; Podolsky, D.K. Evaluation of a serologic marker, ca19-9, in the diagnosis of pancreatic cancer. *Ann. Intern. Med.* **1989**, *110*, 704–709. [CrossRef] [PubMed]
33. Ćwik, G.; Wallner, G.; Skoczylas, T.; Ciechański, A.; Zinkiewicz, K. Cancer antigens 19-9 and 125 in the differential diagnosis of pancreatic mass lesions. *Arch. Surg.* **2006**, *141*, 968–973. [CrossRef] [PubMed]
34. Paganuzzi, M.; Onetto, M.; Marroni, P.; Barone, D.; Conio, M.; Aste, H.; Pugliese, V. Ca 19-9 and Ca 50 in benign and malignant pancreatic and biliary diseases. *Cancer* **1988**, *61*, 2100–2108. [CrossRef]
35. Maithel, S.K.; Maloney, S.; Winston, C.; Gönen, M.; D'Angelica, M.I.; DeMatteo, R.P.; Jarnagin, W.R.; Brennan, M.F.; Allen, P.J. Preoperative ca 19-9 and the yield of staging laparoscopy in patients with radiographically resectable pancreatic adenocarcinoma. *Ann. Surg. Oncol.* **2008**, *15*, 3512–3520. [CrossRef] [PubMed]
36. Bartley, A.N.; Washington, M.K.; Colasacco, C.; Ventura, C.B.; Ismaila, N.; Benson, A.B., 3rd; Carrato, A.; Gulley, M.L.; Jain, D.; Kakar, S.; et al. HER2 testing and clinical decision making in gastroesophageal adenocarcinoma: Guideline from the college of american pathologists, american society for clinical pathology, and the american society of clinical oncology. *J. Clin. Oncol.* **2017**, *35*, 446–464. [CrossRef] [PubMed]
37. Park, J.-B.; Rhim, J.S.; Park, S.-C.; Kimm, S.-W.; Kraus, M.H. Amplification, overexpression, and rearrangement of the *erb*B-2 protooncogene in primary human stomach carcinomas. *Cancer Res.* **1989**, *49*, 6605–6609. [PubMed]
38. Yonemura, Y.; Ninomiya, I.; Ohoyama, S.; Kimura, H.; Yamaguchi, A.; Fushida, S.; Kosaka, T.; Miwa, K.; Miyazaki, I.; Endou, Y.; et al. Expression of c-erbB-2 oncoprotein in gastric carcinoma. Immunoreactivity for c-erbB-2 protein is an independent indicator of poor short-term prognosis in patients with gastric carcinoma. *Cancer* **1991**, *67*, 2914–2918. [CrossRef]

39. Yonemura, Y.; Yamaguchi, A.; Fushida, S.; Kimura, H.; Ohoyama, S.; Miyazaki, I.; Endou, Y.; Tanaka, M.; Sasaki, T. Evaluation of immunoreactivity for erbB-2 protein as a marker of poor short term prognosis in gastric cancer. *Cancer Res.* **1991**, *51*, 1034–1038. [PubMed]
40. Yoon, H.H.; Shi, Q.; Sukov, W.R.; Wiktor, A.E.; Khan, M.; Sattler, C.A.; Grothey, A.; Wu, T.T.; Diasio, R.B.; Jenkins, R.B.; et al. Association of HER2/ERBB2 expression and gene amplification with pathologic features and prognosis in esophageal adenocarcinomas. *Clin. Cancer Res.* **2012**, *18*, 546–554. [CrossRef] [PubMed]
41. Hu, Y.; Bandla, S.; Godfrey, T.E.; Tan, D.; Luketich, J.D.; Pennathur, A.; Qiu, X.; Hicks, D.G.; Peters, J.H.; Zhou, Z. HER2 amplification, overexpression and score criteria in esophageal adenocarcinoma. *Mod. Pathol.* **2011**, *24*, 899–907. [CrossRef] [PubMed]
42. Di Renzo, M.F.; Olivero, M.; Giacomini, A.; Porte, H.; Chastre, E.; Mirossay, L.; Nordlinger, B.; Bretti, S.; Bottardi, S.; Giordano, S.; et al. Overexpression and amplification of the MET/HGF receptor gene during the progression of colorectal cancer. *Clin. Cancer Res.* **1995**, *1*, 147–154. [PubMed]
43. Bradley, C.A.; Salto-Tellez, M.; Laurent-Puig, P.; Bardelli, A.; Rolfo, C.; Tabernero, J.; Khawaja, H.A.; Lawler, M.; Johnston, P.G.; Van Schaeybroeck, S.; et al. Targeting c-MET in gastrointestinal tumours: Rationale, opportunities and challenges. *Nat. Rev. Clin. Oncol.* **2018**, *15*, 150. [CrossRef] [PubMed]
44. Nakajima, M.; Sawada, H.; Yamada, Y.; Watanabe, A.; Tatsumi, M.; Yamashita, J.; Matsuda, M.; Sakaguchi, T.; Hirao, T.; Nakano, H. The prognostic significance of amplification and overexpression of c-MET and c-ERB b-2 in human gastric carcinomas. *Cancer* **1999**, *85*, 1894–1902. [CrossRef]
45. Yu, S.; Yu, Y.; Zhao, N.; Cui, J.; Li, W.; Liu, T. C-MET as a prognostic marker in gastric cancer: A systematic review and meta-analysis. *PLoS ONE* **2013**, *8*, e79137. [CrossRef] [PubMed]
46. Ueki, T.; Fujimoto, J.; Suzuki, T.; Yamamoto, H.; Okamoto, E. Expression of hepatocyte growth factor and its receptor, the c-met proto-oncogene, in hepatocellular carcinoma. *Hepatology* **1997**, *25*, 619–623. [CrossRef] [PubMed]
47. Zucali, P.; Santoro, A.; Rodriguez-Lope, C.; Simonelli, M.; Camacho, L.; Senzer, N.; Bolondi, L.; Lamar, M.; Abbadessa, G.; Schwartz, B. Final results from ARQ 197-114: A phase ib safety trial evaluating ARQ 197 in cirrhotic patients (PTS) with hepatocellular carcinoma (HCC). *J. Clin. Oncol.* **2010**, *28*, 4137. [CrossRef]
48. Rimassa, L.; Porta, C.; Borbath, I.; Daniele, B.; Salvagni, S.; Van Laethem, J.L.; Van Vlieberghe, H.; Trojan, J.; Kolligs, F.T.; Weiss, A. Tivantinib (ARQ 197) versus placebo in patients (PTS) with hepatocellular carcinoma (HCC) who failed one systemic therapy: Results of a randomized controlled phase II trial (RCT). *Am. Soc. Clin. Oncol.* **2012**. [CrossRef]
49. Goyal, L.; Muzumdar, M.D.; Zhu, A.X. Targeting the HGF/C-met pathway in hepatocellular carcinoma. *Clin. Cancer Res.* **2013**, *19*, 2310–2318. [CrossRef] [PubMed]
50. Weekes, C.D.; Clark, J.W.; Zhu, A.X. Tivantinib for advanced hepatocellular carcinoma: Is met still a viable target? *Lancet Oncol.* **2018**, *19*, 591–592. [CrossRef]
51. Rimassa, L.; Assenat, E.; Peck-Radosavljevic, M.; Pracht, M.; Zagonel, V.; Mathurin, P.; Rota Caremoli, E.; Porta, C.; Daniele, B.; Bolondi, L.; et al. Tivantinib for second-line treatment of met-high, advanced hepatocellular carcinoma (metiv-HCC): A final analysis of a phase 3, randomised, placebo-controlled study. *Lancet Oncol.* **2018**, *19*, 682–693. [CrossRef]
52. Souglakos, J.; Philips, J.; Wang, R.; Marwah, S.; Silver, M.; Tzardi, M.; Silver, J.; Ogino, S.; Hooshmand, S.; Kwak, E.; et al. Prognostic and predictive value of common mutations for treatment response and survival in patients with metastatic colorectal cancer. *Br. J. Cancer* **2009**, *101*, 465–472. [CrossRef] [PubMed]
53. Andreyev, H.J.; Norman, A.R.; Cunningham, D.; Oates, J.R.; Clarke, P.A. Kirsten ras mutations in patients with colorectal cancer: The multicenter "rascal" study. *J. Natl. Cancer Inst.* **1998**, *90*, 675–684. [CrossRef] [PubMed]
54. Yoon, H.H.; Tougeron, D.; Shi, Q.; Alberts, S.R.; Mahoney, M.R.; Nelson, G.D.; Nair, S.G.; Thibodeau, S.N.; Goldberg, R.M.; Sargent, D.J.; et al. KRAS codon 12 and 13 mutations in relation to disease-free survival in braf–wild-type stage III colon cancers from an adjuvant chemotherapy trial (n0147 alliance). *Clin. Cancer Res.* **2014**, *20*, 3033–3043. [CrossRef] [PubMed]
55. Misale, S.; Yaeger, R.; Hobor, S.; Scala, E.; Janakiraman, M.; Liska, D.; Valtorta, E.; Schiavo, R.; Buscarino, M.; Siravegna, G.; et al. Emergence of kras mutations and acquired resistance to anti-EGFR therapy in colorectal cancer. *Nature* **2012**, *486*, 532–536. [CrossRef] [PubMed]

56. Tejpar, S.; Stintzing, S.; Ciardiello, F.; Tabernero, J.; Van Cutsem, E.; Beier, F.; Esser, R.; Lenz, H.J.; Heinemann, V. Prognostic and predictive relevance of primary tumor location in patients with ras wild-type metastatic colorectal cancer: Retrospective analyses of the crystal and fire-3 trials. *JAMA Oncol.* **2016**. [CrossRef] [PubMed]
57. Papadopoulos, N.; Nicolaides, N.C.; Wei, Y.F.; Ruben, S.M.; Carter, K.C.; Rosen, C.A.; Haseltine, W.A.; Fleischmann, R.D.; Fraser, C.M.; Adams, M.D.; et al. Mutation of a mutl homolog in hereditary colon cancer. *Science* **1994**, *263*, 1625–1629. [CrossRef] [PubMed]
58. Chung, D.C.; Rustgi, A.K. DNA mismatch repair and cancer. *Gastroenterology* **1995**, *109*, 1685–1699. [CrossRef]
59. Farris, A.B., III; Demicco, E.G.; Le, L.P.; Finberg, K.E.; Miller, J.; Mandal, R.; Fukuoka, J.; Cohen, C.; Gaissert, H.A.; Zukerberg, L.R. Clinicopathologic and molecular profiles of microsatellite unstable barrett esophagus-associated adenocarcinoma. *Am. J. Surg. Pathol.* **2011**, *35*, 647–655. [CrossRef] [PubMed]
60. Smyth, E.C.; Wotherspoon, A.; Peckitt, C.; Gonzalez, D.; Hulkki-Wilson, S.; Eltahir, Z.; Fassan, M.; Rugge, M.; Valeri, N.; Okines, A.; et al. Mismatch repair deficiency, microsatellite instability, and survival: An exploratory analysis of the medical research council adjuvant gastric infusional chemotherapy (magic) trial. *JAMA Oncol.* **2017**, *3*, 1197–1203. [CrossRef] [PubMed]
61. Nakata, B.; Wang, Y.Q.; Yashiro, M.; Nishioka, N.; Tanaka, H.; Ohira, M.; Ishikawa, T.; Nishino, H.; Hirakawa, K. Prognostic value of microsatellite instability in resectable pancreatic cancer. *Clin. Cancer Res.* **2002**, *8*, 2536–2540. [PubMed]
62. De la Chapelle, A. Microsatellite instability. *N. Engl. J. Med.* **2003**, *349*, 209–210. [CrossRef] [PubMed]
63. Ribic, C.M.; Sargent, D.J.; Moore, M.J.; Thibodeau, S.N.; French, A.J.; Goldberg, R.M.; Hamilton, S.R.; Laurent-Puig, P.; Gryfe, R.; Shepherd, L.E.; et al. Tumor microsatellite-instability status as a predictor of benefit from fluorouracil-based adjuvant chemotherapy for colon cancer. *N. Engl. J. Med.* **2003**, *349*, 247–257. [CrossRef] [PubMed]
64. Sargent, D.J.; Marsoni, S.; Monges, G.; Thibodeau, S.N.; Labianca, R.; Hamilton, S.R.; French, A.J.; Kabat, B.; Foster, N.R.; Torri, V.; et al. Defective mismatch repair as a predictive marker for lack of efficacy of fluorouracil-based adjuvant therapy in colon cancer. *J. Clin. Oncol.* **2010**, *28*, 3219–3226. [CrossRef] [PubMed]
65. Viale, G.; Trapani, D.; Curigliano, G. Mismatch repair deficiency as a predictive biomarker for immunotherapy efficacy. *BioMed Res. Int.* **2017**, *2017*. [CrossRef] [PubMed]
66. FDA Approves First Cancer Treatment for Any Solid Tumor with a Specific Genetic Feature. Available online: https://www.fda.gov/newsevents/newsroom/pressannouncements/ucm560167.htm (accessed on 27 July 2018).
67. Diaz, L.A.; Le, D.T.; Yoshino, T.; Andre, T.; Bendell, J.C.; Koshiji, M.; Zhang, Y.; Kang, S.P.; Lam, B.; Jaeger, D. Phase 3, open-label, randomized study of first-line pembrolizumab (pembro) vs. investigator-choice chemotherapy for mismatch repair-deficient (dmmr) or microsatellite instability-high (MSI-H) metastatic colorectal carcinoma (MCRC): Keynote-177. *J. Clin. Oncol.* **2017**, *35*. [CrossRef]
68. Frank, A.S.; Qian, S.; Andrew, B.N.; Mody, K.; Levasseur, A.; Dueck, A.C.; Asha, R.D.; Christopher, H.L.; Deirdre, J.C.; Federico, I.R.; et al. Randomized trial of folfox alone or combined with atezolizumab as adjuvant therapy for patients with stage III colon cancer and deficient DNA mismatch repair or microsatellite instability (atomic, alliance a021502). *J. Clin. Oncol.* **2017**, *35*. [CrossRef]
69. Dong, H.; Strome, S.E.; Salomao, D.R.; Tamura, H.; Hirano, F.; Flies, D.B.; Roche, P.C.; Lu, J.; Zhu, G.; Tamada, K.; et al. Tumor-associated B7-H1 promotes T-cell apoptosis: A potential mechanism of immune evasion. *Nat. Med.* **2002**, *8*, 793–800. [CrossRef] [PubMed]
70. Patel, S.P.; Kurzrock, R. PD-L1 expression as a predictive biomarker in cancer immunotherapy. *Mol. Cancer Ther.* **2015**, *14*, 847–856. [CrossRef] [PubMed]
71. Pardoll, D.M. The blockade of immune checkpoints in cancer immunotherapy. *Nat. Rev. Cancer* **2012**, *12*, 252–264. [CrossRef] [PubMed]
72. Wu, C.; Zhu, Y.; Jiang, J.; Zhao, J.; Zhang, X.G.; Xu, N. Immunohistochemical localization of programmed death-1 ligand-1 (PD-l1) in gastric carcinoma and its clinical significance. *Acta Histochem.* **2006**, *108*, 19–24. [CrossRef] [PubMed]
73. Powles, T.; Eder, J.P.; Fine, G.D.; Braiteh, F.S.; Loriot, Y.; Cruz, C.; Bellmunt, J.; Burris, H.A.; Petrylak, D.P.; Teng, S.-L. MPDL3280A (anti-PD-L1) treatment leads to clinical activity in metastatic bladder cancer. *Nature* **2014**, *515*, 558–562. [CrossRef] [PubMed]

74. Herbst, R.S.; Soria, J.-C.; Kowanetz, M.; Fine, G.D.; Hamid, O.; Gordon, M.S.; Sosman, J.A.; McDermott, D.F.; Powderly, J.D.; Gettinger, S.N.; et al. Predictive correlates of response to the anti-PD-L1 antibody MPDL3280A in cancer patients. *Nature* **2014**, *515*, 563–567. [CrossRef] [PubMed]
75. Zheng, L. PD-L1 expression in pancreatic cancer. *JNCI J. Natl. Cancer Inst.* **2017**, *109*. [CrossRef] [PubMed]
76. Lutz, E.R.; Wu, A.A.; Bigelow, E.; Sharma, R.; Mo, G.; Soares, K.; Solt, S.; Dorman, A.; Wamwea, A.; Yager, A.; et al. Immunotherapy converts nonimmunogenic pancreatic tumors into immunogenic foci of immune regulation. *Cancer Immunol. Res.* **2014**, *2*, 616–631. [CrossRef] [PubMed]
77. Herbst, R.S.; Baas, P.; Kim, D.W.; Felip, E.; Perez-Gracia, J.L.; Han, J.Y.; Molina, J.; Kim, J.H.; Arvis, C.D.; Ahn, M.J.; et al. Pembrolizumab versus docetaxel for previously treated, PD-L1-positive, advanced non-small-cell lung cancer (keynote-010): A randomised controlled trial. *Lancet* **2016**, *387*, 1540–1550. [CrossRef]
78. Carbone, D.P.; Reck, M.; Paz-Ares, L.; Creelan, B.; Horn, L.; Steins, M.; Felip, E.; van den Heuvel, M.M.; Ciuleanu, T.-E.; Badin, F.; et al. First-line nivolumab in stage iv or recurrent non–small-cell lung cancer. *N. Engl. J. Med.* **2017**, *376*, 2415–2426. [CrossRef] [PubMed]
79. Gandhi, L.; Rodríguez-Abreu, D.; Gadgeel, S.; Esteban, E.; Felip, E.; De Angelis, F.; Domine, M.; Clingan, P.; Hochmair, M.J.; Powell, S.F.; et al. Pembrolizumab plus chemotherapy in metastatic non–small-cell lung cancer. *N. Engl. J. Med.* **2018**. [CrossRef] [PubMed]
80. Eggermont, A.M.M.; Blank, C.U.; Mandala, M.; Long, G.V.; Atkinson, V.; Dalle, S.; Haydon, A.; Lichinitser, M.; Khattak, A.; Carlino, M.S.; et al. Adjuvant pembrolizumab versus placebo in resected stage iii melanoma. *N. Engl. J. Med.* **2018**, *378*, 1789–1801. [CrossRef] [PubMed]
81. Hellmann, M.D.; Ciuleanu, T.-E.; Pluzanski, A.; Lee, J.S.; Otterson, G.A.; Audigier-Valette, C.; Minenza, E.; Linardou, H.; Burgers, S.; Salman, P.; et al. Nivolumab plus ipilimumab in lung cancer with a high tumor mutational burden. *N. Engl. J. Med.* **2018**, *378*, 2094–2104. [CrossRef] [PubMed]
82. Fuchs, C.S.; Doi, T.; Jang, R.W.; Muro, K.; Satoh, T.; Machado, M.; Sun, W.; Jalal, S.I.; Shah, M.A.; Metges, J.P.; et al. Safety and efficacy of pembrolizumab monotherapy in patients with previously treated advanced gastric and gastroesophageal junction cancer: Phase 2 clinical keynote-059 trial. *JAMA Oncol.* **2018**, *4*, e180013. [CrossRef] [PubMed]
83. FDA Grants Accelerated Approval to Pembrolizumab for Advanced Gastric Cancer. Available online: https://www.fda.gov/Drugs/InformationOnDrugs/ApprovedDrugs/ucm577093.htm (accessed on 27 July 2018).
84. Mahalingam, D. The coming of age: Immunotherapy in gastrointestinal malignancies. *J. Gastrointest. Oncol.* **2018**, *9*, 140–142. [CrossRef] [PubMed]
85. El-Khoueiry, A.B.; Sangro, B.; Yau, T.; Crocenzi, T.S.; Kudo, M.; Hsu, C.; Kim, T.-Y.; Choo, S.-P.; Trojan, J.; Welling, T.H.; et al. Nivolumab in patients with advanced hepatocellular carcinoma (checkmate 040): An open-label, non-comparative, phase 1/2 dose escalation and expansion trial. *Lancet* **2017**, *389*, 2492–2502. [CrossRef]
86. Zhang, J.; Wolfgang, C.L.; Zheng, L. Precision immuno-oncology: Prospects of individualized immunotherapy for pancreatic cancer. *Cancers (Basel)* **2018**, *10*, 39. [CrossRef] [PubMed]
87. Wang, X.; Yang, Z.; Tian, H.; Li, Y.; Li, M.; Zhao, W.; Zhang, C.; Wang, T.; Liu, J.; Zhang, A.; et al. Circulating MIC-1/GDF15 is a complementary screening biomarker with cea and correlates with liver metastasis and poor survival in colorectal cancer. *Oncotarget* **2017**, *8*, 24892–24901. [CrossRef] [PubMed]
88. Tsao, M.; Kerr, K.; Yatabe, Y.; Hirsch, F.R. PL 03.03 blueprint 2: PD-L1 immunohistochemistry comparability study in real-life, clinical samples. *J. Thorac. Oncol.* **2017**, *12*, S1606. [CrossRef]
89. Galon, J.; Costes, A.; Sanchez-Cabo, F.; Kirilovsky, A.; Mlecnik, B.; Lagorce-Pagès, C.; Tosolini, M.; Camus, M.; Berger, A.; Wind, P.; et al. Type, density, and location of immune cells within human colorectal tumors predict clinical outcome. *Science* **2006**, *313*, 1960–1964. [CrossRef] [PubMed]
90. Zhang, L.; Conejo-Garcia, J.R.; Katsaros, D.; Gimotty, P.A.; Massobrio, M.; Regnani, G.; Makrigiannakis, A.; Gray, H.; Schlienger, K.; Liebman, M.N.; et al. Intratumoral T cells, recurrence, and survival in epithelial ovarian cancer. *N. Engl. J. Med.* **2003**, *348*, 203–213. [CrossRef] [PubMed]
91. Fridman, W.H.; Pages, F.; Sautes-Fridman, C.; Galon, J. The immune contexture in human tumours: Impact on clinical outcome. *Nat. Rev. Cancer* **2012**, *12*, 298–306. [CrossRef] [PubMed]
92. Amsen, D.; van Gisbergen, K.P.J.M.; Hombrink, P.; van Lier, R.A.W. Tissue-resident memory T cells at the center of immunity to solid tumors. *Nat. Immunol.* **2018**, *19*, 538–546. [CrossRef] [PubMed]

93. Iseki, Y.; Shibutani, M.; Maeda, K.; Nagahara, H.; Fukuoka, T.; Matsutani, S.; Kashiwagi, S.; Tanaka, H.; Hirakawa, K.; Ohira, M. A new method for evaluating tumor-infiltrating lymphocytes (TILs) in colorectal cancer using hematoxylin and eosin (he)-stained tumor sections. *PLoS ONE* **2018**, *13*, e0192744. [CrossRef] [PubMed]
94. Seo, A.N.; Kang, B.W.; Kwon, O.K.; Park, K.B.; Lee, S.S.; Chung, H.Y.; Yu, W.; Bae, H.I.; Jeon, S.W.; Kang, H. Intratumoural PD-L1 expression is associated with worse survival of patients with epstein–barr virus-associated gastric cancer. *Br. J. Cancer* **2017**, *117*, 1753. [CrossRef] [PubMed]
95. Yao, W.; He, J.-C.; Yang, Y.; Wang, J.-M.; Qian, Y.-W.; Yang, T.; Ji, L. The prognostic value of tumor-infiltrating lymphocytes in hepatocellular carcinoma: A systematic review and meta-analysis. *Sci. Rep.* **2017**, *7*, 7525. [CrossRef] [PubMed]
96. Gataa, I.; Mezquita, L.; Auclin, E.; Le Moulec, S.; Alemany, P.; Kossai, M.; Massé, J.; Caramella, C.; Remon Masip, J.; Lahmar, J.; et al. 112PPathological evaluation of tumor infiltrating lymphocytes and the benefit of nivolumab in advanced non-small cell lung cancer (NSCLC). *Ann. Oncol.* **2017**, *28*. [CrossRef]
97. Wallden, B.; Pekker, I.; Popa, S.; Dowidar, N.; Sullivan, A.; Hood, T.; Danaher, P.; Mashadi-Hossein, A.; Lunceford, J.K.; Marton, M.J.; et al. Development and analytical performance of a molecular diagnostic for anti-PD1 response on the ncounter dx analysis system. *J. Clin. Oncol.* **2016**, *34*.
98. Ayers, M.; Lunceford, J.; Nebozhyn, M.; Murphy, E.; Loboda, A.; Kaufman, D.R.; Albright, A.; Cheng, J.D.; Kang, S.P.; Shankaran, V.; et al. Ifn-γ–related mrna profile predicts clinical response to PD-1 blockade. *J. Clin. Investig.* **2017**, *127*, 2930–2940. [CrossRef] [PubMed]
99. Stromnes, I.M.; Hulbert, A.; Pierce, R.H.; Greenberg, P.D.; Hingorani, S.R. T-cell localization, activation, and clonal expansion in human pancreatic ductal adenocarcinoma. *Cancer Immunol. Res.* **2017**, *5*, 978–991. [CrossRef] [PubMed]
100. DeNardo, D.G.; Brennan, D.J.; Rexhepaj, E.; Ruffell, B.; Shiao, S.L.; Madden, S.F.; Gallagher, W.M.; Wadhwani, N.; Keil, S.D.; Junaid, S.A.; et al. Leukocyte complexity predicts breast cancer survival and functionally regulates response to chemotherapy. *Cancer Discov.* **2011**, *1*, 54–67. [CrossRef] [PubMed]
101. Ruffell, B.; Chang-Strachan, D.; Chan, V.; Rosenbusch, A.; Ho, C.M.; Pryer, N.; Daniel, D.; Hwang, E.S.; Rugo, H.S.; Coussens, L.M. Macrophage IL-10 blocks CD8+ T cell-dependent responses to chemotherapy by suppressing IL-12 expression in intratumoral dendritic cells. *Cancer Cell* **2014**, *26*, 623–637. [CrossRef] [PubMed]
102. Ugel, S.; De Sanctis, F.; Mandruzzato, S.; Bronte, V. Tumor-induced myeloid deviation: When myeloid-derived suppressor cells meet tumor-associated macrophages. *J. Clin. Investig.* **2015**, *125*, 3365–3376. [CrossRef] [PubMed]
103. Wang, L.; Chang, E.W.; Wong, S.C.; Ong, S.M.; Chong, D.Q.; Ling, K.L. Increased myeloid-derived suppressor cells in gastric cancer correlate with cancer stage and plasma s100a8/a9 proinflammatory proteins. *J. Immunol.* **2013**, *190*, 794–804. [CrossRef] [PubMed]
104. Porembka, M.R.; Mitchem, J.B.; Belt, B.A.; Hsieh, C.-S.; Lee, H.-M.; Herndon, J.; Gillanders, W.E.; Linehan, D.C.; Goedegebuure, P. Pancreatic adenocarcinoma induces bone marrow mobilization of myeloid-derived suppressor cells which promote primary tumor growth. *Cancer Immunol. Immunother.* **2012**, *61*, 1373–1385. [CrossRef] [PubMed]
105. Gabitass, R.F.; Annels, N.E.; Stocken, D.D.; Pandha, H.A.; Middleton, G.W. Elevated myeloid-derived suppressor cells in pancreatic, esophageal and gastric cancer are an independent prognostic factor and are associated with significant elevation of the TH2 cytokine interleukin-13. *Cancer Immunol. Immunother.* **2011**, *60*, 1419–1430. [CrossRef] [PubMed]
106. Iwata, T.; Kondo, Y.; Kimura, O.; Morosawa, T.; Fujisaka, Y.; Umetsu, T.; Kogure, T.; Inoue, J.; Nakagome, Y.; Shimosegawa, T. PD-L1+mdscs are increased in HCC patients and induced by soluble factor in the tumor microenvironment. *Sci. Rep.* **2016**, *6*, 39296. [CrossRef] [PubMed]
107. Michor, F.; Iwasa, Y.; Lengauer, C.; Nowak, M.A. Dynamics of colorectal cancer. *Semin. Cancer Biol.* **2005**, *15*, 484–493. [CrossRef] [PubMed]
108. Park, J.H.; Richards, C.H.; McMillan, D.C.; Horgan, P.G.; Roxburgh, C.S.D. The relationship between tumour stroma percentage, the tumour microenvironment and survival in patients with primary operable colorectal cancer. *Ann. Oncol.* **2014**, *25*, 644–651. [CrossRef] [PubMed]

109. Lee, D.; Ham, I.-H.; Son, S.Y.; Han, S.-U.; Kim, Y.-B.; Hur, H. Intratumor stromal proportion predicts aggressive phenotype of gastric signet ring cell carcinomas. *Gastric Cancer* **2017**, *20*, 591–601. [CrossRef] [PubMed]
110. Huijbers, A.; Tollenaar, R.A.E.M.; Pelt, G.W.; Zeestraten, E.C.M.; Dutton, S.; McConkey, C.C.; Domingo, E.; Smit, V.T.H.B.M.; Midgley, R.; Warren, B.F.; et al. The proportion of tumor-stroma as a strong prognosticator for stage II and III colon cancer patients: Validation in the victor trial. *Ann. Oncol.* **2013**, *24*, 179–185. [CrossRef] [PubMed]
111. Wang, K.; Ma, W.; Wang, J.; Yu, L.; Zhang, X.; Wang, Z.; Tan, B.; Wang, N.; Bai, B.; Yang, S.; et al. Tumor-stroma ratio is an independent predictor for survival in esophageal squamous cell carcinoma. *J. Thorac. Oncol.* **2012**, *7*, 1457–1461. [CrossRef] [PubMed]
112. Wu, Y.; Grabsch, H.; Ivanova, T.; Tan, I.B.; Murray, J.; Ooi, C.H.; Wright, A.I.; West, N.P.; Hutchins, G.G.A.; Wu, J.; et al. Comprehensive genomic meta-analysis identifies intra-tumoural stroma as a predictor of survival in patients with gastric cancer. *Gut* **2013**, *62*, 1100–1111. [CrossRef] [PubMed]
113. Tauriello, D.V.F.; Palomo-Ponce, S.; Stork, D.; Berenguer-Llergo, A.; Badia-Ramentol, J.; Iglesias, M.; Sevillano, M.; Ibiza, S.; Cañellas, A.; Hernando-Momblona, X.; et al. TGFB drives immune evasion in genetically reconstituted colon cancer metastasis. *Nature* **2018**, *554*, 538–543. [CrossRef] [PubMed]
114. Zehir, A.; Benayed, R.; Shah, R.H.; Syed, A.; Middha, S.; Kim, H.R.; Srinivasan, P.; Gao, J.; Chakravarty, D.; Devlin, S.M.; et al. Mutational landscape of metastatic cancer revealed from prospective clinical sequencing of 10,000 patients. *Nat. Med.* **2017**, *23*, 703–713. [CrossRef] [PubMed]
115. Lowery, M.A.; Jordan, E.J.; Basturk, O.; Ptashkin, R.N.; Zehir, A.; Berger, M.F.; Leach, T.; Herbst, B.; Askan, G.; Maynard, H.; et al. Real-time genomic profiling of pancreatic ductal adenocarcinoma: Potential actionability and correlation with clinical phenotype. *Clin. Cancer Res.* **2017**, *23*, 6094–6100. [CrossRef] [PubMed]
116. Forde, P.M.; Chaft, J.E.; Smith, K.N.; Anagnostou, V.; Cottrell, T.R.; Hellmann, M.D.; Zahurak, M.; Yang, S.C.; Jones, D.R.; Broderick, S.; et al. Neoadjuvant PD-1 blockade in resectable lung cancer. *N. Engl. J. Med.* **2018**. [CrossRef] [PubMed]
117. Salem, M.E.; Xiu, J.; Weinberg, B.A.; El-Deiry, W.S.; Weiner, L.M.; Gatalica, Z.; Liu, Z.; El Ghazaly, H.; Xiao, N.; Hwang, J.J.; et al. Characterization of tumor mutation burden (TMB) in gastrointestinal (GI) cancers. *J. Clin. Oncol.* **2017**, *35*, 530. [CrossRef]
118. Llosa, N.J.; Cruise, M.; Tam, A.; Wick, E.C.; Hechenbleikner, E.M.; Taube, J.M.; Blosser, L.; Fan, H.; Wang, H.; Luber, B.; et al. The vigorous immune microenvironment of microsatellite instable colon cancer is balanced by multiple counter-inhibitory checkpoints. *Cancer Discov.* **2015**, *5*, 43–51. [CrossRef] [PubMed]
119. Yang, M.; Forbes, M.E.; Bitting, R.L.; O'Neill, S.S.; Chou, P.C.; Topaloglu, U.; Miller, L.D.; Hawkins, G.A.; Grant, S.C.; DeYoung, B.R.; et al. Incorporating blood-based liquid biopsy information into cancer staging: Time for a tnmb system? *Ann. Oncol.* **2018**, *29*, 311–323. [CrossRef] [PubMed]
120. Diaz, L.A., Jr.; Bardelli, A. Liquid biopsies: Genotyping circulating tumor DNA. *J. Clin. Oncol.* **2014**, *32*, 579–586. [CrossRef] [PubMed]
121. Thiele, J.-A.; Bethel, K.; Králíčková, M.; Kuhn, P. Circulating tumor cells: Fluid surrogates of solid tumors. *Annu. Rev.Pathol.* **2017**, *12*, 419–447. [CrossRef] [PubMed]
122. Reinert, T.; Scholer, L.V.; Thomsen, R.; Tobiasen, H.; Vang, S.; Nordentoft, I.; Lamy, P.; Kannerup, A.S.; Mortensen, F.V.; Stribolt, K.; et al. Analysis of circulating tumour DNA to monitor disease burden following colorectal cancer surgery. *Gut* **2016**, *65*, 625–634. [CrossRef] [PubMed]
123. Jiang, P.; Chan, C.W.; Chan, K.C.; Cheng, S.H.; Wong, J.; Wong, V.W.; Wong, G.L.; Chan, S.L.; Mok, T.S.; Chan, H.L.; et al. Lengthening and shortening of plasma DNA in hepatocellular carcinoma patients. *Proc. Natl. Acad. Sci. USA* **2015**, *112*, E1317–E1325. [CrossRef] [PubMed]
124. Siravegna, G.; Mussolin, B.; Buscarino, M.; Corti, G.; Cassingena, A.; Crisafulli, G.; Ponzetti, A.; Cremolini, C.; Amatu, A.; Lauricella, C.; et al. Clonal evolution and resistance to EGFR blockade in the blood of colorectal cancer patients. *Nat. Med.* **2015**, *21*, 795–801. [CrossRef] [PubMed]
125. Cabel, L.; Riva, F.; Servois, V.; Livartowski, A.; Daniel, C.; Rampanou, A.; Lantz, O.; Romano, E.; Milder, M.; Buecher, B.; et al. Circulating tumor DNA changes for early monitoring of anti-pd1 immunotherapy: A proof-of-concept study. *Ann. Oncol.* **2017**, *28*, 1996–2001. [CrossRef] [PubMed]
126. Yao, J.; Zang, W.; Ge, Y.; Weygant, N.; Yu, P.; Li, L.; Rao, G.; Jiang, Z.; Yan, R.; He, L.; et al. RAS/BRAF circulating tumor DNA mutations as a predictor of response to first-line chemotherapy in metastatic colorectal cancer patients. *Can. J. Gastroenterol. Hepatol.* **2018**, *2018*, 10. [CrossRef] [PubMed]

127. Balic, M.; Dandachi, N.; Hofmann, G.; Samonigg, H.; Loibner, H.; Obwaller, A.; van der Kooi, A.; Tibbe, A.G.; Doyle, G.V.; Terstappen, L.W.; et al. Comparison of two methods for enumerating circulating tumor cells in carcinoma patients. *Cytom. B Clin. Cytom.* **2005**, *68*, 25–30. [CrossRef] [PubMed]
128. Hiroya, T.; Yuko, K. Circulating tumor cells in gastrointestinal cancer. *J. Hepato-Biliary-Pancreat. Sci.* **2010**, *17*, 577–582.
129. Li, Y.; Gong, J.; Zhang, Q.; Lu, Z.; Gao, J.; Li, Y.; Cao, Y.; Shen, L. Dynamic monitoring of circulating tumour cells to evaluate therapeutic efficacy in advanced gastric cancer. *Br. J. Cancer* **2016**, *114*, 138–145. [CrossRef] [PubMed]
130. Sotelo, M.J.; Sastre, J.; Maestro, M.L.; Veganzones, S.; Viéitez, J.M.; Alonso, V.; Grávalos, C.; Escudero, P.; Vera, R.; Aranda, E.; et al. Role of circulating tumor cells as prognostic marker in resected stage iii colorectal cancer. *Ann. Oncol.* **2015**, *26*, 535–541. [CrossRef] [PubMed]
131. Allard, W.J.; Matera, J.; Miller, M.C.; Repollet, M.; Connelly, M.C.; Rao, C.; Tibbe, A.G.J.; Uhr, J.W.; Terstappen, L.W.M.M. Tumor cells circulate in the peripheral blood of all major carcinomas but not in healthy subjects or patients with nonmalignant diseases. *Clin. Cancer Res.* **2004**, *10*, 6897–6904. [CrossRef] [PubMed]
132. Hong, X.; Sullivan, R.J.; Kalinich, M.; Kwan, T.T.; Giobbie-Hurder, A.; Pan, S.; LiCausi, J.A.; Milner, J.D.; Nieman, L.T.; Wittner, B.S.; et al. Molecular signatures of circulating melanoma cells for monitoring early response to immune checkpoint therapy. *Proc. Natl. Acad. Sci. USA* **2018**, *115*, 2467–2472. [CrossRef] [PubMed]
133. Merker, J.D.; Oxnard, G.R.; Compton, C.; Diehn, M.; Hurley, P.; Lazar, A.J.; Lindeman, N.; Lockwood, C.M.; Rai, A.J.; Schilsky, R.L.; et al. Circulating tumor DNA analysis in patients with cancer: American society of clinical oncology and college of american pathologists joint review. *J. Clin. Oncol.* **2018**, *36*, 1631–1641. [CrossRef] [PubMed]
134. Ignatiadis, M.; Lee, M.; Jeffrey, S.S. Circulating tumor cells and circulating tumor DNA: Challenges and opportunities on the path to clinical utility. *Clin. Cancer Res.* **2015**, *21*, 4786–4800. [CrossRef] [PubMed]
135. Tkach, M.; Théry, C. Communication by extracellular vesicles: Where we are and where we need to go. *Cell* **2016**, *164*, 1226–1232. [CrossRef] [PubMed]
136. Melo, S.A.; Luecke, L.B.; Kahlert, C.; Fernandez, A.F.; Gammon, S.T.; Kaye, J.; LeBleu, V.S.; Mittendorf, E.A.; Weitz, J.; Rahbari, N.; et al. Glypican-1 identifies cancer exosomes and detects early pancreatic cancer. *Nature* **2015**, *523*, 177–182. [CrossRef] [PubMed]
137. Yoshioka, Y.; Kosaka, N.; Konishi, Y.; Ohta, H.; Okamoto, H.; Sonoda, H.; Nonaka, R.; Yamamoto, H.; Ishii, H.; Mori, M.; et al. Ultra-sensitive liquid biopsy of circulating extracellular vesicles using exoscreen. *Nat. Commun.* **2014**, *5*, 3591. [CrossRef] [PubMed]
138. Heitzer, E.; Ulz, P.; Geigl, J.B. Circulating tumor DNA as a liquid biopsy for cancer. *Clin. Chem.* **2015**, *61*, 112–123. [CrossRef] [PubMed]
139. Kidess-Sigal, E.; Liu, H.E.; Triboulet, M.M.; Che, J.; Ramani, V.C.; Visser, B.C.; Poultsides, G.A.; Longacre, T.A.; Marziali, A.; Vysotskaia, V.; et al. Enumeration and targeted analysis of kras, BRAF and PIK3CA mutations in ctcs captured by a label-free platform: Comparison to ctdna and tissue in metastatic colorectal cancer. *Oncotarget* **2016**, *7*, 85349–85364. [CrossRef] [PubMed]
140. Hardingham, J.E.; Grover, P.; Winter, M.; Hewett, P.J.; Price, T.J.; Thierry, B. Detection and clinical significance of circulating tumor cells in colorectal cancer—20 years of progress. *Mol. Med.* **2015**, *21*, S25–S31. [CrossRef] [PubMed]
141. Lastraioli, E.; Iorio, J.; Arcangeli, A. Ion channel expression as promising cancer biomarker. *Biochim. Biophys. Acta BBA* **2015**, *1848*, 2685–2702. [CrossRef] [PubMed]
142. Nagaraju, G.P.; Basha, R.; Rajitha, B.; Alese, O.B.; Alam, A.; Pattnaik, S.; El-Rayes, B. Aquaporins: Their role in gastrointestinal malignancies. *Cancer Lett.* **2016**, *373*, 12–18. [CrossRef] [PubMed]
143. Pelagalli, A.; Squillacioti, C.; Mirabella, N.; Meli, R. Aquaporins in Health and Disease: An Overview Focusing on the Gut of Different Species. *Int. J. Mol. Sci.* **2016**, *17*, 1213. [CrossRef] [PubMed]

© 2018 by the authors. Licensee MDPI, Basel, Switzerland. This article is an open access article distributed under the terms and conditions of the Creative Commons Attribution (CC BY) license (http://creativecommons.org/licenses/by/4.0/).

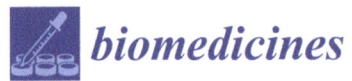

Review

Utilizing Peptide Ligand GPCRs to Image and Treat Pancreatic Cancer

Gail L. Matters [1],* and John F. Harms [2]

1. Department of Biochemistry and Molecular Biology, The Pennsylvania State University College of Medicine, Hershey, PA 17033, USA
2. Department of Biological Sciences, Messiah College, Mechanicsburg, PA 17055, USA; jharms@messiah.edu
* Correspondence: gmatters@pennstatehealth.psu.edu; Tel.: +1-717-531-4098

Received: 15 May 2018; Accepted: 28 May 2018; Published: 2 June 2018

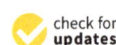

Abstract: It is estimated that early detection of pancreatic ductal adenocarcinoma (PDAC) could increase long-term patient survival by as much as 30% to 40% (Seufferlein, T. et al., *Nat. Rev. Gastroenterol. Hepatol.* **2016**, *13*, 74–75). There is an unmet need for reagents that can reliably identify early cancerous or precancerous lesions through various imaging modalities or could be employed to deliver anticancer treatments specifically to tumor cells. However, to date, many PDAC tumor-targeting strategies lack selectivity and are unable to discriminate between tumor and nontumor cells, causing off-target effects or unclear diagnoses. Although a variety of approaches have been taken to identify tumor-targeting reagents that can effectively direct therapeutics or imaging agents to cancer cells (Liu, D. et al., *J. Controlled Release* **2015**, *219*, 632–643), translating these reagents into clinical practice has been limited, and it remains an area open to new methodologies and reagents (O'Connor, J.P. et al., *Nat. Rev. Clin. Oncol.* **2017**, *14*, 169–186). G protein–coupled receptors (GPCRs), which are key target proteins for drug discovery and comprise a large proportion of currently marketed therapeutics, hold significant promise for tumor imaging and targeted treatment, particularly for pancreatic cancer.

Keywords: G protein–coupled receptors; cholecystokinin; gastrin; gastrin-releasing peptide; bombesin; neurokinin; neurotensin; somatostatin

---

1. Introduction

The utility of reagents to enhance tumor imaging or direct treatment often relies on tumor-targeting ligands that bind to proteins that are overexpressed on the surface of malignant cells [1–3]. Tumor-directed targeting can make use of antibodies, peptides, small molecules, or other moieties, and can result in a higher cargo concentration either within or on the surface of tumor cells than would be attained without targeting [4]. In pancreatic ductal adenocarcinoma (PDAC), development of targeted therapies has focused on receptor tyrosine kinases (RTKs) or their downstream pathways, with limited efficacy [5]. G protein-coupled receptors (GPCRs) represent an opportunity to develop new targeted therapeutics and imaging agents for pancreatic cancer [6] (Figure 1).

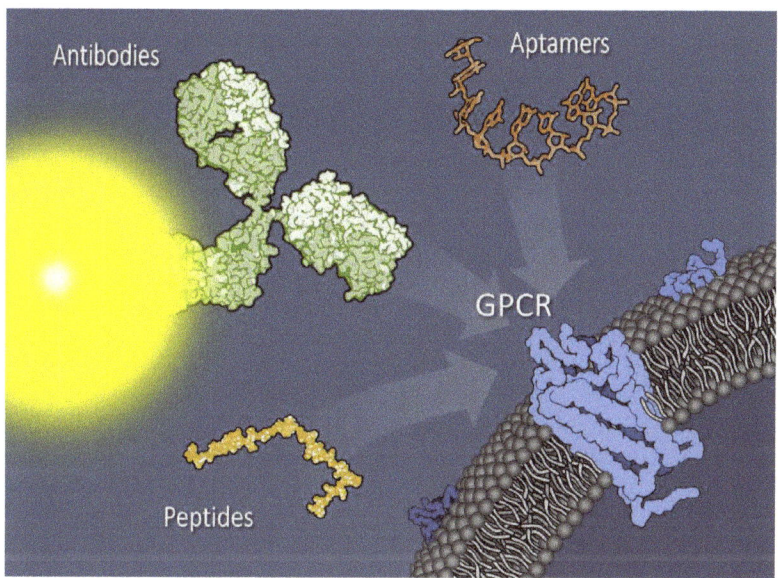

Figure 1. Pancreatic tumor cell surface membrane with G protein–coupled receptors (GPCRs) can be targeted with a variety of reagents, including antibodies (depicted as dye-conjugated) or antibody fragments, aptamers, or small peptides. Additionally, novel bi- or multivalent combinations of targeting agents exhibit promise as tools for imaging and treatment. Targeting agents are not drawn to scale.

2. G Protein-Coupled Receptors

GPCRs are plasma membrane proteins composed of seven transmembrane-spanning α-helices linked by three intracellular and three extracellular loop regions, an extracellular amino-terminal domain, and an intracellular carboxyl-terminal domain. Classical GPCR signaling is initiated by a ligand interacting with extracellular receptor loop/transmembrane domain residues, which form a ligand-binding pocket. This interaction triggers a conformational change in the receptor that initiates binding and activation of intracellular heterotrimeric G proteins. The exchange of guanosine diphosphate (GDP) for guanosine triphosphate (GTP) on the G alpha subunit dissociates G alpha from the G beta/gamma subunits and activates numerous downstream effector pathways [7,8]. Receptor activation is followed by desensitization and internalization. Once activated, GPCRs are phosphorylated by G protein kinases (GPKs), and cytosolic β-arrestins can then bind to the GPCRs, competing with the GPCR-G protein interaction and downregulating G protein-mediated signaling. The GPCR/β-arrestin complex can follow one of the endocytic pathways [9], in which GPCRs can either be recycled back to the plasma membrane or sent to the lysosomes for degradation [10].

GPCRs play an important role in cancer progression, and these proteins have been utilized as therapeutic and imaging targets. Since many chemotherapeutic agents are only active intracellularly, transmembrane transport of targeted cargos is a key issue. Unlike single transmembrane spanning proteins, which are often cleaved by proteases such as matrix metalloproteases (MMPs) to release their ectodomains [11,12], ligand-induced GPCR internalization improves intracellular bioavailability of the cargo. GPCR recycling also provides cell membrane–associated targets for additional rounds of internalization. Increased expression and activity of GPCRs is evident at all stages of PDAC tumor development, and GPCRs contribute to tumor cell proliferation, tumor progression through stimulation of angiogenic and metastatic cascades, and the creation of a proinflammatory tumor microenvironment and evasion of immune cell recognition [13].

Recent evidence suggests that mutations in GPCRs and their associated G proteins are common in tumors—approximately 20% of all cancers contain mutated GPCRs or G alpha subunits [14]. For example, defects that impact GPCR trafficking can contribute to receptor retention at the cell surface and altered downstream signaling. Activating mutations in GPCR-associated proteins, particularly *GNAS*, which encodes the Gs-alpha subunit, can be present in up to 12% of pancreatic tumors [10,14]. Reduced GTPase activity leads to constitutive signaling that can drive tumor progression. In addition, crosstalk between GPCR and RTK signaling pathways can stimulate receptor transactivation and has been linked to oncogenic Kras activation in early-stage PDAC [15,16].

GPCRs mediate a broad range of autocrine and paracrine responses in cancer cells. They bind to a diverse group of ligands, including small peptides (e.g., gastrointestinal hormones), lipids (e.g., sphingosine-1-phosphate, prostaglandins), and proteins (e.g., chemokines) [8]. The density of GPCRs on the cell surface is typically 10^3–10^4 receptors/cell, which should be adequate to ensure ample uptake of the targeted drug cargo or to bind sufficient imaging reagents to achieve quality images [17,18]. Herein, we focus on the peptide hormone–ligand subfamily of GPCRs and their use in developing reagents to identify and treat pancreatic cancer.

3. CCKRs

The peptides gastrin and cholecystokinin (CCK) activate two structurally related G protein-coupled receptors, the CCK1 receptor (CCK1R) and CCK2 receptor (CCK2R), which are expressed by many PDAC tumors [19]. Although highly homologous, with 50% overall identity, these receptors differ in their ligand-binding specificities and inhibitor profiles [20]. CCK1R binds with high affinity to CCK-8 amide with a sulfated tyrosine. CCK2R binds gastrin and CCK with similar affinity and does not discriminate between sulfated and nonsulfated CCK, as binding is directed by the final four amino acids of these peptides (Trp-Met-Asp-Phe-NH$_2$, although leucine or norleucine can be interchanged for methionine to improve stability without altering binding affinity) [21]. Functionally, CCK2R expressed on pancreatic tumors plays a role in tumor cell proliferation and angiogenesis [22].

Beginning in the late 1990s, many groups explored the use of CCK1R and CCK2R for tumor imaging and treatment. While anti-CCK2R antibodies have been developed [23,24], most targeting reagents have been peptide analogs of either CCK or gastrin. With a radionuclide chelator attached to the N-terminus of CCK or gastrin peptide analogs, a variety of reagents have been created for tumor imaging and radiotherapy, including CCK-8, gastrin 10, mini-gastrin, gastrin dimers, and cyclic gastrin analogs [25–31]. Although tumor uptake relative to other tissues was good, the ability of the peptide-targeted constructs to deliver cargo to tumors was limited by high proteolytic turnover in serum, often with less than 10% of the reagent remaining in circulation 10 minutes post-injection [32]. One approach to extending the half-life of gastrin- or CCK-based reagents has been to inhibit the activity of the protease responsible for gastrin/CCK degradation, neutral endopeptidase (NEP). Co-injection of the NEP inhibitor phosphoramidon with gastrin analogs increased their half-life in circulation and improved tumor uptake [33–35]. Finally, nanoparticles can be bioconjugated with gastrin peptide to improve tumor-specific uptake. Attaching gastrin 10 to fluorescent dye–loaded calcium phosphosilicate nanoparticles enhanced particle uptake by orthotopic pancreatic tumors in a murine model [36].

4. GRP/Bombesin Receptors

This family of peptide receptors contains gastrin-releasing peptide receptor (GRPR), neuromedin B receptor (NMBR), and bombesin receptor subtype 3 (BRS3), which are overexpressed by a number of cancers, including PDAC [37]. PDAC cells have previously been targeted with a GRPR ligand radiolabeled for positron emission tomography (PET) imaging, or conjugated with Gd^{3+} for magnetic resonance imaging (MRI) [38,39]. Human gastrin releasing peptide (GRP) as well as mammalian bombesin (BN), which differ by only 1 out of 10 amino acids, have been utilized for GRP- or BN-drug conjugates with paclitaxel or docetaxel. Compared to free drug, the peptide-drug conjugates resulted in enhanced cytotoxicity in vitro [40–42]. However, the efficacy of these compounds against pancreatic tumors in vivo remains unclear [43].

5. Neurokinin Receptors

The neurokinin-1 receptor (NK1R) and its peptide ligand, substance P (SP), regulate many tumor cell processes, including proliferation, angiogenesis, migration, invasion, and metastasis [44]. NK1R is upregulated in human pancreatic tumors, especially in advanced tumors with poor prognosis, and has recently been implicated in perineural invasion of PDAC tumors [45]. In mice, a subpopulation of PanIN epithelial cells express NK1R. Evidence suggests that these are acinar cell–derived neoplastic PanIN epithelial cells, opening the potential for using NK1R-targeted imaging for detection of early lesions [46]. Tumor imaging using an NK1R-targeted fluorescent dye has been used during surgery to facilitate identification and resection of NK1R-positive lesions [47,48]. In PET imaging, ^{64}Cu-NK1R-NOTA is a promising reagent for identifying NK1R-expressing tumors [49], and NK1R-targeted cytotoxic drugs are also under development [50].

6. Neurotensin Receptors

Neurotensin receptor (NTS1) has been identified on several PDAC cells lines, in human PDAC tissues, and in late-stage PanINs and PDAC liver metastases, with lower expression in chronic pancreatitis [51,52]. NTS1 binding of the ligand neurotensin (NT) activates mitogenic signaling, while a selective NTS1 antagonist, SR 48692, reduces PDAC cell proliferation [53,54]. Because NT interacts with the NTS1 receptor with high affinity and only the six C-terminal amino acids of NT are required for receptor binding, bioconjugation of NT peptide to a variety of reagents holds potential for improving their delivery to NTS1-expressing tumors [17]. Biodistribution studies using NT-targeted probes in PDAC tumor–bearing mice showed high tumor-specific uptake of ^{68}Ga-labeled NT peptides in vivo [55]. In addition to NT peptides, NTS1 small-molecule antagonists labeled with ^{18}F and ^{177}Lu also demonstrated tumor cell internalization and retention in vivo with low kidney and liver uptake [56,57]. Liposomes functionalized with a branched neurotensin peptide, NT4, and loaded with doxorubicin have been assessed for antitumor cell efficacy in vitro [58].

Interestingly, recent evidence shows that there is crosstalk between the insulin/IGF-1 receptor and NT/NTS1 signaling pathways, which leads to activation of the oncogenic YAP/TAZ pathway. Stimulation of PDAC cells with both insulin and neurotensin results in nuclear localization of YAP, decreased YAP phosphorylation, and increased expression of YAP/TEAD-regulated genes, while treatment with either insulin or neurotensin alone only modestly induced the expression of these genes [59]. This suggests that either antagonism of NTS1 or blockade of downstream signaling pathways connecting to YAP could a be promising therapeutic target for PDAC [60].

7. Somatostatin Receptors

Somatostatin receptor (SSTR) subtypes SSTR2, SSTR3, and SSTR5 are present in human PDAC tumors based on mRNA expression [61,62]. The short half-life of somatostatin (SST) prompted the development of several peptide analogs for therapeutic and imaging purposes, the most clinically relevant of which is octreotide (OCT). This eight-amino-acid peptide binds to SSTR2 with high affinity and triggers receptor endocytosis [18,63,64]. OCT-drug conjugates, created by direct coupling of camptothecin or paclitaxel to the N-terminus of the peptide, were cytotoxic to cancer cell lines that overexpressed SSTR2 [65] and induced regression of subcutaneous CFPAC-1 tumors in athymic mice [66]. More recently, a reagent that combined MRI/optical imaging capability and a synthetic peptide (PTR86) with high affinity for somatostatin receptors showed efficient imaging and targeting of pancreatic tumors [67]. An SST analog dual-labeled with a radionuclide and fluorescent dye has recently been evaluated in a preclinical colon cancer model system [68].

Interestingly, a PDAC-specific interaction between two GPCRs, the mu opioid receptor (MOR) and SSTR2, has recently been identified [69]. The presence of this GPCR heterodimer correlated with increased oncogenic signaling and tumor progression and antagonists to either receptor triggered heterodimer internalization. This suggests that the MOR-SSTR2 heterodimer may represent a unique PDAC-specific target. Investigation of other novel GPCR heterodimers in PDAC may uncover new opportunities for therapeutic targeting with higher tumor cell specificity.

8. Dual-Targeted Agents

A challenge for the development of tumor-targeted drug delivery or imaging is the level at which the target protein is expressed. It is well documented that PDAC tumors and metastatic lesions are heterogeneous with regard to their expression of GPCRs and other cell-surface receptors [70]. Dual-targeted reagents are capable of targeting different GPCRs simultaneously, or a GPCR and another extracellular protein. These reagents can achieve better specificity than targeting the proteins individually. Dual-targeting agents also can provide better sensitivity through a greater number of potential tumor cell binding sites, thus enabling clearer visualization of cancerous lesions or improved drug delivery [71].

Simultaneous targeting of two independent GPCRs was achieved using a peptide that combined ligands for the CCK2 receptor and the melanocortin 1 receptor (also known as MC1R) [72]. This bivalent reagent joins seven amino acids from melanocortin to the CCK-4 tetrapeptide via a synthetic fluorescently tagged linker. In vitro, the hybrid ligand was able to bind both cell-surface receptors, demonstrating a 12-fold higher specificity for cells expressing both receptors. The ability of the bivalent ligand to improve the imaging of tumors in vivo was confirmed using tumor cell lines engineered to express either the MSH receptor, CCK2 receptor, or both.

Dual targeting can also exploit a target protein on a nonmalignant cell type within the tumor microenvironment (TME) in addition to a tumor-cell GPCR. Demonstrating this strategy, bombesin was fused to an RGD peptide motif, thereby targeting both a GPCR and integrin $\alpha v \beta 3$ on tumor endothelial cells [73]. The resulting ^{68}Ga-labeled heterodimeric peptide has been successfully employed in PET imaging. A second example, while not targeting a GPCR, demonstrates the utility of bivalent targeting. Pancreatic tumor xenografts were imaged using a heterodimer of antibody fragments targeting CD105 on the tumor vasculature and tissue factor (TF) on tumor cells [74,75]. Further explorations of multivalent combinations of a GPCR-targeted ligand with other TME targets would constitute novel advancements.

9. Nonpeptide Targeting to GPCRs: Aptamers

RNA and DNA aptamers are single-stranded, structured oligonucleotides that have promise for both targeted tumor imaging and drug delivery while avoiding some of the common disadvantages of peptide and antibody targeting [76]. Targeting with antibodies can be associated with a risk of inappropriate immune response, while peptides are typically susceptible to proteolytic degradation in the systemic circulation, making them unsuitable for many in vivo applications. Small molecules such as antagonists, while having a well-defined chemical structure and good stability, can have low target selectivity or rapid clearance in vivo [3]. Aptamers have a reproducible structure and can be easily modified to resist nucleases, can be synthesized at a lower cost, are stable to changes in temperature and pH, and can refold spontaneously once conditions normalize. They have fewer nonspecific interactions in the systemic circulation, are less immunogenic, and display high binding affinity to targets with dissociation constant (Kd) values in the nanomolar range. Due to their low molecular weight (25–70 nucleotides is equivalent to 8–20 kDa), aptamers can also penetrate tumor tissues more efficiently than antibodies or Fab fragments [77,78].

Aptamers can be attached to a variety of payloads, including small interfering RNAs (siRNAs), cytotoxic drugs, or nanoparticles, which improves the selective delivery and efficacy of the cargo [79–82]. Tumor-targeting aptamers have been selected for cell-adhesion molecules such as EpCAM, tyrosine kinase receptors, mucins, and other cell-surface proteins [83]. For example, EGFR-targeted aptamers conjugated to gold nanospheres have been successfully used to image head and neck tumors [84]. Aptamer-based imaging agents and aptamer-targeted therapeutics are now moving into clinical trials [85].

Our research team has identified and characterized aptamers against the GPCR CCK2R. Using a SELEX-based library selection protocol, we selected aptamers that bound to both a synthetic peptide contained within the extracellular N-terminal domain of the CCK2R and PDAC cells expressing CCK2R in its native conformation. Negative selection with non–CCK2R-expressing cells ruled out nonspecific interactors. Overall, we identified a pool of >100 high-affinity DNA aptamers that specifically recognized the extracellular N terminus of the human CCK2R [86]. Quantitatively, we have shown that one of the selected CCK2R aptamers (AP1153) has a 300-fold higher affinity for CCK2R than its native peptide ligand, gastrin. As evidence for its utility as a pancreatic tumor targeting agent, we demonstrated that AP1153 was internalized by PDAC cells in a receptor-mediated fashion, and that bioconjugation of AP1153 to the surface of fluorescent nanoparticles enhanced whole-animal optical detection of PDAC tumors in vivo. Others have identified aptamers that bind to the GPCR NTS1, although their further development for diagnostic or therapeutic use has not yet been shown [87].

Finally, aptamers can have direct therapeutic benefit as antitumor reagents. A variety of RNA aptamers that bind to β2-adrenoceptor (β2AR), a non–peptide-liganded GPCR, have been shown to stabilize this receptor in active, inactive, or ligand-specific conformations [88]. Similar to neutralizing antibodies, aptamers can block the interaction between ligand and receptor. Although not directed toward a GPCR, anti–PD-L1 aptamers block the PD-1/PD-L1 signaling axis, reducing tumor growth and improving immune surveillance [89]. An anti–CTLA-4 aptamer has also shown promise for delivering siRNA cargo. The lack of therapeutic efficacy of siRNA-mediated gene silencing is due in part to low siRNA internalization by tumor cells [90]. Conjugation of an anti–CTLA-4 aptamer to a STAT3 siRNA helped to overcome this limitation and achieved STAT3 gene silencing in both tumor-associated T cells and tumor cells [91,92]. GPCR-binding aptamers that disrupt ligand-receptor interactions and abrogate downstream GPCR signaling, or that improve delivery of either siRNAs or drug-loaded nanoparticles to tumors, could have application as new PDAC therapeutics [76].

10. Conclusions

Earlier detection and targeted therapies for pancreatic cancer will undoubtedly improve patient survival [93,94]. However, developing reagents capable of specifically targeting tumors for imaging and drug delivery remains a significant challenge. GPCRs represent a class of tumor cell surface proteins with well-characterized ligands, well-understood pathways for internalization and recycling, and well-documented signaling capabilities, including crosstalk with other oncogenic signaling pathways. Identifying and validating GPCR-specific imaging or therapeutic reagents could provide new tools to make clinically significant improvements in PDAC patient care and achieve the goal of improving survival rates for patients battling this disease.

Author Contributions: G.L.M. and J.F.H. contributed to writing, editing, and graphic design.

Funding: The Matters laboratory was supported by NIH R01 CA167535 and R21 CA170121. The content is solely the responsibility of the authors and does not necessarily represent the official views of the National Institutes of Health. Matters has also received funding from the Pennsylvania Department of Health's Tobacco CURE fund. The Department of Health specifically disclaims responsibility for any analysis, interpretations, or conclusions.

Acknowledgments: We thank Christopher McGovern for critical readings of the manuscript.

Conflicts of Interest: The authors declare no conflict of interest.

References

1. Liu, D.; Auguste, D.T. Cancer targeted therapeutics: From molecules to drug delivery vehicles. *J. Control. Release* **2015**, *219*, 632–643. [CrossRef] [PubMed]

2. O'Connor, J.P.; Aboagye, E.O.; Adams, J.E.; Aerts, H.J.; Barrington, S.F.; Beer, A.J.; Boellaard, R.; Bohndiek, S.E.; Brady, M.; Brown, G.; et al. Imaging biomarker roadmap for cancer studies. *Nat. Rev.. Clin. Oncol.* **2017**, *14*, 169–186. [CrossRef] [PubMed]
3. Srinivasarao, M.; Galliford, C.V.; Low, P.S. Principles in the design of ligand-targeted cancer therapeutics and imaging agents. *Nat. Rev. Drug Discov.* **2015**, *14*, 203–219. [CrossRef] [PubMed]
4. Hussain, S.; Rodriguez-Fernandez, M.; Braun, G.B.; Doyle, F.J.; Ruoslahti, E. Quantity and accessibility for specific targeting of receptors in tumours. *Sci. Rep.* **2014**, *4*, 5232. [CrossRef] [PubMed]
5. Mosquera, C.; Maglic, D.; Zervos, E.E. Molecular targeted therapy for pancreatic adenocarcinoma: A review of completed and ongoing late phase clinical trials. *Cancer Genet.* **2016**, *209*, 567–581. [CrossRef] [PubMed]
6. Sriram, K.; Insel, P.A. G protein-coupled receptors as targets for approved drugs: How many targets and how many drugs? *Mol. Pharmacol.* **2018**, *93*, 251–258. [CrossRef] [PubMed]
7. Dorsam, R.T.; Gutkind, J.S. G-protein-coupled receptors and cancer. *Nat. Rev. Cancer* **2007**, *7*, 79–94. [CrossRef] [PubMed]
8. O'Hayre, M.; Degese, M.S.; Gutkind, J.S. Novel insights into g protein and g protein-coupled receptor signaling in cancer. *Curr. Opin. Cell Biol.* **2014**, *27*, 126–135. [CrossRef] [PubMed]
9. Kang, D.S.; Tian, X.; Benovic, J.L. Role of beta-arrestins and arrestin domain-containing proteins in g protein-coupled receptor trafficking. *Curr. Opin. Cell Biol.* **2014**, *27*, 63–71. [CrossRef] [PubMed]
10. Nieto Gutierrez, A.; McDonald, P.H. Gpcrs: Emerging anti-cancer drug targets. *Cell. Signal.* **2018**, *41*, 65–74. [CrossRef] [PubMed]
11. Sanderson, M.P.; Keller, S.; Alonso, A.; Riedle, S.; Dempsey, P.J.; Altevogt, P. Generation of novel, secreted epidermal growth factor receptor (EGFR/ERBB1) isoforms via metalloprotease-dependent ectodomain shedding and exosome secretion. *J. Cell. Biochem.* **2008**, *103*, 1783–1797. [CrossRef] [PubMed]
12. Miller, M.A.; Sullivan, R.J.; Lauffenburger, D.A. Molecular pathways: Receptor ectodomain shedding in treatment, resistance, and monitoring of cancer. *Clin. Cancer Res.* **2017**, *23*, 623–629. [CrossRef] [PubMed]
13. Heasley, L.E. Autocrine and paracrine signaling through neuropeptide receptors in human cancer. *Oncogene* **2001**, *20*, 1563–1569. [CrossRef] [PubMed]
14. O'Hayre, M.; Vazquez-Prado, J.; Kufareva, I.; Stawiski, E.W.; Handel, T.M.; Seshagiri, S.; Gutkind, J.S. The emerging mutational landscape of g proteins and g-protein-coupled receptors in cancer. *Nat. Rev. Cancer* **2013**, *13*, 412–424. [CrossRef] [PubMed]
15. Natarajan, K.; Berk, B.C. Crosstalk coregulation mechanisms of g protein-coupled receptors and receptor tyrosine kinases. *Methods Mol. Biol.* **2006**, *332*, 51–77. [PubMed]
16. Logsdon, C.D.; Lu, W. The significance of ras activity in pancreatic cancer initiation. *Int. J. Biol. Sci.* **2016**, *12*, 338–346. [CrossRef] [PubMed]
17. Bird, J.L.; Simpson, R.; Vllasaliu, D.; Goddard, A.D. Neurotensin receptor 1 facilitates intracellular and transepithelial delivery of macromolecules. *Eur. J. Pharm. Biopharm.* **2017**, *119*, 300–309. [CrossRef] [PubMed]
18. Accardo, A.; Aloj, L.; Aurilio, M.; Morelli, G.; Tesauro, D. Receptor binding peptides for target-selective delivery of nanoparticles encapsulated drugs. *Int. J. Nanomed.* **2014**, *9*, 1537–1557.
19. Smith, J.P.; Fonkoua, L.K.; Moody, T.W. The role of gastrin and cck receptors in pancreatic cancer and other malignancies. *Int. J. Biol. Sci.* **2016**, *12*, 283–291. [CrossRef] [PubMed]
20. Dockray, G.J.; Moore, A.; Varro, A.; Pritchard, D.M. Gastrin receptor pharmacology. *Curr. Gastroenterol. Rep.* **2012**, *14*, 453–459. [CrossRef] [PubMed]
21. Foucaud, M.; Archer-Lahlou, E.; Marco, E.; Tikhonova, I.G.; Maigret, B.; Escrieut, C.; Langer, I.; Fourmy, D. Insights into the binding and activation sites of the receptors for cholecystokinin and gastrin. *Regul. Pept.* **2008**, *145*, 17–23. [CrossRef] [PubMed]
22. Goetze, J.P.; Nielsen, F.C.; Burcharth, F.; Rehfeld, J.F. Closing the gastrin loop in pancreatic carcinoma: Coexpression of gastrin and its receptor in solid human pancreatic adenocarcinoma. *Cancer* **2000**, *88*, 2487–2494. [CrossRef]
23. Tohidkia, M.R.; Asadi, F.; Barar, J.; Omidi, Y. Selection of potential therapeutic human single-chain fv antibodies against cholecystokinin-b/gastrin receptor by phage display technology. *BioDrugs Clin. Immunother. Biopharm. Gene Ther.* **2013**, *27*, 55–67. [CrossRef] [PubMed]
24. Jo, M.; Jung, S.T. Engineering therapeutic antibodies targeting g-protein-coupled receptors. *Exp. Mol. Med.* **2016**, *48*, e207. [CrossRef] [PubMed]

25. Laverman, P.; Roosenburg, S.; Gotthardt, M.; Park, J.; Oyen, W.J.; de Jong, M.; Hellmich, M.R.; Rutjes, F.P.; van Delft, F.L.; Boerman, O.C. Targeting of a CCK(2) receptor splice variant with (111)In-labelled cholecystokinin-8 (CCK8) and (111)In-labelled minigastrin. *Eur. J. Nucl. Med. Mol. Imaging* **2008**, *35*, 386–392. [CrossRef] [PubMed]
26. Sosabowski, J.K.; Matzow, T.; Foster, J.M.; Finucane, C.; Ellison, D.; Watson, S.A.; Mather, S.J. Targeting of cck-2 receptor-expressing tumors using a radiolabeled divalent gastrin peptide. *J. Nucl. Med.* **2009**, *50*, 2082–2089. [CrossRef] [PubMed]
27. Brom, M.; Joosten, L.; Laverman, P.; Oyen, W.J.; Behe, M.; Gotthardt, M.; Boerman, O.C. Preclinical evaluation of 68ga-dota-minigastrin for the detection of cholecystokinin-2/gastrin receptor-positive tumors. *Mol. Imaging* **2011**, *10*, 144–152. [CrossRef] [PubMed]
28. Behr, T.M.; Behe, M.; Angerstein, C.; Gratz, S.; Mach, R.; Hagemann, L.; Jenner, N.; Stiehler, M.; Frank-Raue, K.; Raue, F.; et al. Cholecystokinin-B/gastrin receptor binding peptides: Preclinical development and evaluation of their diagnostic and therapeutic potential. *Clin. Cancer Res.* **1999**, *5*, 3124s–3138s. [CrossRef] [PubMed]
29. Aloj, L.; Caraco, C.; Panico, M.; Zannetti, A.; Del Vecchio, S.; Tesauro, D.; De Luca, S.; Arra, C.; Pedone, C.; Morelli, G.; et al. In vitro and in vivo evaluation of 111In-DTPAGLU-G-CCK8 for cholecystokinin-B receptor imaging. *J. Nucl. Med.* **2004**, *45*, 485–494. [PubMed]
30. Nock, B.A.; Maina, T.; Behe, M.; Nikolopoulou, A.; Gotthardt, M.; Schmitt, J.S.; Behr, T.M.; Macke, H.R. CCK-2/gastrin receptor-targeted tumor imaging with (99m)Tc-labeled minigastrin analogs. *J. Nucl. Med.* **2005**, *46*, 1727–1736. [PubMed]
31. Kaloudi, A.; Nock, B.A.; Krenning, E.P.; Maina, T.; De Jong, M. Radiolabeled gastrin/cck analogs in tumor diagnosis: Towards higher stability and improved tumor targeting. *Q. J. Nucl. Med. Mol. Imaging* **2015**, *59*, 287–302. [PubMed]
32. Breeman, W.A.; Froberg, A.C.; de Blois, E.; van Gameren, A.; Melis, M.; de Jong, M.; Maina, T.; Nock, B.A.; Erion, J.L.; Macke, H.R.; et al. Optimised labeling, preclinical and initial clinical aspects of cck-2 receptor-targeting with 3 radiolabeled peptides. *Nucl. Med. Biol.* **2008**, *35*, 839–849. [CrossRef] [PubMed]
33. Kaloudi, A.; Nock, B.A.; Lymperis, E.; Krenning, E.P.; de Jong, M.; Maina, T. Improving the in vivo profile of minigastrin radiotracers: A comparative study involving the neutral endopeptidase inhibitor phosphoramidon. *Cancer Biother. Radiopharm.* **2016**, *31*, 20–28. [CrossRef] [PubMed]
34. Kaloudi, A.; Nock, B.A.; Lymperis, E.; Sallegger, W.; Krenning, E.P.; de Jong, M.; Maina, T. In vivo inhibition of neutral endopeptidase enhances the diagnostic potential of truncated gastrin (111)In-radioligands. *Nucl. Med. Biol.* **2015**, *42*, 824–832. [CrossRef] [PubMed]
35. Kaloudi, A.; Nock, B.A.; Lymperis, E.; Valkema, R.; Krenning, E.P.; de Jong, M.; Maina, T. Impact of clinically tested NEP/ACE inhibitors on tumor uptake of [(111)In-DOTA]MG11-first estimates for clinical translation. *EJNMMI Res.* **2016**, *6*, 15. [CrossRef] [PubMed]
36. Barth, B.M.; Sharma, R.; Altinoglu, E.I.; Morgan, T.T.; Shanmugavelandy, S.S.; Kaiser, J.M.; McGovern, C.O.; Matters, G.L.; Smith, J.P.; Kester, M.; et al. Bioconjugation of calcium phosphosilicate composite nanoparticles for selective targeting of huan breast and pancreatic cancers in vivo. *ACS Nano* **2010**, *4*, 1279–1287. [CrossRef] [PubMed]
37. Szepeshazi, K.; Schally, A.V.; Nagy, A.; Halmos, G. Inhibition of growth of experimental human and hamster pancreatic cancers in vivo by a targeted cytotoxic bombesin analog. *Pancreas* **2005**, *31*, 275–282. [CrossRef] [PubMed]
38. Sancho, V.; Di Florio, A.; Moody, T.W.; Jensen, R.T. Bombesin receptor-mediated imaging and cytotoxicity: Review and current status. *Curr. Drug Deliv.* **2011**, *8*, 79–134. [CrossRef] [PubMed]
39. Yu, Z.; Ananias, H.J.; Carlucci, G.; Hoving, H.D.; Helfrich, W.; Dierckx, R.A.; Wang, F.; de Jong, I.J.; Elsinga, P.H. An update of radiolabeled bombesin analogs for gastrin-releasing peptide receptor targeting. *Curr. Pharm. Des.* **2013**, *19*, 3329–3341. [CrossRef] [PubMed]
40. Safavy, A.; Raisch, K.P.; Matusiak, D.; Bhatnagar, S.; Helson, L. Single-drug multiligand conjugates: Synthesis and preliminary cytotoxicity evaluation of a paclitaxel-dipeptide "scorpion" molecule. *Bioconjug. Chem.* **2006**, *17*, 565–570. [CrossRef] [PubMed]
41. Nagy, A.; Armatis, P.; Cai, R.Z.; Szepeshazi, K.; Halmos, G.; Schally, A.V. Design, synthesis, and in vitro evaluation of cytotoxic analogs of bombesin-like peptides containing doxorubicin or its intensely potent derivative, 2-pyrrolinodoxorubicin. *Proc. Natl. Acad. Sci. USA* **1997**, *94*, 652–656. [CrossRef] [PubMed]

42. Moody, T.W.; Sun, L.C.; Mantey, S.A.; Pradhan, T.; Mackey, L.V.; Gonzales, N.; Fuselier, J.A.; Coy, D.H.; Jensen, R.T. In vitro and in vivo antitumor effects of cytotoxic camptothecin-bombesin conjugates are mediated by specific interaction with cellular bombesin receptors. *J. Pharmacol. Exp. Ther.* **2006**, *318*, 1265–1272. [CrossRef] [PubMed]
43. Ramos-Alvarez, I.; Moreno, P.; Mantey, S.A.; Nakamura, T.; Nuche-Berenguer, B.; Moody, T.W.; Coy, D.H.; Jensen, R.T. Insights into bombesin receptors and ligands: Highlighting recent advances. *Peptides* **2015**, *72*, 128–144. [CrossRef] [PubMed]
44. Munoz, M.; Covenas, R. Involvement of substance p and the nk-1 receptor in pancreatic cancer. *World J. Gastroenterol.* **2014**, *20*, 2321–2334. [CrossRef] [PubMed]
45. Li, X.; Ma, G.; Ma, Q.; Li, W.; Liu, J.; Han, L.; Duan, W.; Xu, Q.; Liu, H.; Wang, Z.; et al. Neurotransmitter substance p mediates pancreatic cancer perineural invasion via NK-1R in cancer cells. *Mol. Cancer Res.* **2013**, *11*, 294–302. [CrossRef] [PubMed]
46. Sinha, S.; Fu, Y.Y.; Grimont, A.; Ketcham, M.; Lafaro, K.; Saglimbeni, J.A.; Askan, G.; Bailey, J.M.; Melchor, J.P.; Zhong, Y.; et al. Panin neuroendocrine cells promote tumorigenesis via neuronal crosstalk. *Cancer Res.* **2017**, *77*, 1868–1879. [CrossRef] [PubMed]
47. Kanduluru, A.K.; Srinivasarao, M.; Low, P.S. Design, synthesis, and evaluation of a neurokinin-1 receptor-targeted near-IR dye for fluorescence-guided surgery of neuroendocrine cancers. *Bioconjug. Chem.* **2016**, *27*, 2157–2165. [CrossRef] [PubMed]
48. Low, P.S.; Singhal, S.; Srinivasarao, M. Fluorescence-guided surgery of cancer: Applications, tools and perspectives. *Curr. Opin. Chem. Biol.* **2018**, *45*, 64–72. [CrossRef] [PubMed]
49. Zhang, H.; Kanduluru, A.K.; Desai, P.; Ahad, A.; Carlin, S.; Tandon, N.; Weber, W.A.; Low, P.S. Synthesis and evaluation of a novel (64)Cu- and (67)Ga-labeled neurokinin 1 receptor antagonist for in vivo targeting of NK1R-positive tumor xenografts. *Bioconjug. Chem.* **2018**, *29*, 1319–1326. [CrossRef] [PubMed]
50. Kanduluru, A.K.; Low, P.S. Development of a ligand-targeted therapeutic agent for neurokinin-1 receptor expressing cancers. *Mol. Pharm.* **2017**, *14*, 3859–3865. [CrossRef] [PubMed]
51. Korner, M.; Waser, B.; Strobel, O.; Buchler, M.; Reubi, J.C. Neurotensin receptors in pancreatic ductal carcinomas. *EJNMMI Res.* **2015**, *5*, 17. [CrossRef] [PubMed]
52. Yin, X.; Wang, M.; Wang, H.; Deng, H.; He, T.; Tan, Y.; Zhu, Z.; Wu, Z.; Hu, S.; Li, Z. Evaluation of neurotensin receptor 1 as a potential imaging target in pancreatic ductal adenocarcinoma. *Amino Acids* **2017**, *49*, 1325–1335. [CrossRef] [PubMed]
53. Guha, S.; Lunn, J.A.; Santiskulvong, C.; Rozengurt, E. Neurotensin stimulates protein kinase c-dependent mitogenic signaling in human pancreatic carcinoma cell line PANC-1. *Cancer Res.* **2003**, *63*, 2379–2387. [PubMed]
54. Wang, J.G.; Li, N.N.; Li, H.N.; Cui, L.; Wang, P. Pancreatic cancer bears overexpression of neurotensin and neurotensin receptor subtype-1 and SR 48692 counteracts neurotensin induced cell proliferation in human pancreatic ductal carcinoma cell line PANC-1. *Neuropeptides* **2011**, *45*, 151–156. [CrossRef] [PubMed]
55. Maschauer, S.; Einsiedel, J.; Hubner, H.; Gmeiner, P.; Prante, O. (18)F- and (68)Ga-labeled neurotensin peptides for PET imaging of neurotensin receptor 1. *J. Med. Chem.* **2016**, *59*, 6480–6492. [CrossRef] [PubMed]
56. Maschauer, S.; Prante, O. Radiopharmaceuticals for imaging and endoradiotherapy of neurotensin receptor-positive tumors. *J. Label. Compd. Radiopharm.* **2018**, *61*, 309–325. [CrossRef] [PubMed]
57. Schulz, J.; Rohracker, M.; Stiebler, M.; Goldschmidt, J.; Grosser, O.S.; Osterkamp, F.; Pethe, A.; Reineke, U.; Smerling, C.; Amthauer, H. Comparative evaluation of the biodistribution profiles of a series of nonpeptidic neurotensin receptor-1 antagonists reveals a promising candidate for theranostic applications. *J. Nucl. Med.* **2016**, *57*, 1120–1123. [CrossRef] [PubMed]
58. Falciani, C.; Brunetti, J.; Lelli, B.; Accardo, A.; Tesauro, D.; Morelli, G.; Bracci, L. Nanoparticles exposing neurotensin tumor-specific drivers. *J. Pept. Sci.* **2013**, *19*, 198–204. [CrossRef] [PubMed]
59. Hao, F.; Xu, Q.; Zhao, Y.; Stevens, J.V.; Young, S.H.; Sinnett-Smith, J.; Rozengurt, E. Insulin receptor and GPCR crosstalk stimulates YAP via PI3K and PKD in pancreatic cancer cells. *Mol. Cancer Res.* **2017**, *15*, 929–941. [CrossRef] [PubMed]
60. Rozengurt, E.; Sinnett-Smith, J.; Eibl, G. Yes-associated protein (YAP) in pancreatic cancer: At the epicenter of a targetable signaling network associated with patient survival. *Signal Transduct. Targeted Ther.* **2018**, *3*, 11. [CrossRef] [PubMed]

61. Shahbaz, M.; Ruliang, F.; Xu, Z.; Benjia, L.; Cong, W.; Zhaobin, H.; Jun, N. Mrna expression of somatostatin receptor subtypes SSTR-2, SSTR-3, and SSTR-5 and its significance in pancreatic cancer. *World J. Surg. Oncol.* **2015**, *13*, 46. [CrossRef] [PubMed]
62. Chalabi-Dchar, M.; Cassant-Sourdy, S.; Duluc, C.; Fanjul, M.; Lulka, H.; Samain, R.; Roche, C.; Breibach, F.; Delisle, M.B.; Poupot, M.; et al. Loss of somatostatin receptor subtype 2 promotes growth of KRAS-induced pancreatic tumors in mice by activating PI3K signaling and overexpression of CXCL16. *Gastroenterology* **2015**, *148*, 1452–1465. [CrossRef] [PubMed]
63. De Jong, M.; Breeman, W.A.; Kwekkeboom, D.J.; Valkema, R.; Krenning, E.P. Tumor imaging and therapy using radiolabeled somatostatin analogues. *Acc. Chem. Res.* **2009**, *42*, 873–880. [CrossRef] [PubMed]
64. Wolin, E.M. The expanding role of somatostatin analogs in the management of neuroendocrine tumors. *Gastrointest. Cancer Res.* **2012**, *5*, 161–168. [PubMed]
65. Sun, L.C.; Coy, D.H. Somatostatin receptor-targeted anti-cancer therapy. *Curr. Drug Deliv.* **2011**, *8*, 2–10. [CrossRef] [PubMed]
66. Sun, L.C.; Mackey, L.V.; Luo, J.; Fuselier, J.A.; Coy, D.H. Targeted chemotherapy using a cytotoxic somatostatin conjugate to inhibit tumor growth and metastasis in nude mice. *Clin. Med. Oncol.* **2008**, *2*, 491–499. [CrossRef] [PubMed]
67. Ahmadi, Y.; Kostenich, G.; Oron-Herman, M.; Wadsak, W.; Mitterhauser, M.; Orenstein, A.; Mirzaei, S.; Knoll, P. In vivo magnetic resonance imaging of pancreatic tumors using iron oxide nanoworms targeted with PTR86 peptide. *Colloids Surf. B Biointerfaces* **2017**, *158*, 423–430. [CrossRef] [PubMed]
68. Ghosh, S.C.; Hernandez Vargas, S.; Rodriguez, M.; Kossatz, S.; Voss, J.; Carmon, K.S.; Reiner, T.; Schonbrunn, A.; Azhdarinia, A. Synthesis of a fluorescently labeled (68)Ga-DOTA-TOC analog for somatostatin receptor targeting. *ACS Med. Chem. Lett.* **2017**, *8*, 720–725. [CrossRef] [PubMed]
69. Jorand, R.; Biswas, S.; Wakefield, D.L.; Tobin, S.J.; Golfetto, O.; Hilton, K.; Ko, M.; Ramos, J.W.; Small, A.R.; Chu, P.; et al. Molecular signatures of mu opioid receptor and somatostatin receptor 2 in pancreatic cancer. *Mol. Biol. Cell* **2016**, *27*, 3659–3672. [CrossRef] [PubMed]
70. Maddipati, R.; Stanger, B.Z. Pancreatic cancer metastases harbor evidence of polyclonality. *Cancer Discov.* **2015**, *5*, 1086–1097. [CrossRef] [PubMed]
71. Ehlerding, E.B.; Sun, L.; Lan, X.; Zeng, D.; Cai, W. Dual-targeted molecular imaging of cancer. *J. Nucl. Med.* **2018**, *59*, 390–395. [CrossRef] [PubMed]
72. Xu, L.; Josan, J.S.; Vagner, J.; Caplan, M.R.; Hruby, V.J.; Mash, E.A.; Lynch, R.M.; Morse, D.L.; Gillies, R.J. Heterobivalent ligands target cell-surface receptor combinations in vivo. *Proc. Natl. Acad. Sci. USA* **2012**, *109*, 21295–21300. [CrossRef] [PubMed]
73. Zhang, J.; Niu, G.; Lang, L.; Li, F.; Fan, X.; Yan, X.; Yao, S.; Yan, W.; Huo, L.; Chen, L.; et al. Clinical translation of a dual integrin alphavbeta3- and gastrin-releasing peptide receptor-targeting pet radiotracer, 68ga-BBN-RGD. *J. Nucl. Med.* **2017**, *58*, 228–234. [CrossRef] [PubMed]
74. Luo, H.; England, C.G.; Goel, S.; Graves, S.A.; Ai, F.; Liu, B.; Theuer, C.P.; Wong, H.C.; Nickles, R.J.; Cai, W. Immunopet and near-infrared fluorescence imaging of pancreatic cancer with a dual-labeled bispecific antibody fragment. *Mol. Pharm.* **2017**, *14*, 1646–1655. [CrossRef] [PubMed]
75. Luo, H.; England, C.G.; Shi, S.; Graves, S.A.; Hernandez, R.; Liu, B.; Theuer, C.P.; Wong, H.C.; Nickles, R.J.; Cai, W. Dual targeting of tissue factor and cd105 for preclinical pet imaging of pancreatic cancer. *Clin. Cancer Res.* **2016**, *22*, 3821–3830. [CrossRef] [PubMed]
76. Rothlisberger, P.; Gasse, C.; Hollenstein, M. Nucleic acid aptamers: Emerging applications in medical imaging, nanotechnology, neurosciences, and drug delivery. *Int. J. Mol. Sci.* **2017**, *18*, 2430. [CrossRef] [PubMed]
77. Tawiah, K.D.; Porciani, D.; Burke, D.H. Toward the selection of cell targeting aptamers with extended biological functionalities to facilitate endosomal escape of cargoes. *Biomedicines* **2017**, *5*, 51. [CrossRef] [PubMed]
78. Xiang, D.; Zheng, C.; Zhou, S.F.; Qiao, S.; Tran, P.H.; Pu, C.; Li, Y.; Kong, L.; Kouzani, A.Z.; Lin, J.; et al. Superior performance of aptamer in tumor penetration over antibody: Implication of aptamer-based theranostics in solid tumors. *Theranostics* **2015**, *5*, 1083–1097. [CrossRef] [PubMed]
79. Yoon, S.; Rossi, J.J. Emerging cancer-specific therapeutic aptamers. *Curr. Opin. Oncol.* **2017**, *29*, 366–374. [CrossRef] [PubMed]

80. Hori, S.I.; Herrera, A.; Rossi, J.J.; Zhou, J. Current advances in aptamers for cancer diagnosis and therapy. *Cancers* **2018**, *10*, 9. [CrossRef] [PubMed]
81. Li, X.; Zhao, Q.; Qiu, L. Smart ligand: Aptamer-mediated targeted delivery of chemotherapeutic drugs and sirna for cancer therapy. *J. Control. Release* **2013**, *171*, 152–162. [CrossRef] [PubMed]
82. Catuogno, S.; Esposito, C.L.; de Franciscis, V. Aptamer-mediated targeted delivery of therapeutics: An update. *Pharmaceuticals* **2016**, *9*, 69. [CrossRef] [PubMed]
83. Alshaer, W.; Ababneh, N.; Hatmal, M.; Izmirli, H.; Choukeife, M.; Shraim, A.; Sharar, N.; Abu-Shiekah, A.; Odeh, F.; Al Bawab, A.; et al. Selection and targeting of epcam protein by ssdna aptamer. *PLoS ONE* **2017**, *12*, e0189558. [CrossRef] [PubMed]
84. Melancon, M.P.; Zhou, M.; Zhang, R.; Xiong, C.; Allen, P.; Wen, X.; Huang, Q.; Wallace, M.; Myers, J.N.; Stafford, R.J.; et al. Selective uptake and imaging of aptamer- and antibody-conjugated hollow nanospheres targeted to epidermal growth factor receptors overexpressed in head and neck cancer. *ACS Nano* **2014**, *8*, 4530–4538. [CrossRef] [PubMed]
85. Pei, X.; Zhang, J.; Liu, J. Clinical applications of nucleic acid aptamers in cancer. *Mol. Clin. Oncol.* **2014**, *2*, 341–348. [CrossRef] [PubMed]
86. Clawson, G.A.; Abraham, T.; Pan, W.; Tang, X.; Linton, S.S.; McGovern, C.O.; Loc, W.S.; Smith, J.P.; Butler, P.J.; Kester, M.; et al. A cholecystokinin b receptor-specific DNA aptamer for targeting pancreatic ductal adenocarcinoma. *Nucleic Acid Ther.* **2016**, *27*, 23–35. [CrossRef] [PubMed]
87. Daniels, D.A.; Sohal, A.K.; Rees, S.; Grisshammer, R. Generation of rna aptamers to the g-protein-coupled receptor for neurotensin, NTS-1. *Anal. Biochem.* **2002**, *305*, 214–226. [CrossRef] [PubMed]
88. Kahsai, A.W.; Wisler, J.W.; Lee, J.; Ahn, S.; Cahill Iii, T.J.; Dennison, S.M.; Staus, D.P.; Thomsen, A.R.; Anasti, K.M.; Pani, B.; et al. Conformationally selective rna aptamers allosterically modulate the beta2-adrenoceptor. *Nat. Chem. Biol.* **2016**, *12*, 709–716. [CrossRef] [PubMed]
89. Lai, W.Y.; Huang, B.T.; Wang, J.W.; Lin, P.Y.; Yang, P.C. A novel pd-l1-targeting antagonistic DNA aptamer with antitumor effects. *Mol. Ther. Nucleic Acids* **2016**, *5*, e397. [CrossRef] [PubMed]
90. Shi, K.; Zhao, Y.; Miao, L.; Satterlee, A.; Haynes, M.; Luo, C.; Musetti, S.; Huang, L. Dual functional lipomet mediates envelope-type nanoparticles to combinational oncogene silencing and tumor growth inhibition. *Mol. Ther. J. Am. Soc. Gene Ther.* **2017**, *25*, 1567–1579. [CrossRef] [PubMed]
91. Herrmann, A.; Priceman, S.J.; Swiderski, P.; Kujawski, M.; Xin, H.; Cherryholmes, G.A.; Zhang, W.; Zhang, C.; Lahtz, C.; Kowolik, C.; et al. Ctla4 aptamer delivers stat3 sirna to tumor-associated and malignant T cells. *J. Clin. Investig.* **2014**, *124*, 2977–2987. [CrossRef] [PubMed]
92. Huang, B.T.; Lai, W.Y.; Chang, Y.C.; Wang, J.W.; Yeh, S.D.; Lin, E.P.; Yang, P.C. A ctla-4 antagonizing DNA aptamer with antitumor effect. *Mol. Ther. Nucleic Acids* **2017**, *8*, 520–528. [CrossRef] [PubMed]
93. Seufferlein, T.; Mayerle, J. Pancreatic cancer in 2015: Precision medicine in pancreatic cancer—Fact or fiction? *Nat. Rev. Gastroenterol. Hepatol.* **2016**, *13*, 74–75. [CrossRef] [PubMed]
94. Kenner, B.J.; Chari, S.T.; Maitra, A.; Srivastava, S.; Cleeter, D.F.; Go, V.L.; Rothschild, L.J.; Goldberg, A.E. Early detection of pancreatic cancer-a defined future using lessons from other cancers: A white paper. *Pancreas* **2016**, *45*, 1073–1079. [CrossRef] [PubMed]

 © 2018 by the authors. Licensee MDPI, Basel, Switzerland. This article is an open access article distributed under the terms and conditions of the Creative Commons Attribution (CC BY) license (http://creativecommons.org/licenses/by/4.0/).

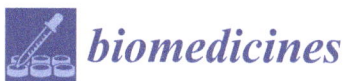

Review

Molecular Characterization of Gastric Carcinoma: Therapeutic Implications for Biomarkers and Targets

Lionel Kankeu Fonkoua [1] and Nelson S. Yee [2,*]

[1] Department of Medicine, Penn State Health Milton S. Hershey Medical Center, Hershey, PA 17033, USA; lkankeufonkoua@pennstatehealth.psu.edu

[2] Division of Hematology-Oncology, Department of Medicine, Penn State Health Milton S. Hershey Medical Center, Experimental Therapeutics Program, Penn State Cancer Institute, Pennsylvania State University College of Medicine, Hershey, PA 17033, USA

* Correspondence: nyee@pennstatehealth.psu.edu; Tel.: +1-717-531-0003

Received: 1 January 2018; Accepted: 5 March 2018; Published: 9 March 2018

Abstract: Palliative chemotherapy is the mainstay of treatment of advanced gastric carcinoma (GC). Monoclonal antibodies including trastuzumab, ramucirumab, and pembrolizumab have been shown to provide additional benefits. However, the clinical outcomes are often unpredictable and they can vary widely among patients. Currently, no biomarker is available for predicting treatment response in the individual patient except human epidermal growth factor receptor 2 (HER2) amplification and programmed death-ligand 1 (PD-L1) expression for effectiveness of trastuzumab and pembrolizumab, respectively. Multi-platform molecular analysis of cancer, including GC, may help identify predictive biomarkers to guide selection of therapeutic agents. Molecular classification of GC by The Cancer Genome Atlas Research Network and the Asian Cancer Research Group is expected to identify therapeutic targets and predictive biomarkers. Complementary to molecular characterization of GC is molecular profiling by expression analysis and genomic sequencing of tumor DNA. Initial analysis of patients with gastroesophageal carcinoma demonstrates that the ratio of progression-free survival (PFS) on molecular profile (MP)-based treatment to PFS on treatment prior to molecular profiling exceeds 1.3, suggesting the potential value of MP in guiding selection of individualized therapy. Future strategies aiming to integrate molecular classification and profiling of tumors with therapeutic agents for achieving the goal of personalized treatment of GC are indicated.

Keywords: Asian Cancer Research Group (ACRG); gastric carcinoma; molecular profiling; precision therapy; pembrolizumab; predictive biomarkers; ramucirumab; The Cancer Genome Atlas (TCGA); therapeutic targets; trastuzumab

---

1. Introduction

With about a million diagnosed cases and over 700,000 deaths recorded annually, gastric carcinoma (GC) is the third most common cause of cancer deaths worldwide [1]. While 80 to 90% of tumors develop sporadically, hereditary factors also contribute to gastric carcinogenesis [2]. The incidence is strongly influenced by ethnicity, diet, and infectious agents [3–6]. In particular, *Helicobacter pylori* (*H. pylori*) and human papilloma virus (HPV) are involved in multi-step processes causing chronic gastritis, intestinal metaplasia, and invasive carcinoma [7–9]. Population-based screening and treatment of *H. pylori* and HPV would be a logical strategy for prevention of some types of GC, but no randomized trial to date has shown a clear benefit of this approach [10]. Until a preventive intervention is implemented, it is imperative that effective and tolerable therapies are developed in attempt to attenuate the global burden of GC.

Systemic chemotherapy and targeted therapy play important roles in the multi-disciplinary management of GC. With the exception of GC diagnosed at T1 stage, chemotherapy is employed in the neoadjuvant and adjuvant settings, or concurrent with radiation therapy. Palliative combination chemotherapy and targeted therapy are the only treatment options for patients with advanced or metastatic GC. Selection of chemotherapeutic drugs is typically based on performance status, medical comorbidities, and medical oncologist's experience or preference. There are no valid biomarkers predictive of treatment response of GC to therapeutic agents. Exceptions are, amplification of human epidermal growth factor receptor 2 (HER2) and expression of programmed death-ligand 1 (PD-L1), for which trastuzumab and pembrolizumab, respectively, have been demonstrated to produce clinical benefit [11,12]. Preliminary evidence has indicated that variable responses to treatment can be attributed to tumor heterogeneity with regard to molecular alterations [13]. Recently, two classification systems of GC using multi-platforms of molecular analyses have been developed, and they provide new insights into tumor heterogeneity of GC.

The genomic characterization of GC has led to the development of two new classifications of GC by The Cancer Genome Atlas (TCGA) Research Network [14] and the Asian Cancer Research Group (ACRG) [15]. These may serve as a valuable diagnostic companion to the conventionally used classification systems of GC based on histopathology by World Health Organization [16] and Lauren [17]. Importantly, TCGA and ACRG are expected to facilitate the development of personalized prognostication and treatment, as well as improved patient stratification for clinical trial design. Moreover, molecular profiling of GC has been accomplished through immunohistochemistry (IHC), in situ hybridization (ISH), genomic DNA sequencing, proteomics, and microRNA expression. The tumor molecular profiles can potentially be developed into predictive biomarkers of treatment that could help guide selection of cytotoxic drugs and targeted therapeutics.

The goal of this article is to provide a critical review of the molecular characterization of GC, and elaborate on the molecular features that can be translated into therapeutic biomarkers and targets for clinical use. First, we provide an overview of the conventionally used systemic chemotherapy and targeted therapeutics of GC. The data on molecular classification of GC by TCGA and ACRG as well as molecular profiling of GC are examined. The potential of translating the molecular classification and profiling of GC into therapeutic targets and predictive biomarkers are discussed. We hope that this article will help identify the opportunity and challenge of developing strategies towards the goal of precision medicine in GC by improving therapeutic efficacy and minimizing treatment-related toxicity.

2. Systemic Treatment of Gastric Carcinoma

Systemic chemotherapy is employed for treatment of patients with localized GC as well as for those with advanced GC. Surgical resection with pre- and post-operative chemotherapy and/or radiation therapy represents the primary curative treatment of early-stage GC with 5-year survival rate of less than 30% [18–20]. For patients with advanced unresectable or metastatic disease, palliative systemic therapy and chemoradiation therapy are the standard treatment options. The chemotherapeutic regimens used for patients with advanced or metastatic GC are essentially the same as those for peri-operative treatment of patients with localized GC. In addition, for advanced or metastatic GC, trastuzumab is indicated to use in combination with HER2 amplified GC as first-line treatment; ramucirumab either as monotherapy or in combination with paclitaxel is indicated as second-line treatment; pembrolizumab has recently been approved as 3rd-line treatment for GC expressing PD-L1. A number of targeted therapeutics is being investigated in clinical studies.

2.1. Chemotherapy

Chemotherapeutic regimens currently being used for GC consist of anthracycline, fluoropyrimidine, taxane, and platinum-based agents. For advanced or metastatic GC, first-line combinations such as EOX (epirubicin, oxaliplatin, capecitabine) and DCF (docetaxel, cisplatin, 5-fluorouracil (5-FU)) have produced limited survival benefits, with median survival not exceeding one year (Table 1). Second-line agents such as docetaxel or irinotecan can lead to slight improvement of survival. For most patients, GC may initially respond to chemotherapy. However, the tumors will typically become resistant, such that the prognosis of patients with advanced disease remains poor. Currently, there is no clinically available predictor of tumor response to the empiric use of these drug combinations [21].

Table 1. Major phase III clinical trials of first-line cytotoxic agents in metastatic/advanced gastric carcinoma.

Treatment	Patients (*n*)	RR (%)	PFS (months)	OS (months)	Reference
CF vs. DCF	224 vs. 221	25 vs. 37	3.7 vs. 5.6 (* $p < 0.001$)	8.6 vs. 9.2 (* $p < 0.02$)	[22]
ECF vs. ECX vs. EOF vs. EOX	263 vs. 250 vs. 245 vs. 244	38 vs. 41 vs. 40 vs. 47	6.2 vs. 6.7 vs. 6.5 vs. 7.0 (NS)	9.9 vs. 9.9 vs. 9.3 vs. 11.2 (NS)	[23]
5-FU + LV + cisplatin vs. 5-FU + LV + oxaliplatin	112 vs. 106	25 vs. 34	3.9 vs. 5.8 (NS)	8.8 vs. 10.7 (NS)	[24]
Cisplatin + 5-FU vs. Cisplatin + S-1	508 vs. 521	31 vs. 29	5.6 vs. 5.3 (NS)	7.9 vs. 8.6 (NS)	[25]

CF, cisplatin/5-fluorouracil (5-FU); DCF, docetaxel/cisplatin/5-FU; ECF, epirubicin/cisplatin/5-FU; ECX, epirubicin/cisplatin/capecitabine; EOF, epirubicin/oxaliplatin/5-FU; EOX, epirubicin/oxaliplatin/ capecitabine; LV, leucovorin; NS, not statistically significant; OS, overall survival; * $p < 0.05$, statistically significant; PFS, progression-free survival; RR, response rate.

2.2. Targeted Therapy

Despite the clinical heterogeneity and molecular complexity of GC, targeted therapeutics directed against the genetic mutations and signaling pathways that drive tumor growth and invasion have been developed and clinically investigated. Targeted therapies currently in clinical use include trastuzumab, ramucirumab, and pembrolizumab. Other targeted therapeutics directed against the signaling pathways of mitogenesis, angiogenesis, and immune checkpoints are under clinical investigation for treatment of GC.

2.2.1. Mitogenic Signaling Pathways as Therapeutic Targets

Human epidermal growth factor receptor (HER2, also known as ErbB2) is a transmembrane tyrosine kinase receptor of the ErbB family. The ErbB members play important roles in regulation of cellular functions including proliferation, growth, survival, adhesion, migration, and differentiation. HER2 acts by heterodimerization with other ErbB family receptors leading to activation of the RAS-MAPK (mitogen-activated protein kinase) and PI3K-AKT (phosphatidylinositol 3-kinase—AKT) pathways. HER2 has been found to be over-expressed in 20% to 30% of GC depending on the tumor subtype and location.

Several HER2-targeting agents have been developed and evaluated in phase III trials for patients with advanced HER2-positive gastroesophageal junction carcinoma (GEJC)/GC. Trastuzumab is a humanized IgG1 monoclonal antibody (mAb) directed against the extracellular domain of HER2, and it prevents dimerization of the HER2 receptors. This triggers receptor internalization and mediates antibody-dependent cell-mediated cytotoxicity (ADCC), resulting in inhibition of tumor growth [26]. In the phase III ToGA trial, the combination of trastuzumab and cisplatin/fluoropyrimidine-based chemotherapy was compared to chemotherapy alone as first-line therapy for advanced HER2-positive GEJC/GC. Results of this study indicated a significant improvement in the overall response rate (ORR; 47% vs. 35%; $p < 0.01$) as well as prolonged progression-free survival (PFS; 6.7 months vs. 5.5 months, $p < 0.01$) and overall survival (OS; 13.8 months vs. 11.1 months; $p < 0.01$) [11]. Based on the results of this study, the combination of trastuzumab with platinum/fluoropyrimidine-based chemotherapy has become the standard of care for advanced HER2-positive GEJC/GC. However, the treatment response was not durable, as the benefit from trastuzumab was noted to have diminished considerably in an updated survival analysis, with an increased hazard ratio (HR) from 0.73 to 0.80, and narrowed OS difference to 1.4 months. These data suggest considerable heterogeneity among patients with HER2-positive GEJC/GC, possible treatment resistance, and need to refine and optimize biomarker selection criteria for future clinical trials. A recent report shows that trastuzumab conjugated with nanoparticle albumin-bound paclitaxel produced enhanced anti-tumor effect in a mouse xenograft of

HER2-positive gastric cancer cells [27]. Further investigation of this antibody-nanoparticle conjugate in patients may raise hope for a novel form of targeted therapy in HER2-positive GC.

2.2.2. Signaling Pathways in Angiogenesis as Therapeutic Targets

Several signaling pathways are involved in tumor-associated angiogenesis, such as those activated by vascular endothelial growth factor (VEGF) [28], angiopoietins and angiopoietin-like proteins [29,30], platelet-derived growth factor (PDGF) [31], basic fibroblast growth factor (FGF) [32], fibroblast activation protein and hepatocyte growth factor [33], and Wingless-related integration site (WNT) [34]. These growth factors and their receptors have been investigated for therapeutic targeting in various types of malignant tumors. Antibodies directed against VEGF and VEGF receptor (VEGFR) have been shown to produce anti-tumor efficacy and they are used in combination with cytotoxic chemotherapy as standard first- or second-line treatment of certain solid tumors.

VEGF is a growth factor secreted by the tumor to stimulate formation of new blood vessels in response to hypoxia and nutrient depletion. When it binds to VEGFR, a complex cascade of downstream signaling pathways is activated, resulting in neovascularization, vasodilation, and increased vascular permeability [28]. Blockade of VEGF and/or VEGFR impedes these pathways and thereby inhibits tumor survival, migration, and invasion. VEGF and its receptors are over-expressed in approximately 30% to 40% of all GEJC/GC [35,36], and anti-angiogenic agents targeting VEGF and VEGFR have shown therapeutic efficacy in GEJC/GC.

Ramucirumab is a recombinant humanized monoclonal antibody (mAb) that binds to VEGF-R2 and prevents its activation by VEGF. In contrast to bevacizumab (anti-VEGFA mAb), it has shown clinical efficacy as a single agent (REGARD trial) and in combination with paclitaxel (RAINBOW trial). Based on the results of these studies, ramucirumab either alone or in combination with paclitaxel has become standard second-line treatments for advanced GEJC/GC. In the REGARD trial, ramucirumab was associated with a significant improvement in OS (5.2 months vs. 3.8 months, $p = 0.0473$) and PFS (2.1 months vs. 1.3 months, $p < 0.0001$) in patients previously treated with first-line platinum- or fluoro-pyrimidine-based therapy [37]. In the RAINBOW study, the combination of ramucirumab and paclitaxel produced significant improvement in OS (9.6 months vs. 7.4 months, $p = 0.0169$), PFS (4.4 months vs. 2.9 months, $p < 0.0001$), and ORR (28% vs. 16%, $p = 0.0001$) compared with those treated with paclitaxel alone [38]. However, the clinical benefit of ramucirumab with or without paclitaxel is limited, and there is no biomarker available to predict tumor response to these treatments.

2.2.3. Immune Checkpoint Molecules as Targets for Therapy

The programmed death-ligand 1 (PD-L1) and 2 (PD-L2) are normally expressed on antigen-presenting cells (APC) and also on tumor cells. Binding of PD-L1 and PD-L2 to their receptors (PD-1) on activated T cells leads to downregulation of cytotoxic T-cell activity and causing immunosuppression. PD-L1 is expressed in 15% to 70% of GCs, and they are associated with poor prognosis [39]. Pembrolizumab and nivolumab are humanized mAbs directed against PD-1, and they enhance the ability of the immune system to detect and destroy cancer cells. By blocking the interaction between PD-1 and PD-L1/L2, pembrolizumab or nivolumab counters the tumor's immune-escaping tactic.

In the phase Ib KEYNOTE-012 trial, the activity and safety of pembrolizumab were evaluated in a cohort of 39 patients with advanced GEJC/GC. Pembrolizumab produced an ORR of 22.2%, 6-month PFS rate 24%, and OS rate 69% [40,41]. An association between higher levels of PD-L1 expression and ORR ($p = 0.102$), PFS ($p = 0.162$), and OS ($p = 0.124$) was observed. In a phase II study (KEYNOTE-059) of 259 patients, pembrolizumab monotherapy showed clinical efficacy in previously treated advanced GEJC/GC [12]. For patients with PD-L1 positive tumors, pembrolizumab produced an ORR of 15.5%, whereas in patients with PD-L1 negative tumors, 6.4%. In patients with microsatellite-high (MSI-H), ORR was 57.1%; in those with non-MSI-H tumors, ORR 9.0%. These data demonstrate the value of PD-L1 and MSI-H as predictive biomarkers for efficacy of pembrolizumab. In the cohort 2 of this study, the efficacy and safety of pembrolizumab in combination with cisplatin and 5-fluorouracil (5-FU) will be assessed.

3. Molecular Classification and Profiling of Gastric Carcinoma

Advances in next-generation sequencing (NGS) technologies and improved understanding of cancer biology have unlocked opportunities to characterize the genomic landscape of cancer including GC. Using multi-platform analyses, molecular profiling of GC has enabled The Cancer Genome Atlas (TCGA) Research Network and the Asian Cancer Research Group (ACRG) to classify GC into subtypes. The new molecular classification of GC is complementary to the conventionally used system of subtyping GC based on histopathology. Importantly, molecular classification of GC helps identify molecular alterations that may be targeted for therapy. Furthermore, molecular profiling of GC collected from individual patients using a multi-platform approach has offered new opportunity to identify biomarkers that may be predictive of tumor response to treatment [42–44].

3.1. TCGA Sub-Typing of Gastric Carcinoma: Potential Therapeutic Targets

Molecular classification of GC by the TCGA Research Network utilized six distinct platforms, including exome sequencing, copy number analysis, methylation, expression of miRNA and mRNA. Based on TCGA molecular data, GC were divided into four groups: Epstein–Barr virus-positive (EBV; 9%), microsatellite instability (MSI; 22%), chromosomal instability (CIN; 50%), genomically stable (GS; 20%) (Figure 1). Each of these GC subtypes is characterized by distinct features that provide prognostic information and suggest potential benefit of targeted therapy.

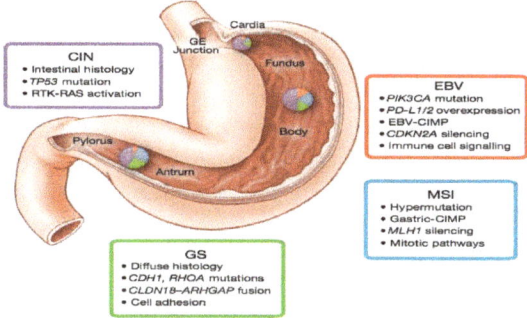

Figure 1. The four molecular subtypes described in the TCGA study, their mutational patterns, and location. CIN, chromosomal instability; EBV, Epstein–Barr virus; GE, gastroesophageal junction; GS, genomically stable; MSI, microsatellite instability. This figure is reproduced from reference [14] with permission from the Nature Publishing Group.

The EBV-positive tumors were found to be mainly located in the gastric fundus or body. They exhibited higher prevalence of DNA promoter hypermethylation, A to C transversions, *PIK3CA* mutation, recurrent JAK2 and ERBB2 amplifications, interleukin-12 (IL-12) mediated signaling, and PD-L1/2 overexpression. The presence of viral antigens such as EBV (a hallmark of 9% of GCs) has been shown to result in increased neo-epitope presentation [14], which might contribute to an anti-tumor immune response. Moreover, the strength of IL-12 mediated signaling signature suggests a robust immune cell presence, which when coupled with evidence of PD-L1/2 overexpression, provides support for targeted immunotherapy. PD-L1/2 may therefore represent promising targets in these tumors and initial promising results have been reported with pembrolizumab [40,41]. In addition, the strong predilection for mutation in *PIK3CA* (80%) suggests that inhibition of PI3K warrants further evaluation in EBV-positive GC.

The MSI tumors, characterized by genomic instability due to a deficient DNA mismatch repair system, lacked targetable amplifications. This subtype of tumors was noted to have hypermethylation in the *MLH1* promoter region (leading to MLH1 silencing), and targetable hotspot mutations in *PIK3CA*, *ERBB3*, *ERBB2*, and *EGFR*. Of note, the $BRAF^{V600E}$ mutation commonly seen in MSI colorectal cancer was absent. However, gastric MSI tumors had a high rate of PD-L1 expression. In particular, recent evidence shows that enhanced anti-PD-1 responsiveness of mismatch repair-deficient tumors is related to the high number of mutation-associated neoantigens [45].

The CIN tumors were more frequent in the gastro-esophageal junction/cardia. They were noted to have the highest frequency of *TP53* mutations (71%), as well as genomic amplifications of RTKs and cell cycle mediators. Phosphorylation of EGFR was significantly elevated. Recurrent amplification of the gene encoding ligand VEGFA was also notable. Additionally, frequent amplifications of cell cycle mediators (*CCNE1*, *CCND1* and *CDK6*) were present. Alterations of these genes have been confirmed in a cohort of 116 advanced/metastatic GC cases [44].

The GS tumors, which lack either chromosomal alteration or microsatellite instability, exhibited elevated expression of molecules in the cell adhesion and angiogenesis-related pathways. Previous studies had demonstrated loss of the tumor-suppressor gene *CDH1* encoding the cell adhesion molecule E-cadherin in hereditary diffuse gastric cancer [6]. The TCGA data also revealed recurrent mutations in *RHOA* (Ras homolog gene family, member A) and fusion of *CLDN18-ARHGAP6* or 26 (30% of cases). RHOA modulates programmed cell death and actomyosin-dependent cell contractility and motility [46–48], while *CLDN18* and *ARHGAP6* are involved in intercellular tight junction structure and Rho signaling activation, respectively. Thus, alterations in either *RHOA* or *CLDN18-ARHGAP6* might contribute to lack of cellular cohesion, dispersed growth, and resistance to programmed cell death.

The TCGA data indicate that each of the four defined molecular subtypes displays distinct but overlapping candidate therapeutic targets. These suggest the potential of targeted therapeutics in each subtype of GC (Table 2). The discovery of mutations in the *RHOA* and *CLDN18* gene products could be exploited to develop new therapeutic strategies in the genomically stable subtype.

Table 2. TCGA molecular subtypes of gastric carcinoma and the associated targets and targeted agents.

Subtypes	Targets	Targeted Agents
EBV	PIK3CA	Idelalisib, Taselisib
	PD-L1/L2	Pembrolizumab, Nivolumab, Durvalumab, Avelumab, Atezolizumab
MSI	MLH1 silencing	Pembrolizumab, Nivolumab, Durvalumab, Avelumab, Atezolizumab
	PIK3CA	Idelalisib, Taselisib
	EGFR	Erlotinib, Gefitinib
	ERBB2	Trastuzumab
	ERBB3	Pertuzumab
	PD-L1	Pembrolizumab, Nivolumab, Durvalumab, Avelumab, Atezolizumab
CIN	EGFR	Erlotinib, Gefitinib
	VEGFA	Bevacizumab, Ramucirumab
	CCNE1, CCND1, CDK6	Palbociclib, Ribociclib, Abemaciclib
GS	RHOA	-
	CLDN18	-

CDK, cyclin-dependent kinase; CCND, cyclin D; CCNE, cyclin E; CIN, chromosomal instability; CLDN, claudin; EBV, Epstein–Barr virus; EGFR, epidermal growth factor receptor; GS, genomically stable; MLH1, MutL homolog 1; MSI, microsatellite instability; PD-L1/L2, programmed death ligand 1/ligand 2; PIK3CA, phosphatidylinositol-4,5-bisphosphate 3-kinase catalytic subunit alpha; VEGF, vascular endothelial growth factor

3.2. ACRG Sub-Typing of Gastric Carcinoma: Potential Prognostic Biomarkers

Complementary to the TCGA data, the ACRG proposed a classification of GC that correlates four molecular subtypes with distinct patterns of molecular alterations, disease progression and prognosis. The molecular analyses include principal component analysis (PCA) [49] of expression data and compared the association of the first three principal components with a small pre-defined set of gene expression signatures relevant to biology of GC. These include epithelial-to-mesenchymal transition (EMT) [50], microsatellite instability (MSI) [51], cytokine signaling [52], cell proliferation [53], DNA methylation [54], p53 activity [55], and gastric tissue [56]. Of the 300 specimens of GC being analyzed, the MSI subtype accounts for 23%, MSS/EMT 20%, MSS/TP53+ (mutated) 26%, and MSS/TP53− (wild-type) 36% (Figure 2). *TP53* is the most frequently mutated gene in GC, and the status of p53 activation is based on a two-gene (CDKN1A and MDM2) p53-activity signature.

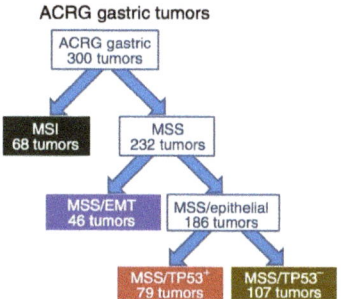

Figure 2. Illustration of the Asian Cancer Research Group (ACRG) classification tree. EMT, epithelia-to-mesenchymal transition; MSI, microsatellite instability; MSS, microsatellite stability. This figure is reproduced from reference [15] with permission from the Nature Publishing Group.

The MSI tumors, as in the TCGA cohort, were found to be hypermutated [57,58] intestinal-subtype tumors occurring in the antrum. It is associated with the best overall prognosis and the lowest frequency of recurrence (22%) of the four subtypes. They exhibited mutations in genes such as *KRAS* (23.3%), the PI3K-PTEN-mTOR pathway (42%), *ALK* (16.3%) and *ARID1A* (44.2%) [46].

The MSS/TP53+ phenotype is associated with a better prognosis, and a higher prevalence of mutations in *APC*, *ARID1A*, *KRAS*, *PIK3CA* and *SMAD4*, compared to the MSS/TP53− phenotype. Consistent with these observations, mutations in *TP53* (54%), *APC* (10%), *SMAD4* (5.9%), *KRAS* (5.9%), and *PIK3CA* (5.1%) were present at a high rate in a large cohort of 666 specimens of GC [42]. The MSS/TP53− phenotype exhibited the highest prevalence of *TP53* and *RHOA* mutations, as well as recurrent focal amplifications in *ERBB2*, *CCNE1* and *CCND1*.

The MSS/EMT phenotype includes tumors of the diffuse-subtype. It is associated with the worst prognosis, tendency to occur at an earlier age, and the highest recurrence frequency (63%) of the four subtypes. The MSS/EMT subtype also includes a large set of signet ring cell carcinomas and showed loss of *CDH1* expression.

The ACRG subtyping of GC could be complementary to the TCGA system for molecular classification of GC. The ACRG data are potentially important for generating prognostic biomarkers in GC. The validity of these biomarkers for prognosis of patients with GC will need to be investigated in prospective clinical studies.

3.3. Comparison of TCGA and ACRG Data

TCGA and ACRG integrated the results of a wide scale molecular analysis into two different and partially overlapping models encompassing four molecular subtypes with distinct salient genomic features (Table 3). They both identified a MSI subtype characterized by high mutation frequency and best prognosis. While CIN and GS TCGA subtypes tumors were present across all ACRG subtypes, TCGA GS, EBV+, and CIN subtypes were enriched in ACRG MSS/EMT, MSS/TP53+, and TP53− subtypes, respectively. However, CDH1 and RHOA mutations were highly prevalent in the TCGA GS subtype but infrequent in the ACRG MSS/EMT subtype, these two subtypes were deemed not equivalent. Similarly, MSS/TP53 did not overlap with the TCGA EBV subtype, as EBV+ tumors represented a small proportion of samples in the MSS/TP53+ subtype.

Table 3. Distribution of key genomic alterations across molecular subtypes of gastric carcinoma from TCGA and ACRG data.

Genetic Alteration	TCGA				ACRG			
	MSI	EBV	GS	CIN	MSI	MSS/EMT	MSS/TP53+	MSS/TP53−
HER2 amp	0	12	3	22	0	0	3.0	17.4
HER2 mut	11	4	3	3	16.3	2.8	0	4.7
MET amp	2	0	0	7	1.6	0	3.0	3.5
PIK3CA amp	3	8	2	7	0	0	0	1.1
PIK3CA mut	42	77	10	3	32.6	8.3	16.9	4.7
KRAS mut	23	4	9	5	23.3	0	8.5	3.5
RHOA mut	5	8	14	2	0	2.8	6.8	3.5
CDH1 mut	8	0	34	3	7.0	2.8	1.7	3.5
FGFR2 amp	0	0	7	7	0	4.9	3.0	1.2
BRAF mut	22	8	0	0	11.6	2.8	1.7	3.5
ALK mut	9	0	5	2	16.3	0	0	2.4
ARID1A mut	84	54	16	9	44.2	13.9	18.6	5.9
TP53 mut	39	4	14	70	25.6	33.3	23.7	60
PTEN mut	25	15	2	1	14	5.6	3.4	3.5
MTOR mut	30	4	3	1	14	0	1.7	3.5
APC mut	36	0	3	12	16.3	2.8	15.3	8.2
FBXW7 mut	34	0	5	1	16.3	2.8	1.7	2.4
SMAD4 mut	8	12	9	7	4.7	2.8	8.5	2.4

MSI, microsatellite instability; EBV, Epstein–Barr virus; GS, genomically stable; CIN, chromosome instability; MSS, microsatellite stability; EMT, epithelial-mesenchymal transition; amp, amplification; mut, mutation; Numbers refer to % of samples with the genomic alteration.

Possible reasons for the partial overlap of these two classifications include differences related to the patient population (Korea in ACRG vs. USA and Western Europe in TCGA), tumor sampling (predominantly intestinal diffuse type in ACRG), and technological platforms (six distinct molecular platforms in TCGA including exome sequencing, copy number analysis, methylation, miRNA and mRNA expression vs. reliance upon mRNA expression in ACRG). Despite these differences, these two classification schemes not only clarified and simplified the genomic and epigenomic heterogeneity of GC, but also revealed distinct salient genomic features among gastric cancer subtypes linked to clinical outcomes. These molecular classification systems of GC lay the groundwork for targeted therapies, patient stratification for clinical trials and treatment, and improved prognostication.

4. Molecular Profiling of Gastric Carcinoma: Therapeutic Targets and Predictive Biomarkers

Complementary to molecular classification of GC, analysis of molecular profiles of tumors collected from individual patients using a multi-platform approach has led to identification of targets for therapy as well as biomarkers that may be predictive of tumor response to treatment.

4.1. Therapeutic Targets

Molecular profiling of tumors including GC has been employed with the hope of identifying actionable and predictive biomarkers. In one study, 666 specimens of GC were analyzed by immunohistochemistry, in-situ hybridization, and genomic DNA sequencing [42]. Some of the analyzed molecules included ribonucleotide reductase regulatory subunit M1 (RRM1), O-6-methylguanine-DNA-methyltransferase (MGMT), phosphatase and tensin homolog deleted on chromosome ten (PTEN), topoisomerase (TOP), thymidine synthase (TS), and excision repair cross-complementing 1 (ERCC1).

Negative expression of three non-NCCN (National Comprehensive Cancer Network) compendium actionable targets including RRM1 (62%), MGMT (45%), and PTEN (58%) was identified in more than 40% of the tumor specimens. These data suggest potential sensitivity to gemcitabine, temozolomide, or PI3K inhibitors, respectively. Negative RRM1 expression is associated with higher response rates to gemcitabine-based chemotherapy regimens [59–61]. Therefore, stratifying patients based on RRM1 expression may increase the likelihood of gemcitabine efficacy.

In the HER2-positive cohort, co-expression of TOP2A occurred most frequently (93%), suggesting potential sensitivity to a combined anthracycline/trastuzumab approach to treatment. Furthermore, 50% of patients demonstrated possible benefit from a combination of trastuzumab with 5FU/capecitabine based on concurrent low TS, 53% with irinotecan (high TOPO1), 63% with cisplatin (low ERCC1) and 55% with gemcitabine (low RRM1).

4.2. Predictive Biomarkers

The potential of these biochemical markers to predict treatment response of tumors to chemotherapy was examined. Molecular profiling of tumor specimens from 27 patients with gastroesophageal carcinoma was conducted by the Caris Molecular Intelligence® service (Phoenix, AZ, USA). These included eleven GC, nine EGJC, and seven esophageal carcinoma (EC) [13]. The frequencies of actionable targets (Table 4) and mutations including *TP53* (33%), *APC* (7.4%), *SMAD4* (7.4%), and *PIK3CA* (7.4%), were consistent with those in a cohort of 666 specimens of GC [42].

Table 4. Frequency of actionable targets tested by immunohistochemistry along with the associated therapeutic agents.

Biomarker	Number of Specimens (%)	Beneficial Agents
TS (−)	19 (70.4)	Fluorouracil, Capecitabine
TOPO1 (+) *	16 (59.3)	Irinotecan, Topotecan
PTEN (−)	11 (40.7)	Trastuzumab, anti-EGFR
ERCC1 (−) *	11 (40.7)	Cisplatin, Carboplatin, Oxaliplatin
TOP2A (+) *	11 (40.7)	Doxorubicin, Epirubicin
RRM1 (−)	10 (37.0)	Gemcitabine
MGMT (−)	9 (33.3)	Temozolomide, Dacarbazine
TUBB3 (−)	8 (29.6)	Docetaxel, *nab*-paclitaxel, paclitaxel
cMET (+)	7 (25.9)	Anti-MET
TLE3 (+)	6 (22.2)	Docetaxel, Paclitaxel
SPARC Mono (+)	5 (18.5)	*nab*-Paclitaxel
SPARC Poly (+)	4 (14.8)	*nab*-Paclitaxel
HER2 (+) *	4 (14.8)	Trastuzumab, Lapatinib
PGP (−) *	4 (14.8)	Taxane

* Biomarker with associated agent on the National Comprehensive Cancer Network (NCCN) compendium. ERCC1, excision repair cross-complementation group 1; HER2, human epidermal growth factor receptor 2; cMET, hepatocyte growth factor receptor; MGMT, O-6-methylguanine-DNA methyltransferase; PGP, p-glycoprotein; PTEN, phosphatase and tensin homolog; RRM1, ribonucleotide reductase subunit M1; SPARC, secreted protein acidic and rich in cysteine; TLE3, transducin-like enhancer of split 3; TOPO1, topoisomerase 1; TOP2A, topoisomerase 2A; TS, thymidylate synthase; TUBB3, tubulin beta 3. The data are modified from [13].

In several cases, the PFS based on tumor molecular profile (MP) was compared to that on therapy prior to molecular profiling. A ratio of PFS-MP to PFS prior to MP greater than 1.3 is considered clinically significant. As shown in the three cases in Table 5, the ratio of PFS on MP-based treatment to PFS on treatment prior to molecular profiling exceeds 1.3, suggesting the potential value of MP in guiding selection of individualized therapy [13,62]. These results support further investigation using large sets of data from patients to correlate treatment response with tumor MP, and testing the hypothesis that tumor MP guides the selection of optimal therapeutic regimen for individualized treatment.

Table 5. Progression-free survival on molecular profile-matched therapy vs. on prior therapy.

Biomarker	Method	Beneficial Agent	Treatment Prior to MP	MP-Based Treatment	PFS Ratio
HER2/Neu amplification	FISH, IHC	Trastuzumab	Docetaxel + Irinotecan PFS = 2.2 months	Trastuzumab + Docetaxel + Irinotecan PFS = 6.3 months	2.9
Topoisomerase 1 positive	IHC	Irinotecan, Topotecan	Epirubicin + Oxaliplatin + Capecitabine PFS = 2.3 months	Docetaxel + Irinotecan PFS = 4.5 months	2.0
SPARC Monoclonal positive	IHC	nab-Paclitaxel	Docetaxel + Irinotecan PFS = 1.9 months	Gemcitabine + nab-Paclitaxel PFS = 3.6 month	1.9

FISH, fluorescent in situ hybridization; HER2, human epidermal growth factor receptor 2; IHC, immunohistochemistry; MP, molecular profile; PFS, progression-free survival; PFS ratio, PFS on MP-matched therapy vs. PFS on prior therapy; SPARC, secreted protein acidic and rich in cysteine.

5. Conclusions and Perspectives

Systemic treatment plays important roles in the multi-disciplinary management of gastric carcinoma. Cytotoxic drugs, targeted agents, and immunotherapeutics have been shown to provide clinical benefit though to a limited extent. With the exception of trastuzumab for HER2-amplified and PD-L1-expressing GC, a clinical tool to predict the treatment response and outcomes of the currently used systemic therapy is lacking. Moreover, tumor heterogeneity and molecular evolution of tumor during treatment contribute to therapeutic resistance. Clinically tested and validated biomarkers for predicting tumor response to systemic treatment will be needed for patients to derive maximal benefit and avoid unnecessary toxic side effects.

Molecular classification and profiling of GC generate potential targets for therapy as well as prognostic and predictive biomarkers. The TCGA and ACRG data have not only revealed the molecular and etiologic differences across the various subtypes of GC, but also yielded many potentially targetable genomic changes. In addition, molecular profiling of GC by analysis of proteomics [63–65] and microRNA [66] as well as detection of circulating tumor DNA in plasma and exosomes of patients with GC [67] have been reported. These platforms may help identify therapeutic biomarkers and targets that are complementary to tumor molecular profiling by genomic and immunohistochemical analyses as described above.

Development of therapeutic agents targeting some of those molecular alterations as defined to the subtyping and profiling of GC are undergoing pre-clinical and clinical investigation. Identification and validation of prognostic and predictive biomarkers by correlation of molecular profiles of tumors with clinical outcomes such as tumor response, progression-free survival, and overall survival are indicated. Future studies aiming to identify and validate predictive tumor biomarkers through molecular profiling in large data sets are indicated. Results of these studies are expected to facilitate selection of optimal chemotherapy regimen individualized for the patients, and the development of novel targeted therapies.

While the molecular data brings the possible hope of developing precision therapies, many challenges must be overcome to fully understand and realize their clinical impact. First, it is imperative to design and implement clinical trials that take into account the molecular heterogeneity across the various subtypes of GC and develop protocols specific for each of these entities. The Personalized Antibodies from Gastro-Esophageal Adenocarcinoma (PANGEA) "umbrella trial" is one such innovative trial in which patients are assigned to different treatment arms by matching the molecular characteristics of a single tumor type to a specific drug [68,69]. Considering that the tumor mutational profiles can evolve over time and in response to treatment, the adaptive design of this trial, which allows modifications of some aspects to be made while the trial is ongoing, would be very beneficial by matching the right drugs to the right patients in a time-sensitive fashion.

Secondly, targeted therapy guided by molecular profiling will need to be tested in patient-derived tumor xenografts (PDX) and genetically-engineered mouse (GEM) models. The development and characterization of these realistic model systems represent the complex molecular heterogeneity of GC. They will be helpful for validating the genomic alterations in the molecular subtypes of GC and facilitating drug and biomarker development. Finally, development of novel therapies combining immunotherapeutics, cytotoxic chemotherapeutic agents, and molecularly-targeted therapeutics is expected to offer durable clinical benefits and maximize survival in patients with GC.

By integrating the various molecular and clinical data, we hope to develop strategies that will enable clinicians and scientists to better characterize and classify these tumors, develop targeted therapies, and identify prognostic and predictive biomarkers for achieving the goal of precision therapy in patients with this malignant disease.

Author Contributions: Lionel Kankeu Fonkoua and Nelson S. Yee conceived and designed the study and reviewed the literature; Lionel Kankeu Fonkoua and Nelson S. Yee collected and analyzed the data; Lionel Kankeu Fonkoua and Nelson S. Yee wrote the paper.

Conflicts of Interest: The authors declare no conflict of interest.

References

1. International Agency for Research on Cancer. Stomach Cancer. Estimated Incidence, Mortality and Prevalence Worldwide in 2012. Available online: http://globocan.iarc.fr/old/FactSheets/cancers/stomach-new.asp (accessed on 28 October 2017).
2. Colvin, H.; Yamamoto, K.; Wada, N.; Mori, M. Hereditary gastric cancer syndromes. *Surg. Oncol. Clin. N. Am.* **2015**, *24*, 765–777. [CrossRef] [PubMed]
3. Lunet, N.; Valbuena, C.; Virira, A.; Lopes, C.; Lopes, C.; David, L.; Careneiro, F.; Barros, H. Fruit and vegetable consumption and gastric cancer by location and histological type: Case-control and meta-analysis. *Eur. J. Cancer Prev.* **2007**, *16*, 312–327. [CrossRef] [PubMed]
4. Ladeiras-Lopes, R.; Pereira, A.; Nogueira, A.; Pinheiro-Torres, T.; Pinto, I.; Santos-Pereira, R.; Lunet, N. Smoking and gastric cancer: Systemic review and meta-analysis of cohort studies. *Cancer Causes Control.* **2008**, *19*, 689–701. [CrossRef] [PubMed]
5. Yang, P.; Zhou, Y.; Chen, B.; Wan, H.W.; Jia, G.Q.; Bai, H.L.; Wu, X.T. Overweight, obesity and gastric cancer risk: Results from a meta-analysis of cohort studies. *Eur. J. Cancer* **2009**, *45*, 2867–2873. [CrossRef] [PubMed]
6. Oliveira, C.; Pinheiro, H.; Figueiredo, J.; Seruca, R.; Carneiro, F. Familial gastric cancer: Genetic susceptibility, pathology, and implications for management. *Lancet Oncol.* **2015**, *16*, e60–e70. [CrossRef]
7. Crew, K.D.; Neugut, A.I. Epidemiology of gastric cancer. *World J. Gastroenterol.* **2006**, *12*, 354–362. [CrossRef] [PubMed]
8. Wang, H.H.; Wu, M.S.; Shun, C.T.; Wang, H.P.; Lin, C.C.; Lin, J.T. Lymphoepithelioma-like carcinoma of the stomach: A subset of gastric carcinoma with distinct clinicopathological features and high prevalence of Epstein-Barr virus infection. *Hepatogastroenterology* **1999**, *46*, 1214–1219. [CrossRef] [PubMed]
9. Wu, M.S.; Shun, C.T.; Wu, C.C.; Hsu, T.Y.; Lin, M.T.; Chang, M.C.; Wang, H.P.; Lin, J.T. Epstein-Barr virus-associated gastric carcinomas: Relation to H. pylori infection and genetic alterations. *Gastroenterology* **2000**, *118*, 1031–1038. [CrossRef]
10. International Agency for Research on Cancer. IARC Working Group Reports. Helicobacter Pylori: Eradication as A Strategy for Preventing Gastric Cancer. Available online: http://www.iarc.fr/en/publications/pdfs-online/wrk/wrk8 (accessed on 28 October 2017).
11. Bang, Y.J.; Van Cutsem, E.; Feyereislova, A.; Chung, H.C.; Shen, L.; Sawaki, A.; Lordick, F.; Ohtsu, A.; Omuro, Y.; Satoh, T.; et al. Trastuzumab in combination with chemotherapy versus chemotherapy alone for treatment of HER2-positive advanced gastric or gastro-oesophageal junction cancer (ToGA): A phase 3, open-label, randomised controlled trial. *Lancet* **2010**, *376*, 1302. [CrossRef]
12. Fuchs, C.S.; Doi, T.; Woo-Jun Jang, R.; Muro, K.; Satoh, T.; Machado, M. KEYNOTE-059 cohort 1: Efficacy and safety of pembrolizumab (pembro) monotherapy in patients with previously treated advanced gastric cancer. *J. Clin. Oncol.* **2017**, *35* (Suppl. 15), 4003. [CrossRef]
13. Kankeu Fonkoua, L.A.; Liao, J.; Yee, N.S. Molecular profiling-guided therapy in gastroesophageal carcinoma: A single-institution experience. *J. Clin. Oncol.* **2017**, *35* (Suppl. 15), e15582. [CrossRef]
14. The Cancer Genome Atlas Research Network. Comprehensive molecular characterization of gastric adenocarcinoma. *Nature* **2014**, *513*, 202–209. [CrossRef]

15. Cristescu, R.; Lee, J.; Nebozhyn, M.; Kim, K.M.; Ting, J.C.; Wong, S.S.; Liu, J.; Yue, Y.G.; Wang, J.; Yu, K.; et al. Molecular analysis of gastric cancer identifies subtypes associated with distinct clinical outcomes. *Nat. Med.* **2015**, *21*, 449–456. [CrossRef] [PubMed]
16. Bosman, F.T.; Carneiro, F.; Hruban, R.H.; Thiese, N.D. *WHO Classification of Tumors of the Digestive System*, 4th ed.; IARC: Lyon, France, 2010; pp. 44–58.
17. Lauren, P. The two histological main types of gastric carcinoma: Diffuse and so-called intestinal-type carcinoma. An attempt at a histo-clinical classification. *Acta Pathol. Microbiol. Scand.* **1965**, *64*, 31–49. [CrossRef] [PubMed]
18. Ferlay, J.; Shin, H.R.; Bray, F.; Forman, D.; Mathers, C.; Parkin, D.M. Estimates of worldwide burden of cancer in 2008: GLOBOCAN 2008. *Int. J. Cancer* **2010**, *127*, 2893–2917. [CrossRef] [PubMed]
19. Rivera, F.; Vega-Villegas, M.E.; Lopez-Brea, M.F. Chemotherapy of advanced gastric cancer. *Cancer Treat. Rev.* **2007**, *33*, 315–324. [CrossRef] [PubMed]
20. Wesolowski, R.; Lee, C.; Kim, R. Is there a role for second-line chemotherapy in advanced gastric cancer? *Lancet Oncol.* **2009**, *10*, 903–912. [CrossRef]
21. Okines, A.F.; de Castro, D.G.; Cunningham, D.; Chau, I.; Langley, R.E.; Thompson, L.C.; Stenning, S.P.; Saffery, C.; Barbachano, Y.; Coxon, F. Biomarker analysis in oesophagogastric cancer: Results from the REAL3 and TransMAGIC trials. *Eur. J. Cancer* **2013**, *49*, 2116–2125. [CrossRef] [PubMed]
22. Van Cutsem, E.; Moiseyenko, V.; Tjulandin, S.; Majlis, A.; Constenla, M.; Boni, C.; Rodrigues, A.; Fodor, M.; Chao, Y.; Voznyi, E. Phase III study of docetaxel and cisplatin plus fluorouracil compared with cisplatin and fluorouracil as first-line therapy for advanced gastric cancer: A report of the V325 Study Group. *J. Clin. Oncol.* **2006**, *24*, 4991–4997. [CrossRef] [PubMed]
23. Cunningham, D.; Starling, N.; Rao, S.; Iveson, T.; Nicolson, M.; Coxon, F.; Middleton, G.; Daniel, F.; Oates, J.; Norman, A.R. Capecitabine and oxaliplatin for advanced esophagogastric cancer. *N. Engl. J. Med.* **2008**, *358*, 36–46. [CrossRef] [PubMed]
24. Al-Batran, S.; Hartmann, J.; Probst, S.; Schmalenberg, H.; Hollerbach, S.; Hofheinz, R.; Rethwisch, V.; Seipelt, G.; Homann, N.; Wilhelm, G. Phase III trial in metastatic gastroesophageal adenocarcinoma with fluorouracil, leucovorin plus either oxaliplatin or cisplatin: A study of the Arbeitsgemeinschaft Internistische Onkologie. *J. Clin. Oncol.* **2008**, *26*, 1435–1442. [CrossRef] [PubMed]
25. Ajani, J.; Rodriguez, W.; Bodoky, G.; Moiseyenko, V.; Lichinitser, M.; Gorbunova, V.; Vynnychenko, I.; Garin, A.; Lang, I.; Falcon, S. Multicenter phase III comparison of cisplatin/S-1 with cisplatin/infusional fluorouracil in advanced gastric or gastroesophageal adenocarcinoma study: The FLAGS trial. *J. Clin. Oncol.* **2010**, *28*, 1547–1553. [CrossRef] [PubMed]
26. Hudis, C.A. Trastuzumab—Mechanism of action and use in clinical practice. *N. Engl. J. Med.* **2007**, *357*, 39–51. [CrossRef] [PubMed]
27. Xiong, J.; Han, S.; Ding, S.; He, J.; Zhang, H. Antibody-nanoparticle conjugate constructed with trastuzumab and nanoparticle albumin-bound paclitaxel for targeted therapy of human epidermal growth factor receptor 2-positive gastric cancer. *Oncol. Rep.* **2018**, *39*, 1396–1404. [CrossRef] [PubMed]
28. Kowanetz, M.; Ferrara, N. Vascular endothelial growth factor signaling pathways: Therapeutic perspective. *Clin. Cancer Res.* **2006**, *12*, 5018–5022. [CrossRef] [PubMed]
29. Jones, N.; Iljin, K.; Dumont, D.J.; Alitalo, K. Tie receptors: New modulators of angiogenic and lymphangiogenic responses. *Nat. Rev. Mol. Cell Biol.* **2001**, *2*, 257–267. [CrossRef] [PubMed]
30. Carbone, C.; Piro, G.; Merz, V.; Simionato, F.; Santoro, R.; Zecchetto, C.; Tortora, G.; Melisi, D. Angiopoietin-like proteins in angiogenesis, inflammation and cancer. *Int. J. Mol. Sci.* **2018**, *19*, 431. [CrossRef] [PubMed]
31. Heldin, C.-H.; Lennartsson, J.; Westermark, B. Involvement of platelet-derived growth factor ligands and receptors in tumorigenesis. *J. Int. Med.* **2018**, *283*, 16–44. [CrossRef] [PubMed]
32. Ronca, R.; Giacomini, A.; Rusnati, M.; Presta, M. The potential of fibroblast growth factor/fibroblast growth factor receptor signaling as a therapeutic target in tumor angiogenesis. *Expert Opin. Ther. Targets* **2015**, *19*, 1361–1377. [CrossRef] [PubMed]
33. Gao, L.M.; Wang, F.; Zheng, Y.; Fu, Z.Z.; Zheng, L.; Chen, L.L. Roles of fibroblast activation protein and hepatocyte growth factor expressions in angiogenesis and metastasis of gastric cancer. *Pathol. Oncol. Res.* **2017**. [CrossRef] [PubMed]

34. Olsen, J.J.; Other-Gee Pohl, S.; Deshmukh, A.; Visweswaran, M.; Ward, N.C.; Arfuso, F.; Agostino, M.; Dharmarajan, A. The role of Wnt signaling in angiogenesis. *Clin. Biochem. Rev.* **2017**, *38*, 131–142. [PubMed]
35. Tanaka, T.; Ishiguro, H.; Kuwabara, Y.; Kimura, M.; Mitsui, A.; Katada, T.; Shiozaki, M.; Naganawa, Y.; Fujii, Y.; Takeyama, H. Vascular endothelial growth factor C (VEGF-C) in esophageal cancer correlates with lymph node metastasis and poor patient prognosis. *J. Exp. Clin. Cancer Res.* **2010**, *29*, 83. [CrossRef] [PubMed]
36. Omoto, I.; Matsumoto, M.; Okumura, H.; Uchikado, Y.; Setoyama, T.; Kita, Y.; Owaki, T.; Kijima, Y.; Shinchi, H.; Ishigami, S. Expression of vascular endothelial growth factor-C and vascular endothelial growth factor receptor-3 in esophageal squamous cell carcinoma. *Oncol. Lett.* **2014**, *7*, 1027–1032. [CrossRef] [PubMed]
37. Fuchs, C.S.; Tomasek, J.; Yong, C.J.; Dumitru, F.; Passalacqua, R.; Goswami, C.; Safran, H.; Vieira dos Santos, L.; Aprile, G.; Ferry, D. Ramucirumab monotherapy for previously treated advanced gastric or gastro-oesophageal junction adenocarcinoma (REGARD): An international, randomised, multicentre, placebo-controlled, phase 3 trial. *Lancet* **2014**, *383*, 31–39. [CrossRef]
38. Wilke, H.; Muro, K.; Van Cutsem, E.; Oh, S.C.; Bodoky, G.; Shimada, Y.; Hironaka, S.; Sugimoto, N.; Lipatov, O.; Kim, T.Y. Ramucirumab plus paclitaxel versus placebo plus paclitaxel in patients with previously treated advanced gastric or gastro-esophageal junction adenocarcinoma (RAINBOW): A double-blind, randomised phase 3 trial. *Lancet Oncol.* **2014**, *15*, 1224–1235. [CrossRef]
39. Gu, L.; Chen, M.; Guo, D.; Zhu, H.; Zhang, W.; Pan, J.; Zhong, X.; Li, X.; Qian, H.; Wang, X. PD-L1 and gastric cancer prognosis: A systematic review and meta-analysis. *PLoS ONE* **2017**, *12*, e0182692. [CrossRef] [PubMed]
40. Muro, K.; Bang, Y.; Shankaran, V.; Geva, R.; Catenacci, D.V.T.; Gupta, S.; Eder, J.P.; Berger, R.; Gonzalez, E.J.; Pulini, J. A phase 1B study of pembrolizumab (PEMBRO; MK-3475) in patients with advanced gastric cancer. *Ann. Oncol.* **2014**, *25*, 1–41. [CrossRef]
41. Muro, K.; Chung, H.C.; Shankaran, V.; Geva, R., Catenacci, D.; Gupta, S.; Eder, J.P.; Golan, T.; Le, D.T.; Burtness, B.; et al. Pembrolizumab for patients with PD-L1-positive advanced gastric cancer (KEYNOTE-012): A multicenter, open-label, phase 1b trial. *Lancet Oncol.* **2016**, *17*, 717–726. [CrossRef]
42. Miura, J.T.; Xiu, J.; Thomas, J.; George, B.; Carron, B.R.; Tsai, S.; Johnston, F.M.; Turaga, K.K.; Gamblin, T.G. Tumor profiling of gastric and esophageal carcinoma reveal different treatment options. *Cancer Biol. Ther.* **2015**, *16*, 764–769. [CrossRef] [PubMed]
43. Deng, N.; Goh, L.K.; Wang, H.; Das, K.; Tao, J.; Tan, I.B.; Zhang, S.; Lee, M.; Wu, J.; Lim, K.H. A comprehensive survey of genomic alterations in gastric cancer reveals systematic patterns of molecular exclusivity and co-occurrence among distinct therapeutic targets. *Gut* **2012**, *61*, 673–684. [CrossRef] [PubMed]
44. Ali, S.M.; Sanford, E.M.; Klempner, S.J.; Rubinson, D.A.; Wang, K.; Palma, N.A.; Chmielecki, J.; Yelensky, R.; Palmer, G.A.; Morosini, D. Prospective comprehensive genomic profiling of advanced gastric carcinoma cases reveals frequent clinically relevant genomic alterations and new routes for targeted therapies. *Oncologist* **2015**, *20*, 499–507. [CrossRef] [PubMed]
45. Le, D.T.; Uram, J.N.; Wang, H.; Bartlett, B.R.; Kemberling, H.; Eyring, A.D.; Skora, A.D.; Luber, B.S.; Azad, N.S.; Laheru, D. PD-1 blockade in tumors with mismatch-repair deficiency. *N. Engl. J. Med.* **2015**, *373*, 1979. [CrossRef]
46. Wang, K.; Yuen, S.T.; Xu, J.; Lee, S.P.; Yan, H.H.; Shi, S.T.; Siu, H.C.; Deng, S.; Chu, K.M.; Law, S. Whole-genome sequencing and comprehensive molecular profiling identify new driver mutations in gastric cancer. *Nat. Genet.* **2014**, *46*, 573–582. [CrossRef] [PubMed]
47. Ridley, A.J.; Schwartz, M.A.; Burridge, K.; Firtel, R.A.; Ginsberg, M.H.; Borisy, G.; Parsons, J.T.; Horwitz, A.R. Cell migration: Integrating signals from front to back. *Science* **2003**, *302*, 1704–1709. [CrossRef] [PubMed]
48. Thumkeo, D.; Watanabe, S.; Narumiya, S. Physiological roles of Rho and Rho effectors in mammals. *Eur. J. Cell. Biol.* **2013**, *92*, 303–315. [CrossRef] [PubMed]
49. Jolliffe, I. *Principal Component Analysis*; Wiley Online Library: New York, NY, USA, 2002.
50. Loboda, A.; Nebozhyn, M.V.; Watters, J.W.; Buser, C.A.; Shaw, P.M.; Huang, P.S.; Van't Veer, L.; Tollenar, R.A.E.M.; Jackson, D.B.; Agrawal, D. EMT is the dominant program in human colon cancer. *BMC Med. Genom.* **2011**, *4*, 9. [CrossRef] [PubMed]
51. Cancer Genome Atlas Research Network. Comprehensive molecular characterization of human colon and rectal cancer. *Nature* **2012**, *487*, 330–337. [CrossRef]

52. Coppola, D.; Nebozhyn, M.; Khalil, F.; Dai, H.; Yeatman, T.; Loboda, A.; Mule, J.J. Unique ectopic lymph node-like structures present in human primary colorectal carcinoma are identified by immune gene array profiling. *Am. J. Pathol.* **2011**, *179*, 37–45. [CrossRef] [PubMed]
53. Dai, H.; Van't Veer, L.; Lamb, J.; He, Y.D.; Mao, M.; Fine, B.M.; Bernards, R.; Van de Vijver, M.; Deutsch, P.; Sachs, A. A cell proliferation signature is a marker of extremely poor outcome in a subpopulation of breast cancer patients. *Cancer Res.* **2005**, *65*, 4059–4066. [CrossRef] [PubMed]
54. Zouridis, H.; Deng, N.; Ivanova, T.; Zhu, Y.; Wong, B.; Huang, D.; Wu, Y.H.; Wu, Y.; Tan, I.B.; Liem, N.; et al. Methylation subtypes and large-scale epigenetic alterations in gastric cancer. *Sci. Transl. Med.* **2012**, *4*, 156ra140. [CrossRef] [PubMed]
55. The Cancer Genome Atlas Network. Comprehensive molecular portraits of human breast tumours. *Nature* **2012**, *490*, 61–70. [CrossRef]
56. Benita, Y.; Cao, Z.; Giallourakis, C.; Li, C.; Gardet, A.; Xavier, R.J. Gene enrichment profiles reveal T cell development, differentiation, and lineage-specific transcription factors including ZBTB25 as a novel NF-AT repressor. *Blood* **2010**, *115*, 5376–5384. [CrossRef] [PubMed]
57. Mori, Y.; Sato, F.; Selaru, F.M.; Olaru, A.; Perry, K.; Kimos, M.C.; Tamura, G.; Matsubara, N.; Wang, S.; Xu, Y.; et al. Instabilotyping reveals unique mutational spectra in microsatellite unstable gastric cancers. *Cancer Res.* **2002**, *62*, 3641–3645. [PubMed]
58. Mori, Y.; Selaru, F.M.; Sato, F.; Yin, J.; Simms, L.; Xu, Y.; Olaru, A.; Deacu, E.; Wang, S.; Taylor, J.M.; et al. The impact of microsatellite instability on the molecular phenotype of colorectal tumors. *Cancer Res.* **2003**, *63*, 4577–4582. [PubMed]
59. Christman, K.; Kelsen, D.; Saltz, L.; Tarassoff, P.G. Phase II trial of gemcitabine in patients with advanced gastric cancer. *Cancer* **1994**, *73*, 5–7. [CrossRef]
60. De Lange, S.M.; van Groeningen, C.J.; Kroep, J.R.; Van Bochove, A.; Snijders, J.F.; Peters, G.J. Phase II trial of cisplatin and gemcitabine in patients with advanced gastric cancer. *Ann. Oncol.* **2004**, *15*, 484–488. [CrossRef] [PubMed]
61. Dong, X.; Hao, Y.; Wei, Y.; Yin, Q.; Du, J.; Zhao, X. Response to first-line chemotherapy in patients with non-small cell lung cancer according to RRM1 expression. *PLoS ONE* **2014**, *9*, e92320. [CrossRef] [PubMed]
62. Yee, N.S.; Fonkoua, L.A.K.; Liao, J. Molecular Profiling of Gastro-Esophageal Carcinoma as Basis for Precision Cancer Medicine. In Proceedings of the BIT's 8th World Gene Conference—2017, Macao, China, 15 November 2017.
63. Aichler, M.; Luber, B.; Lordick, F.; Walch, A. Proteomic and metabolic prediction of response to therapy in gastric cancer. *World J. Gastroenterol.* **2014**, *14*, 13648–13657. [CrossRef] [PubMed]
64. Balluff, B.; Frese, C.; Maier, S.K.; Schone, C.; Kuster, B.; Schmitt, M.; Aubele, M.; Hofler, H.; Deelder, A.M.; Heck, A.J.R.; et al. De novo discovery of phenotypic intratumor heterogeneity using imaging mass spectrometry. *J. Pathol.* **2015**, *235*, 3–13. [CrossRef] [PubMed]
65. Smith, A.; Piga, I.; Galli, M.; Stella, M.; Denti, V.; Del Puppo, M.; Magni, F. Matrix-assisted laser desorption/ionization mass spectrometry imaging in the study of gastric cancer: A mini review. *Int. J. Mol. Sci.* **2017**, *18*, 2588. [CrossRef] [PubMed]
66. Shrestha, S.; Hsu, S.-D.; Huang, W.-Y.; Huang, H.-Y.; Chen, W.L.; Weng, S.-L.; Huang, H.D. A systematic review of microRNA expression profiling studies in human gastric cancer. *Cancer Med.* **2014**, *3*, 878–888. [CrossRef] [PubMed]
67. Gao, Y.; Zhang, K.; Xi, H.; Cai, A.; Wu, X.; Cui, J.; Li, J.; Qiao, Z.; Wei, B.; Chen, L. Diagnostic and prognostic value of circulating tumor DNA in gastric cancer: A meta-analysis. *Oncotarget* **2017**, *8*, 6330–6340. [CrossRef] [PubMed]
68. Biankin, A.V.; Piantadosi, S.; Hollingsworth, S.J. Patient-centric trials for therapeutic development in precision oncology. *Nature* **2015**, *526*, 361–370. [CrossRef] [PubMed]
69. Catenacci, D.V.T.; Polite, B.N.; Henderson, L.; Xu, P.; Rambo, B.; Liao, W.L.; Hembrough, T.A.; Zhao, L.; Xiao, S.Y.; Hart, J.; et al. Towards personalized treatment for gastroesophageal adenocarcinoma (GEC): Strategies to address tumor heterogeneity. *J. Clin. Oncol.* **2014**, *32*, 66. [CrossRef]

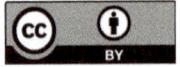

© 2018 by the authors. Licensee MDPI, Basel, Switzerland. This article is an open access article distributed under the terms and conditions of the Creative Commons Attribution (CC BY) license (http://creativecommons.org/licenses/by/4.0/).

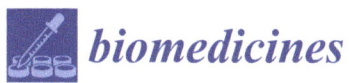

Review

Stereotactic Body Radiation Therapy in the Management of Upper GI Malignancies

Leila Tchelebi *, Nicholas Zaorsky and Heath Mackley

Penn State Health Milton S. Hershey Medical Center, Hershey, PA 17033, USA; nzaorsky@pennstatehealth.psu.edu (N.Z.); hmackley@pennstatehealth.psu.edu (H.M.)
* Correspondence: ltchelebi@pennstatehealth.psu.edu; Tel.: +1-717-531-8024

Received: 8 November 2017; Accepted: 23 December 2017; Published: 3 January 2018

Abstract: The role of external beam radiation therapy (EBRT) in the management of upper gastrointestinal malignancies is constantly evolving. As radiation therapy techniques improve and are able to deliver more ablative doses of radiotherapy while sparing healthy tissue, radiation can be applied to a wider range of clinical scenarios. Stereotactic body radiation therapy (SBRT) allows a high dose of radiation to be delivered to a highly conformal treatment volume in a short amount of time. Another potential advantage of SBRT is its ability to increase tumor immunogenicity, while also having less of an immunosuppressive effect on the patient, as compared to conventionally fractionated radiation therapy. In so doing, SBRT may potentiate the effects of immune therapy when the two treatments are combined, thus improving therapeutic outcomes. This article provides an overview of the role of SBRT in the management of upper gastrointestinal GI malignancies and the emerging data on immune biomarkers and SBRT, with a focus on pancreatic and liver cancer.

Keywords: stereotactic body radiation therapy; immunotherapy; biomarkers

1. Introduction

The role of external beam radiation therapy in the management of upper gastrointestinal (GI) malignancies is constantly evolving. Surgery has historically been the cornerstone of treatment for a majority of these cancers, particularly for pancreatic and hepatobiliary malignancies, with radiation reserved for palliation of symptoms. However, as radiation therapy techniques improve and are able to deliver more ablative doses of radiotherapy while sparing healthy tissue, radiation can be applied to a wider range of clinical scenarios.

Stereotactic body radiation therapy (SBRT) is a technique that allows a high dose of radiation to be delivered to a highly conformal treatment volume in a short amount of time. This results in a number of advantages. First, it allows for treatment of a higher biologically effective dose (BED), thus improving local tumor control. Second, it allows for a shorter overall treatment time which is both more convenient for patients and treating facilities and, more importantly, prevents delays in systemic treatment and/or surgery. Finally, given the highly conformal nature of SBRT, it allows for increased sparing of adjacent organs at risk (OARs) [1]. While the role of SBRT in the treatment of organs organized in series, such as the esophagus, is not well defined, its use in treating those organized in parallel, such as the liver and pancreas, has been established. This article therefore seeks to review the role of SBRT in the management of upper GI malignancies with a focus on pancreatic and liver cancer.

Another potential advantage of SBRT is its ability to increase tumor immunogenicity while having less of an immunosuppressive effect on the patient, as compared to conventionally fractionated radiation therapy [2]. In so doing, SBRT may potentiate the effects of immune therapy when the two treatments are combined, thus improving therapeutic outcomes. While the available data on tumor biomarkers and SBRT is in its infancy, it is hypothesis-generating and will also be reviewed in this article.

2. SBRT for Pancreatic Cancer

Pancreatic cancer is the 4th leading cause of cancer death in the United States [2]. Currently, surgery is considered the only curative treatment; however, less than 20% of patients are operable at the time of diagnosis [3,4]. Radiation therapy, therefore, plays a role in both the preoperative and definitive management of pancreatic malignancies. However, because the pancreas is considered to be radio-resistant, higher radiation doses are required for tumor control [5]. Indeed, studies have shown that delivering a BED of greater than 70 Gy is associated with improved survival for pancreatic cancer [6]. This poses a challenge for standard radiotherapy treatment planning due to the close proximity of highly radiosensitive organs such as the liver, duodenum, and stomach. SBRT in the management of pancreatic cancer is therefore a highly appealing treatment modality which has been well studied [7–27].

2.1. The Neoadjuvant Setting

The close proximity of the pancreas to critical vascular structures makes it technically challenging to achieve microscopically negative (R0) resections. The presence of positive margins following resection is associated with inferior outcomes [27–31]. Radiation therapy has, therefore, been used in the preoperative setting to downsize tumors intimately associated with vascular structures so as to increase the rate of negative margins at the time of surgery. Given the advantages of SBRT outlined above, there is growing interest in utilizing this technique in the neoadjuvant setting.

In 2015, the Moffitt Center published its experience with SBRT for borderline resectable pancreatic cancer [32]. This was a retrospective institutional review of all patients treated neoadjuvantly with SBRT at their institution. It included 159 patients, the majority of which (110) had borderline resectable disease (BRPC), with the remaining patients (49) having locally advanced unresectable pancreatic cancer (LAPC). Patients were treated with multi-agent systemic chemotherapy, followed by SBRT to a median dose of 40 Gy in five fractions and then surgery in patients who were deemed resectable after neoadjuvant therapy.

Ultimately, 51% of BRPC and 10% of LAPC patients were able to undergo surgery. The R0 resection rate in these patients was 96% and 100%, respectively. Seven percent of patients had a pathologic complete response and none of these patients relapsed at a median follow-up of 14 months. The overall survival and progression free survival rates were 19 months and 12 months, respectively, for those with BRPC, and 15 months and 13 months, respectively, for those with LAPC. Remarkably, the overall survival rate for patients who received neoadjuvant treatment and were then able to undergo surgery was 34 months, versus only 14 months for those who received chemotherapy and radiation but remained unresectable. Overall survival rates for up-front resectable pancreatic cancer patients, historically thought to have the best survival outcomes, has not exceeded 30 months in national randomized controlled trials, including the recently published ESPAC-4 trial [33–40]. Treatment was well tolerated in only 7% of cases with Grade 3+ acute or late toxicity. The results of this study were hypothesis-generating and paved the way for prospective trials of neoadjuvant SBRT for borderline resectable pancreatic cancer, including the ongoing ALLIANCE (NCT01992705) and Pancreatic Cancer Research Study (NCT01926197).

2.2. The Definitive Setting

There have been a number of studies investigating the role of SBRT in the definitive setting [10,12–14,16,17,21–26]. Most of these were retrospective series and only two were Phase II studies. The first of these two Phase II studies was published by Hoyer et al. in 2005 [16]. It included 22 patients with T1-3N0 LAPC deemed unresectable by a surgeon measuring up to 6 cm in size. The median PTV volume was 136 cm^3. Patients were treated with SBRT to a total dose of 45 Gy in three fractions. There was no mention of chemotherapy in the trial or a requirement that patients also undergo systemic chemotherapy. Study results were disappointing with only a 57% local control rate at one year and a median survival of 5.4 months. The toxicity profile was unfavorable with 36% of patients experiencing an increase in pain and analgesic use, 23% of patients with severe mucositis or ulceration, and one gastric perforation requiring emergent surgery. There are a number of reasons why this early experience with SBRT yielded such poor outcomes. These include a lack of fiducials for daily set-up and target localization possibly resulting in tumor miss, a lack of OAR constraints, resulting in high toxicity rates, and no specific requirements for systemic chemotherapy in conjunction with SBRT either before or after treatment, which we know today is a key component of treatment for patients with both resectable and especially unresectable disease.

Ten years after the publication of the Hoyer study, Herman et al. published their Phase II trial of SBRT for unresectable pancreatic cancer [21]. In this study, 49 patients with LAPC were treated with three weeks of gemcitabine, followed by a one-week break, followed by SBRT to the tumor to a total dose of 33 Gy in five fractions. The study included 49 patients with a median PTV volume of 71.4 cm^3. Unlike its predecessor study, the results of this trial were encouraging. The freedom from local progression at one year was 78% at one year as compared to 57% in the Moyer study. The median progression free survival was 7.8 months and the median overall survival was 13.9 months—a significant improvement from 5.4 months as reported in the Moyer trial. Ten percent of patients were ultimately able to undergo surgery after completion of SBRT. Overall survival for these patients ranged from 13.6 to 40.2 months. The primary endpoint of the rate of late (>3 months after SBRT) gastritis, fistula, enteritis, or ulcers of Grade 2+ was only seen in 11% of patients.

The superior outcomes reported in the Herman et al. trial as compared to the earlier Moyer trial can be attributed to a number of factors. First, unlike in the Herman trial, and all ongoing protocols, fiducial markers were not required to ensure accurate tumor positioning, which may have led to tumor miss. Second, there was no requirement for gemcitabine-based systemic chemotherapy, unlike in the more recent study, which has been shown to improve survival in patients with locally advanced disease [41–43]. Furthermore, the Moyer trial did not specify OAR constraints, which likely explains the poor toxicity profile. Lastly, tumor margins were large (5 mm axially and 1 cm cranio-caudal) and there was no dose reduction for overlap with the duodenum and stomach as was done in the Herman trial, which likely explains the 20% rate of severe mucositis and ulceration and the case of gastric perforation requiring surgery.

As radiation techniques have improved and we have learned more about tissue tolerance for high dose radiation therapy, SBRT has emerged as an appealing and highly effective treatment modality for LAPC. A meta-analysis of 19 trials of SBRT for LAPC published in 2017 showed that the median overall survival was greater than 12 months in the vast majority of studies and was particularly favorable in the subset of patients who became resectable after receiving SBRT [20]. These studies have paved the way for randomized Phase III trials (NCT01926197), which will hopefully establish the role of SBRT for LAPC.

2.3. The Adjuvant Setting

SBRT in the adjuvant setting for resected pancreatic cancer has not been established. However, there is an ongoing Phase II study examining the role of SBRT in resected T3 and N1 patients, which is currently accruing (NCT02461836).

3. SBRT for Hepatocellular Cancer

Hepatocellular carcinoma (HCC) is the second leading cause of cancer death worldwide [44]. The incidence of HCC is approximately equal to the mortality rate, highlighting the aggressive nature of this fatal malignancy. While relatively uncommon in the Unites States (US), it is the fastest growing cause of cancer death in the US [45]. Like with pancreatic cancer, surgery is considered the only curative treatment but most patients either have unresectable disease due to tumor extent or are inoperable due to underlying liver dysfunction. For the latter group of patients, transplant is the ultimate goal because it can cure both the HCC and the underlying liver disease. However, given the limited supply of healthy livers available for transplant, most patients are unable to undergo the procedure right away, thus requiring local treatment as a bridge to liver transplant when an organ becomes available. SBRT for HCC is, therefore, emerging as a safe and effective treatment modality both in the definitive setting for unresectable cancers and as a bridge to transplant for those with underlying liver disease awaiting organ allocation.

Historically, EBRT has been used with caution in the management of hepatic malignancies due to the low tolerance of the liver for radiation [45]. The challenges facing EBRT for HCC have been delivering a sufficiently high dose of radiation to achieve tumor control in an organ that is highly sensitive to radiation and that moves substantially with breathing, making target localization very difficult. Modern-day SBRT techniques make it possible for external beam radiation to overcome these road-blocks by delivering high doses of radiation in a very conformal manner while accounting, and controlling, for tumor motion. Due to a lack of Level I evidence, SBRT is not currently considered a standard treatment for HCC; however, a number of prospective trials have been completed which show its safety and efficacy in the management of this disease [46–50].

The most notable of these prospective trials was a combined analysis of sequential Phase I and II trials conducted at Princess Margaret Hospital published in 2013 [48]. The study included 102 patients with Child–Turcotte–Pugh Class A disease who were unsuitable for other local liver-directed therapy. Median gross tumor volume was 117 mL with a range of 1.3–1913.4 mL. Patients were treated with 30–54 Gy in six fractions, delivered every other day. The treatment was relatively well-tolerated with Grade 3+ toxicity reported in 30% of cases. Local control at one year was 87% and overall survival was 55%.

SBRT has also been combined with trans-arterial chemo-embolization (TACE) with favorable outcomes in the literature so far. There are a number of advantages to combining SBRT with TACE. TACE can shrink tumors, thus creating a smaller treatment volume for SBRT. The combination of the two treatments allows for ablation of vascular components of the tumor with TACE, while the poorly vascularized, necrotic portions can be targeted by SBRT. Finally, SBRT can be used to recanalize tumors with arterial or portal vein thromboses, rendering TACE more effective. A retrospective study of patients with tumors ≥3 cm compared outcomes among patients who received TACE plus SBRT compared to TACE alone [51]. The authors found that, after censoring for liver transplantation, overall survival was significantly better with TACE plus SBRT compared to TACE alone (33 vs. 20 months, respectively).

In conclusion, modern-day SBRT techniques allow for safe and effective delivery of external beam radiation therapy for hepatocellular carcinoma. While more data is needed, available evidence shows that there is a role for radiation in the management of this disease. Specifically, radiation plays a role for lesions unsuitable for other local therapies, for larger lesions in which TACE is less effective, and in cases with portal vein thrombosis in which other therapies are contra-indicated or ineffective [52]. Indeed, there is a randomized Phase III study underway comparing treatment with Sorafenib with or without SBRT in patients with HCC (NCT01730937).

4. SBRT and Immunomodulatory Biomarkers in Upper GI Malignancies and Therapeutic Implications

In addition to allowing for higher doses of radiation to be delivered to a more precise target in a shorter treatment time, emerging data shows that radiation, specifically SBRT, has advantageous effects on the immune system, which may have therapeutic implications. The immune-stimulatory effects of radiation have been known for some time. Indeed, Demaria et al. first introduced the concept of radiation as an "in situ vaccine" in 2004 [53]. The authors suggest that radiation turns the radiated tumor into a vaccine by priming the immune system to target cancer cells in other sites in addition to treating the disease locally, a concept known as the abscopal effect. Since then, Formenti and colleagues have been able to site clinical data lending credence to this concept in which radiation delivered locally results in tumor response at the site of radiation as well as decreased tumor burden outside the irradiated field, mediated by the patient's immune system [54–57].

While the dose and fractionation needed to optimally prime the immune system is not yet known, SBRT appears to be superior to conventional radiation in terms of its effect on tumor immunogenicity. First, SBRT creates less of an immunosuppressive effect on the host's immune system as compared to conventionally fractionated radiation, both due to the absence of the concomitant chemotherapy and to the relatively smaller volume of irradiated bone marrow [58–60]. In addition, emerging data shows that SBRT has the potential advantage of directly increasing tumor immunogenicity [2,61]. Indeed, numerous pre-clinical models summarized very nicely by Popp et al. have shown that SBRT induces complex changes in the tumor microenvironment [53]. The authors review several preclinical studies showing that SBRT leads to increased recruitment of immune cells, including antigen-presenting-cells and dendritic cells, as well as cytokines and chemokines, which are all involved in the immune response [53]. The authors also summarize existing clinical data demonstrating evidence that SBRT mediates the abscopal effect. However, most of the data they cite involves patients with either melanoma or lung cancer, for which the benefit of immunotherapeutic agents is already widely established [62–64].

There is limited clinical data addressing the role of SBRT and its effects on the immune system for gastrointestinal malignancies; however, studies are emerging. Specifically, studies have shown an increase in tumor infiltrating lymphocytes and in soluble PD-L1, involved in T-cell regulatory pathways, following SBRT in pancreatic and hepatic malignancies [61,65]. The immunogenic effect of SBRT on tumors, coupled with the absence of an immunosuppressive effect on the patient, may allow for novel therapeutic approaches to treating upper GI malignancies by combining SBRT with immunotherapy. The combination of these two therapies may be more effective than either treatment alone.

Tumors have varying degrees of immune activity based on their histology. The tumor environment in pancreatic cancer, for instance, is considered to be immunosuppressive with a low degree of infiltration by T cells [66]. As a result, immunotherapy with immune check-point inhibitors has been investigated in this disease, with disappointing results [67,68]. As Foley et al. detail in their paper on immunotherapy for pancreatic cancer, removing immune suppression without providing a means to activate the immune system is likely responsible for these disappointing outcomes [66].

Emerging data show that SBRT has more of an immunogenic effect on the tumor environment when compared to conventionally fractionated radiation therapy delivered concurrently with chemotherapy for pancreatic cancer. In a recent presentation at the American Society for Radiation Oncology (ASTRO) annual meeting, Chen et al. presented their data on tumor infiltrating cells in pancreatic cancer [65]. They showed that there was a statistically significant difference in the ratio of CD8 T-cells to FOXP3 T-regulatory cells (CD8/FOXP3) detected in tumor cells following SBRT as compared to conventionally fractionated therapy. They also showed that a higher CD8/FOXP3 ratio was associated with improved progression free survival. The authors thus show that SBRT may be more effective in terms of local control as compared to conventional fractionation, in addition to showing that SBRT is more immunogenic than conventional radiation. The combination of SBRT and immunotherapy may, therefore, provide novel therapeutic strategies for this disease. Indeed, there are studies underway looking at the efficacy of combining SBRT with immunotherapy in the treatment of pancreatic cancer (NCT 02648282).

Hepatocellular carcinoma, on the other hand, has been shown to be an immune active malignancy with a high infiltration of T cells [66]. Kim et al. recently presented their data on the effects of radiation on soluble PD-L1 in hepatocellular carcinoma and its therapeutic implications [61]. The authors showed that radiation therapy increases the expression of PD-L1 on tumor cells. This increase was noted both after conventionally fractionated radiation and after SBRT; however, the levels after SBRT continued to rise one month following treatment, which was not true following conventionally fractionated radiation. The authors conclude that this data may provide evidence for a novel therapeutic strategy for patients with HCC that combines SBRT with PD-L1 blockade.

5. Conclusions and Future Directions

SBRT has emerged as a highly promising treatment modality in the management of upper GI malignancies. It allows for more curative doses of radiation to be delivered to a highly conformal treatment volume, in a short amount of time, allowing for effective and expedited treatment for these highly aggressive malignancies.

In the case of pancreatic cancer, SBRT has emerged as an effective neoadjuvant treatment to render tumors which are unresectable upfront, resectable after treatment, thus allowing an increased number of patients to undergo potentially curative resection. In the case of LAPC, SBRT also has the potential advantage of rendering some of these initially unresectable tumors resectable, while also providing reasonable long-term survival rates for patients undergoing definitive treatment. Studies are ongoing for SBRT in the adjuvant setting. In the case of HCC, SBRT has emerged as an effective treatment for patients in which other local therapies either cannot be performed or are ineffective as, for example, for large tumors or those with portal venous invasion.

Finally, the effects of SBRT on the immune system and tumor micro-environment is an area of active research with heretofore promising results. Emerging data shows that SBRT can increase tumor immunogenicity, thus providing a rationale for novel therapeutic approaches combining SBRT and immunotherapeutic agents with the hope that the combination of the two treatments will result in better outcomes than either treatment alone. More data is needed to confirm these initial findings. Prospective trials studying the combination of SBRT and immunotherapy in the management of upper GI malignancies are needed to confirm the therapeutic implications of these retrospective studies, and some are already underway.

Conflicts of Interest: The authors declare no conflict of interest.

References

1. Rosati, L.M.; Kumar, R.; Herman, J.M. Integration of Stereotactic Body Radiation Therapy into the Multidisciplinary Management of Pancreatic Cancer. *Semin. Radiat. Oncol.* **2017**, *27*, 256–267. [CrossRef] [PubMed]
2. Gustafson, M.P.; Bornschlegl, S.; Park, S.S.; Gastineau, D.A.; Roberts, L.R.; Dietz, A.B.; Hallemeier, C.L. Comprehensive assessment of circulating immune cell populations in response to stereotactic body radiation therapy in patients with liver cancer. *Adv. Radiat. Oncol.* **2017**, *2*, 540–547. [CrossRef] [PubMed]
3. Wolfgang, C.L.; Herman, J.M.; Laheru, D.A.; Klein, A.P.; Erdek, M.A.; Fishman, E.K.; Hruban, R.H. Recent progress in pancreatic cancer. *CA Cancer J. Clin.* **2013**, *63*, 318–348. [CrossRef] [PubMed]
4. Siegel, R.L.; Miller, K.D.; Jemal, A. Cancer statistics, 2016. *CA Cancer J. Clin.* **2016**, *66*, 7–30. [CrossRef] [PubMed]
5. Seshacharyulu, P.; Baine, M.J.; Souchek, J.J.; Menning, M.; Kaur, S.; Yan, Y.; Ouellette, M.M.; Jain, M.; Lin, C.; Batra, S.K. Biological determinants of radioresistance and their remediation in pancreatic cancer. *Biochim. Biophys. Acta Rev. Cancer* **2017**, *1868*, 69–92. [CrossRef] [PubMed]
6. Krishnan, S.; Chadha, A.S.; Suh, Y.; Chen, H.C.; Rao, A.; Das, P. Focal Radiation therapy dose escalation improves overall survival in locally advanced pancreatic cancer patients receiving induction chemotherapy and consolidative chemoradiation. *Int. J. Radiat. Oncol.* **2016**, *94*, 755–765. [CrossRef] [PubMed]
7. Su, T.-S.; Liang, P.; Lu, H.-Z.; Liang, J.-N.; Liu, J.-M.; Zhou, Y.; Gao, Y.-C.; Tang, M.-Y. Stereotactic body radiotherapy using CyberKnife for locally advanced unresectable and metastatic pancreatic cancer. *World J. Gastroenterol.* **2015**, *21*, 8156. [CrossRef] [PubMed]
8. Song, Y.; Yuan, Z.; Li, F.; Dong, Y.; Zhuang, H.; Wang, J.; Chen, H.; Wang, P. Analysis of clinical efficacy of CyberKnife® treatment for locally advanced pancreatic cancer. *Onco Targets Ther.* **2015**, *8*, 1427. [CrossRef] [PubMed]

9. Moningi, S.; Dholakia, A.S.; Raman, S.P.; Blackford, A.; Cameron, J.L.; Le, D.T.; De Jesus-Acosta, A.M.C.; Hacker-Prietz, A.; Rosati, L.M.; Assadi, R.K.; et al. The role of stereotactic body radiation therapy for pancreatic cancer: A single-institution experience. *Ann. Surg. Oncol.* **2015**, *22*, 2352–2358. [CrossRef] [PubMed]
10. Rwigema, J.-C.M.; Parikh, S.D.; Heron, D.E.; Howell, M.; Zeh, H.; Moser, A.J.; Bahary, N.; Quinn, A.; Burton, S.A. Stereotactic body radiotherapy in the treatment of advanced adenocarcinoma of the pancreas. *Am. J. Clin. Oncol.* **2011**, *34*, 63–69. [CrossRef] [PubMed]
11. Rajagopalan, M.S.; Heron, D.E.; Wegner, R.E.; Zeh, H.J.; Bahary, N.; Krasinskas, A.M.; Lembersky, B.; Brand, R.; Moser, A.J.; Quinn, A.E.; et al. Pathologic response with neoadjuvant chemotherapy and stereotactic body radiotherapy for borderline resectable and locally-advanced pancreatic cancer. *Radiat. Oncol.* **2013**, *8*, 254. [CrossRef] [PubMed]
12. Polistina, F.; Costantin, G.; Casamassima, F.; Francescon, P.; Guglielmi, R.; Panizzoni, G.; Febbraro, A.; Ambrosino, G. Unresectable Locally Advanced Pancreatic Cancer: A Multimodal Treatment Using Neoadjuvant Chemoradiotherapy (Gemcitabine Plus Stereotactic Radiosurgery) and Subsequent Surgical Exploration. *Ann. Surg. Oncol.* **2010**, *17*, 2092–2101. [CrossRef] [PubMed]
13. Mahadevan, A.; Miksad, R.; Goldstein, M.; Sullivan, R.; Bullock, A.; Buchbinder, E.; Pleskow, D.; Sawhney, M.; Kent, T.; Vollmer, C.; et al. Induction Gemcitabine and Stereotactic Body Radiotherapy for Locally Advanced Nonmetastatic Pancreas Cancer. *Int. J. Radiat. Oncol.* **2011**, *81*, e615–e622. [CrossRef] [PubMed]
14. Lin, J.-C.; Jen, Y.-M.; Li, M.-H.; Chao, H.-L.; Tsai, J.-T. Comparing outcomes of stereotactic body radiotherapy with intensity-modulated radiotherapy for patients with locally advanced unresectable pancreatic cancer. *Eur. J. Gastroenterol. Hepatol.* **2015**, *27*, 259–264. [CrossRef] [PubMed]
15. Kim, C.H.; Ling, D.C.; Wegner, R.E.; Flickinger, J.C.; Heron, D.E.; Zeh, H.; Moser, A.J.; Burton, S.A. Stereotactic body radiotherapy in the treatment of Pancreatic Adenocarcinoma in elderly patients. *Radiat. Oncol.* **2013**, *8*, 240. [CrossRef] [PubMed]
16. Hoyer, M.; Roed, H.; Sengelov, L.; Traberg, A.; Ohlhuis, L.; Pedersen, J.; Nellemann, H.; Berthelsen, A.K.; Eberholst, F.; Engelholm, S.A.; et al. Phase-II study on stereotactic radiotherapy of locally advanced pancreatic carcinoma. *Radiother. Oncol.* **2005**, *76*, 48–53. [CrossRef] [PubMed]
17. Goyal, K.; Einstein, D.; Ibarra, R.A.; Yao, M.; Kunos, C.; Ellis, R.; Brindle, J.; Singh, D.; Hardacre, J.; Zhang, Y.; et al. Stereotactic Body Radiation Therapy for Nonresectable Tumors of the Pancreas. *J. Surg. Res.* **2012**, *174*, 319–325. [CrossRef] [PubMed]
18. Didolkar, M.S.; Coleman, C.W.; Brenner, M.J.; Chu, K.U.; Olexa, N.; Stanwyck, E.; Yu, A.; Neerchal, N.; Rabinowitz, S. Image-Guided Stereotactic Radiosurgery for Locally Advanced Pancreatic Adenocarcinoma Results of First 85 Patients. *J. Gastrointest. Surg.* **2010**, *14*, 1547–1559. [CrossRef] [PubMed]
19. Boone, B.A.; Steve, J.; Krasinskas, A.M.; Zureikat, A.H.; Lembersky, B.C.; Gibson, M.K.; Stoller, R.G.; Zeh, H.J.; Bahary, N. Outcomes with FOLFIRINOX for borderline resectable and locally unresectable pancreatic cancer. *J. Surg. Oncol.* **2013**, *108*, 236–241. [CrossRef] [PubMed]
20. Petrelli, F.; Comito, T.; Ghidini, A.; Torri, V.; Scorsetti, M.; Barni, S. Stereotactic Body Radiation Therapy for Locally Advanced Pancreatic Cancer: A Systematic Review and Pooled Analysis of 19 Trials. *Int. J. Radiat. Oncol.* **2017**, *97*, 313–322. [CrossRef] [PubMed]
21. Herman, J.M.; Chang, D.T.; Goodman, K.A.; Dholakia, A.S.; Raman, S.P.; Hacker-Prietz, A.; Iacobuzio-Donahue, C.A.; Griffith, M.E.; Pawlik, T.M.; Pai, J.S.; et al. Phase 2 multi-institutional trial evaluating gemcitabine and stereotactic body radiotherapy for patients with locally advanced unresectable pancreatic adenocarcinoma. *Cancer* **2015**, *121*, 1128–1137. [CrossRef] [PubMed]
22. Schellenberg, D.; Kim, J.; Christman-Skieller, C.; Chun, C.L.; Columbo, L.A.; Ford, J.M.; Fisher, G.A.; Kunz, P.L.; Van Dam, J.; Quon, A.; et al. Single-Fraction Stereotactic Body Radiation Therapy and Sequential Gemcitabine for the Treatment of Locally Advanced Pancreatic Cancer. *Int. J. Radiat. Oncol.* **2011**, *81*, 181–188. [CrossRef] [PubMed]
23. Koong, A.C.; Le, Q.T.; Ho, A.; Fong, B.; Fisher, G.; Cho, C.; Ford, J.; Poen, J.; Gibbs, I.C.; Mehta, V.K.; et al. Phase I study of stereotactic radiosurgery in patients with locally advanced pancreatic cancer. *Int. J. Radiat. Oncol.* **2004**, *58*, 1017–1021. [CrossRef] [PubMed]
24. Chang, D.T.; Schellenberg, D.; Shen, J.; Kim, J.; Goodman, K.A.; Fisher, G.A.; Ford, J.M.; Desser, T.; Quon, A.; Koong, A.C. Stereotactic radiotherapy for unresectable adenocarcinoma of the pancreas. *Cancer* **2009**, *115*, 665–672. [CrossRef] [PubMed]

25. Mahadevan, A.; Jain, S.; Goldstein, M.; Miksad, R.; Pleskow, D.; Sawhney, M.; Brennan, D.; Callery, M.; Vollmer, C. Stereotactic Body Radiotherapy and Gemcitabine for Locally Advanced Pancreatic Cancer. *Int. J. Radiat. Oncol.* **2010**, *78*, 735–742. [CrossRef] [PubMed]
26. Tozzi, A.; Comito, T.; Alongi, F.; Navarria, P.; Iftode, C.; Mancosu, P.; Reggiori, G.; Clerici, E.; Rimassa, L.; Zerbi, A.; et al. SBRT in unresectable advanced pancreatic cancer: Preliminary results of a mono-institutional experience. *Radiat. Oncol.* **2013**, *8*, 148. [CrossRef] [PubMed]
27. Gurka, M.K.; Collins, S.P.; Slack, R.; Tse, G.; Charabaty, A.; Ley, L.; Berzcel, L.; Lei, S.; Suy, S.; Haddad, N.; et al. Stereotactic body radiation therapy with concurrent full-dose gemcitabine for locally advanced pancreatic cancer: A pilot trial demonstrating safety. *Radiat. Oncol.* **2013**, *8*, 44. [CrossRef] [PubMed]
28. Neoptolemos, J.P.; Stocken, D.D.; Dunn, J.A.; Almond, J.; Beger, H.G.; Pederzoli, P.; Bassi, C.; Dervenis, C.; Fernandez-Cruz, L.; Lacaine, F.; et al. Influence of resection margins on survival for patients with pancreatic cancer treated by adjuvant chemoradiation and/or chemotherapy in the ESPAC-1 randomized controlled trial. *Ann. Surg.* **2001**, *234*, 758–768. [CrossRef] [PubMed]
29. Kinsella, T.J.; Seo, Y.; Willis, J.; Stellato, T.A.; Siegel, C.T.; Harpp, D.; Willson, J.K.; Gibbons, J.; Sanabria, J.R.; Hardacre, J.M.; et al. The Impact of Resection Margin Status and Postoperative CA19-9 Levels on Survival and Patterns of Recurrence after Postoperative High-Dose Radiotherapy With 5-FU—Based Concurrent Chemotherapy for Resectable Pancreatic Cancer. *Am. J. Clin. Oncol.* **2008**, *31*, 446–453. [CrossRef] [PubMed]
30. Chang, D.K.; Johns, A.L.; Merrett, N.D.; Gill, A.J.; Colvin, E.K.; Scarlett, C.J.; Nguyen, N.Q.; Leong, R.W.L.; Cosman, P.H.; Kelly, M.I.; et al. Margin Clearance and Outcome in Resected Pancreatic Cancer. *J. Clin. Oncol.* **2009**, *27*, 2855–2862. [CrossRef] [PubMed]
31. Campbell, F.; Smith, R.A.; Whelan, P.; Sutton, R.; Raraty, M.; Neoptolemos, J.P.; Ghaneh, P. Classification of R1 resections for pancreatic cancer: The prognostic relevance of tumour involvement within 1 mm of a resection margin. *Histopathology* **2009**, *55*, 277–283. [CrossRef] [PubMed]
32. Mellon, E.A.; Hoffe, S.E.; Springett, G.M.; Frakes, J.M.; Strom, T.J.; Hodul, P.J.; Malafa, M.P.; Chuong, M.D.; Shridhar, R. Long-term outcomes of induction chemotherapy and neoadjuvant stereotactic body radiotherapy for borderline resectable and locally advanced pancreatic adenocarcinoma. *Acta Oncol. (Madr)* **2015**, *54*, 979–985. [CrossRef] [PubMed]
33. Hammel, P.; Huguet, F.; van Laethem, J.-L.; Goldstein, D.; Glimelius, B.; Artru, P.; Borbath, I.; Bouche, O.; Shannon, J.; Andre, T.; et al. Effect of Chemoradiotherapy vs. Chemotherapy on Survival in Patients With Locally Advanced Pancreatic Cancer Controlled after 4 Months of Gemcitabine with or without Erlotinib. *JAMA* **2016**, *315*, 1844. [CrossRef] [PubMed]
34. Klinkenbijl, J.H.; Jeekel, J.; Sahmoud, T.; van Pel, R.; Couvreur, M.L.; Veenhof, C.H.; Arnaud, J.P.; Gonzalez, D.G.; de Wit, L.T.; Hennipman, A.; et al. Adjuvant radiotherapy and 5-fluorouracil after curative resection of cancer of the pancreas and periampullary region: Phase III trial of the EORTC gastrointestinal tract cancer cooperative group. *Ann. Surg.* **1999**, *230*, 776. [CrossRef] [PubMed]
35. Kalser, M.H.; Ellenberg, S.S. Pancreatic cancer. Adjuvant combined radiation and chemotherapy following curative resection. *Arch. Surg.* **1985**, *120*, 899–903. [PubMed]
36. Neoptolemos, J.P.; Palmer, D.H.; Ghaneh, P.; Psarelli, E.E.; Valle, J.W.; Halloran, C.M.; Faluyi, O.; O'Reilly, D.A.; Cunningham, D.; Wadsley, J.; et al. Comparison of adjuvant gemcitabine and capecitabine with gemcitabine monotherapy in patients with resected pancreatic cancer (ESPAC-4): A multicentre, open-label, randomised, phase 3 trial. *Lancet (Lond. Engl.)* **2017**, *389*, 1011–1024. [CrossRef]
37. Regine, W.F.; Winter, K.A.; Abrams, R.A.; Safran, H.; Hoffman, J.P.; Konski, A.; Benson, A.B.; Macdonald, J.S.; Kudrimoti, M.R.; Fromm, M.L.; et al. Fluorouracil vs. gemcitabine chemotherapy before and after fluorouracil-based chemoradiation following resection of pancreatic adenocarcinoma: A randomized controlled trial. *JAMA* **2008**, *299*, 1019–1026. [CrossRef] [PubMed]
38. Valle, J.W.; Palmer, D.; Jackson, R.; Cox, T.; Neoptolemos, J.P.; Ghaneh, P.; Rawcliffe, C.L.; Bassi, C.; Stocken, D.D.; Cunningham, D.; et al. Optimal duration and timing of adjuvant chemotherapy after definitive surgery for ductal adenocarcinoma of the pancreas: Ongoing lessons from the ESPAC-3 study. *J. Clin. Oncol.* **2014**, *32*, 504–512. [CrossRef] [PubMed]
39. Oettle, H.; Neuhaus, P.; Hochhaus, A.; Hartmann, J.T.; Gellert, K.; Ridwelski, K.; Niedergethmann, M.; Zulke, C.; Fahlke, J.; Arning, M.B.; et al. Adjuvant chemotherapy with gemcitabine and long-term outcomes among patients with resected pancreatic cancer: The CONKO-001 randomized trial. *JAMA* **2013**, *310*, 1473–1481. [CrossRef] [PubMed]

40. Neoptolemos, J.P.; Stocken, D.D.; Friess, H.; Bassi, C.; Dunn, J.A.; Hickey, H.; Beger, H.; Fernandez-Cruz, L.; Dervenis, C.; Lacaine, F.; et al. A randomized trial of chemoradiotherapy and chemotherapy after resection of pancreatic cancer. *N. Engl. J. Med.* **2004**, *350*, 1200–1210. [CrossRef] [PubMed]
41. Burris, H.A., 3rd; Moore, M.J.; Andersen, J.; Green, M.R.; Rothenberg, M.L.; Modiano, M.R.; Cripps, M.C.; Portenoy, R.K.; Storniolo, A.M.; Tarassoff, P.; et al. Improvements in survival and clinical benefit with gemcitabine as first-line therapy for patients with advanced pancreas cancer: A randomized trial. *J. Clin. Oncol.* **1997**, *15*, 2403–2413. [CrossRef] [PubMed]
42. Moore, M.J.; Hamm, J.; Dancey, J.; Eisenberg, P.D.; Dagenais, M.; Fields, A.; Hagan, K.; Greenberg, B.; Colwell, B.; Zee, B.; et al. Comparison of gemcitabine versus the matrix metalloproteinase inhibitor BAY 12-9566 in patients with advanced or metastatic adenocarcinoma of the pancreas: A phase III trial of the National Cancer Institute of Canada Clinical Trials Group. *J. Clin. Oncol.* **2003**, *21*, 3296–3302. [CrossRef] [PubMed]
43. Ishii, H.; Furuse, J.; Boku, N.; Okusaka, T.; Ikeda, M.; Ohkawa, S.; Fukutomi, A.; Hamamoto, Y.; Nakamura, K.; Fukuda, H.; et al. Phase II study of gemcitabine chemotherapy alone for locally advanced pancreatic carcinoma: JCOG0506. *Jpn. J. Clin. Oncol.* **2010**, *40*, 573–579. [CrossRef] [PubMed]
44. Ferlay, J.; Ferlay, J.; Soerjomataram, I.; Dikshit, R.; Eser, S.; Mathers, C.; Rebelo, M.; Parkin, D.M.; Forman, D.; Bray, F. Cancer incidence and mortality worldwide: Sources, methods and major patterns in GLOBOCAN 2012. *Int. J. Cancer* **2015**, *136*, E359–E386. [CrossRef] [PubMed]
45. Center, M.M.; Jemal, A. International Trends in Liver Cancer Incidence Rates. *Cancer Epidemiol. Biomarkers Prev.* **2011**, *20*, 2362–2368. [CrossRef] [PubMed]
46. Scorsetti, M.; Comito, T.; Cozzi, L.; Clerici, E.; Tozzi, A.; Franzese, C.; Navarria, P.; Fogliata, A.; Tomatis, S.; D'Agostino, G.; et al. The challenge of inoperable hepatocellular carcinoma (HCC): Results of a single-institutional experience on stereotactic body radiation therapy (SBRT). *J. Cancer Res. Clin. Oncol.* **2015**, *141*, 1301–1309. [CrossRef] [PubMed]
47. Lasley, F.D.; Mannina, E.M.; Johnson, C.S.; Perkins, S.M.; Althouse, S.; Maluccio, M.; Kwo, P.; Cardenes, H. Treatment variables related to liver toxicity in patients with hepatocellular carcinoma, Child-Pugh class A and B enrolled in a phase 1-2 trial of stereotactic body radiation therapy. *Pract. Radiat. Oncol.* **2015**, *5*, e443–e449. [CrossRef] [PubMed]
48. Bujold, A.; Massey, C.A.; Kim, J.J.; Brierley, J.; Cho, C.; Wong, R.K.S.; Dinniwell, R.E.; Kassam, Z.; Ringash, J.; Cummings, B.; et al. Sequential Phase I and II Trials of Stereotactic Body Radiotherapy for Locally Advanced Hepatocellular Carcinoma. *J. Clin. Oncol.* **2013**, *31*, 1631–1639. [CrossRef] [PubMed]
49. Kang, J.-K.; Kim, M.-S.; Cho, C.K.; Yang, K.M.; Yoo, H.J.; Kim, J.H.; Bae, S.H.; Jung, D.H.; Kim, K.B.; Lee, D.H.; et al. Stereotactic body radiation therapy for inoperable hepatocellular carcinoma as a local salvage treatment after incomplete transarterial chemoembolization. *Cancer* **2012**, *118*, 5424–5431. [CrossRef] [PubMed]
50. Méndez Romero, A.; Wunderink, W.; Hussain, S.M.; de Pooter, J.A.; Heijmen, B.J.M.; Nowak, P.C.J.M.; Nuyttens, J.J.; Brandwijk, R.P.; Verhoef, C.; Ijzermans, J.N.M.; et al. Stereotactic body radiation therapy for primary and metastatic liver tumors: A single institution phase i-ii study. *Acta Oncol. (Madr)* **2006**, *45*, 831–837. [CrossRef] [PubMed]
51. Jacob, R.; Turley, F.; Redden, D.T.; Saddekni, S.; Aal, A.K.A.; Keene, K.; Yang, E.; Zarzour, J.; Bolus, D.; Smith, J.K.; et al. Adjuvant stereotactic body radiotherapy following transarterial chemoembolization in patients with non-resectable hepatocellular carcinoma tumours of ≥3 cm. *HPB* **2015**, *17*, 140–149. [CrossRef] [PubMed]
52. Klein, J.; Dawson, L.A. Hepatocellular Carcinoma Radiation Therapy: Review of Evidence and Future Opportunities. *Int. J. Radiat. Oncol.* **2013**, *87*, 22–32. [CrossRef] [PubMed]
53. Popp, I.; Grosu, A.L.; Niedermann, G.; Duda, D.G. Immune modulation by hypofractionated stereotactic radiation therapy: Therapeutic implications. *Radiother. Oncol.* **2016**, *120*, 185–194. [CrossRef] [PubMed]
54. Formenti, S.C.; Demaria, S. Combining Radiotherapy and Cancer Immunotherapy: A Paradigm Shift. *J. Natl. Cancer Inst.* **2013**, *105*, 256–265. [CrossRef] [PubMed]
55. Kang, J.; Demaria, S.; Formenti, S. Current clinical trials testing the combination of immunotherapy with radiotherapy. *J. Immunother. Cancer* **2016**, *4*, 51. [CrossRef] [PubMed]
56. Golden, E.B.; Demaria, S.; Schiff, P.B.; Chachoua, A.; Formenti, S.C. An abscopal response to radiation and ipilimumab in a patient with metastatic non-small cell lung cancer. *Cancer Immunol. Res.* **2013**, *1*, 365–372. [CrossRef] [PubMed]

57. Formenti, S.C.; Demaria, S. Radiation therapy to convert the tumor into an in situ vaccine. *Int. J. Radiat. Oncol. Biol. Phys.* **2012**, *84*, 879–880. [CrossRef] [PubMed]
58. Order, S.E. The effects of therapeutic irradiation on lymphocytes and immunity. *Cancer* **1977**, *39*, 737–743. [CrossRef]
59. Uh, S.; Lee, S.M.; Kim, H.T.; Chung, Y.; Kim, Y.H.; Park, C.; Huh, S.J.; Lee, H.B. The effect of radiation therapy on immune function in patients with squamous cell lung carcinoma. *Chest* **1994**, *105*, 132–137. [CrossRef] [PubMed]
60. Sharabi, A.B.; Tran, P.T.; Lim, M.; Drake, C.G.; Deweese, T.L. Stereotactic radiation therapy combined with immunotherapy: Augmenting the role of radiation in local and systemic treatment. *Oncology (Williston Park)* **2015**, *29*, 331–340. [PubMed]
61. Kim, H.J.; Park, S.; Kim, K.J.; Seong, J. The Clinical Implications of Soluble PD-L1 in Hepatocellular Carcinoma Patients Treated With Radiation Therapy. *Int. J. Radiat. Oncol.* **2017**, *99*, S89. [CrossRef]
62. Patel, K.R.; Shoukat, S.; Oliver, D.E.; Chowdhary, M.; Rizzo, M.; Lawson, D.H.; Khosa, F.; Liu, Y.; Khan, M.K. Ipilimumab and Stereotactic Radiosurgery vs. Stereotactic Radiosurgery Alone for Newly Diagnosed Melanoma Brain Metastases. *Am. J. Clin. Oncol.* **2017**, *40*, 444–450. [CrossRef] [PubMed]
63. Kiess, A.P.; Wolchok, J.D.; Barker, C.A.; Postow, M.A.; Tabar, V.; Huse, J.T.; Chan, T.A.; Yamada, Y.; Beal, K. Stereotactic Radiosurgery for Melanoma Brain Metastases in Patients Receiving Ipilimumab: Safety Profile and Efficacy of Combined Treatment. *Int. J. Radiat. Oncol.* **2015**, *92*, 368–375. [CrossRef] [PubMed]
64. Twyman-Saint Victor, C.; Rech, A.J.; Maity, A.; Rengan, R.; Pauken, K.E.; Stelekati, E.; Benci, J.L.; Xu, B.; Dada, H.; Odorizzi, P.M.; et al. Radiation and dual checkpoint blockade activate non-redundant immune mechanisms in cancer. *Nature* **2015**, *520*, 373–377. [CrossRef] [PubMed]
65. Chen, L.; Narang, A.; Thompson, E.; Anders, R.; Waters, K.; Poling, J.; Rosati, L.M.; Huang, C.Y.; Tran, P.T.; Herman, J.M.; et al. Characterizing Tumor Infiltrating Lymphocytes Following Neoadjuvant Chemotherapy and Radiation in Pancreatic Adenocarcinoma. *Int. J. Radiat. Oncol.* **2017**, *99*, S91–S92. [CrossRef]
66. Foley, K.; Kim, V.; Jaffee, E.; Zheng, L. Current progress in immunotherapy for pancreatic cancer. *Cancer Lett.* **2016**, *381*, 244–251. [CrossRef] [PubMed]
67. Brahmer, J.R.; Tykodi, S.S.; Chow, L.Q.M.; Hwu, W.-J.; Topalian, S.L.; Hwu, P.; Drake, C.G.; Camacho, L.H.; Kauh, J.; Odunsi, K.; et al. Safety and Activity of Anti–PD-L1 Antibody in Patients with Advanced Cancer. *N. Engl. J. Med.* **2012**, *366*, 2455–2465. [CrossRef] [PubMed]
68. Royal, R.E.; Levy, C.; Turner, K.; Mathur, A.; Hughes, M.; Kammula, U.S.; Sherry, R.M.; Topalian, S.L.; Yang, J.C.; Lowy, I.; et al. Phase 2 Trial of Single Agent Ipilimumab (Anti-CTLA-4) for Locally Advanced or Metastatic Pancreatic Adenocarcinoma. *J. Immunother.* **2010**, *33*, 828–833. [CrossRef] [PubMed]

© 2018 by the authors. Licensee MDPI, Basel, Switzerland. This article is an open access article distributed under the terms and conditions of the Creative Commons Attribution (CC BY) license (http://creativecommons.org/licenses/by/4.0/).

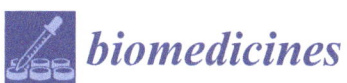

Review

Innovative Disease Model: Zebrafish as an In Vivo Platform for Intestinal Disorder and Tumors

Jeng-Wei Lu [1,*], Yi-Jung Ho [2], Shih-Ci Ciou [3] and Zhiyuan Gong [1,*]

1. Department of Biological Sciences, National University of Singapore, 14 Science Drive 4, Singapore 117543, Singapore
2. School of Pharmacy, National Defense Medical Center, No. 161, Section 6, Minquan East Road, Taipei 114, Taiwan; ejho@mail.ndmctsgh.edu.tw
3. Department of Clinical Laboratory Sciences and Medical Biotechnology, National Taiwan University, No. 1 Chang-Te Street, Taipei 100, Taiwan; scciou@ntu.edu.tw
* Correspondence: dbslujw@nus.edu.sg (J.-W.L.); dbsgzy@nus.edu.sg (Z.G.); Tel.: +65-6516-2860 (Z.G.)

Received: 13 September 2017; Accepted: 29 September 2017; Published: 29 September 2017

Abstract: Colorectal cancer (CRC) is one of the world's most common cancers and is the second leading cause of cancer deaths, causing more than 50,000 estimated deaths each year. Several risk factors are highly associated with CRC, including being overweight, eating a diet high in red meat and over-processed meat, having a history of inflammatory bowel disease, and smoking. Previous zebrafish studies have demonstrated that multiple oncogenes and tumor suppressor genes can be regulated through genetic or epigenetic alterations. Zebrafish research has also revealed that the activation of carcinogenesis-associated signal pathways plays an important role in CRC. The biology of cancer, intestinal disorders caused by carcinogens, and the morphological patterns of tumors have been found to be highly similar between zebrafish and humans. Therefore, the zebrafish has become an important animal model for translational medical research. Several zebrafish models have been developed to elucidate the characteristics of gastrointestinal diseases. This review article focuses on zebrafish models that have been used to study human intestinal disorders and tumors, including models involving mutant and transgenic fish. We also report on xenograft models and chemically-induced enterocolitis. This review demonstrates that excellent zebrafish models can provide novel insights into the pathogenesis of gastrointestinal diseases and help facilitate the evaluation of novel anti-tumor drugs.

Keywords: colorectal cancer; intestinal disorder; intestinal tumors; zebrafish

1. Introduction

Colorectal cancer (CRC) is one of the world's most common cancers. It is also the second-leading cause of cancer deaths in the United States, responsible for more than 50,000 estimated deaths in the world [1]. Although the five-year survival rate for localized CRC is >90%, most CRC patients are asymptomatic; therefore, only 40% of cases are detected at this stage. At the metastatic stage, CRC survival rate falls to 8–12%. There are five stages of CRC: aberrant foci, small adenoma/adenomatous polyps, large adenoma, adenocarcinoma, and invasion/metastasis. Risk factors for CRC include age (>50 years), being overweight, a diet that is high in red and over-processed meat, a history of inflammatory bowel disease, and smoking [1]. In addition, 5–10% of familial CRC cases include mutations in the tumor suppressor gene *APC*, and environmental risk factors have been linked to somatic mutations that can cause CRC. Non-familial cases of CRC are often related to overactivity of epidermal growth factor receptor (*EGFR*), loss of function at *APC*, and activating or allele mutations in *K-RAS*, *N-RAS*, *BRAF*, *PIK3CA*, *WNT*, and TP53 genes. It has been hypothesized that the regulation of different CRC phenotypes could be associated with a balance between anti-proliferation, maintaining genomic stability, and oncogenes. For example, microsatellite instability results in the loss of DNA mismatch repair function, which in turn leads to overactivity of COX-2, EGFR, and/or WNT pathways and results in small adenomas. K-RAS and/or PIK3CA pathway overactivity results in large adenomas; and inactivation of the tumor suppressor gene TP53 and downregulation of TGF-β signaling results in invasive/metastatic carcinomas [2–4]. In non-hereditary sporadic CRC, *APC* is mutated in 85% of cases, TP53 is mutated in 40–50% of cases, *PIK3CA* is mutated in 35% of cases, and *TGFBR2* is mutated in 45–50% of cases [2].

APC mutations activate the WNT pathway by increasing the amount of β-catenin that is translocated into the nucleus and enhancing the transcription of various oncogenes [5]. Causes of *APC* inactivation include hypermethylation of the *APC* promoter, germline mutations, and somatic mutations [6]. The *APC* gene is responsible for approximately 75% of mutations or the loss of heterozygosity (LOH) in CRC. Most *APC* mutations are clustered in the mutation cluster region that is located between codons 1282 and 1581 [7]. Previous studies have demonstrated the effects of *APC* restoration in cancerous mice, whereby tumor cells were replaced by normal cells, and some evidence suggests that *APC* restoration therapy could have similar benefits for humans [8]. Another study showed that, in a CRC cell line, β-catenin activates a set of 162 target genes associated with the WNT pathway; however, no conclusions could be drawn regarding the effect of these genes on cancer prognosis [9].

The first proposed model of genetic events that led to the development of CRC involved point mutations in *K-RAS* [10]. Specifically, point mutations in codons 12, 13, and 61 of *K-RAS* activate an enzyme that increases RAS signaling. Indeed, *K-RAS* has been found to be mutated in 30–40% of CRC cases, and in 60–90% of hyperplastic or non-dysplastic aberrant crypt foci [11,12]. Mutations in codon 12 of *K-RAS* are associated with more advanced tumor stages [13], and RAS signaling further activates the Raf-MEK-ERK pathway, the PI3K/AKT/PKB pathway, and Ral small GTPases [14]. Furthermore, most human CRC cases that involve PI3K gene mutations also involve *K-RAS* mutations [15]. *AKT1* and *AKT2* genes enhance tumor growth by promoting epithelial-to-mesenchymal transition (EMT) through PI3K activation [16,17], and the tumor suppressor gene of the *PTEN* antagonist PI3K/AKT pathway induces AKT-regulated tumor metastasis through loss-of-function mutations [18]. Finally, the MEK/ERK and PI3K/AKT pathways often converge to activate a cap-dependent translation, which can inhibit metastasis through the knockdown of survivin [19].

In the majority of human tumors, TP53 is dysfunctional. Several tumors display a gain of function mutation in TP53, which results in mutated TP53 (mutTP53) proteins [20]. MDM2 can also bind and inactivate the mutTP53 isoform. In CRC tissues, the overexpression of protein and mRNA was observed in the spliced isoform MDM2-B. Protein and mRNA overexpression is mainly associated with the mutTP53 protein as MDM2-B binds to MDM2, which in turn allows mutTP53 to accumulate in cells [21]. Indeed, a previous report showed that a loss-of-function mutation in TP53 affects 44.9% of colorectal adenoma cases, 42.22% of single primary CRC cases, and 43.75% of multiple primary CRC cases [22].

In current clinical practice, the only option to treat unresectable metastatic CRC is conventional chemotherapy. Although chemotherapy tends to relieve initial symptoms, resistance generally develops within six months. Life-extending agents, such as conventional cytotoxics and targeted therapeutics, are frequently used, including 5-fluoracil, capecitabine and topotecan, bevacizumab, cetuximab, and panitumumab [23,24]. Unfortunately, CRC patients who receive these agents also develop a resistance to them, and have a final average survival rate of only 13.3 months [25]. So far, zebrafish has been well used to study several intestinal cancer and disorder. Here we give a broad view to understand how zebrafish involved in those studies.

2. Development and Anatomy of the Gastrointestinal Tract in Zebrafish

The digestive system plays a critical role in vertebrate physiology and the intestinal anatomy among amniotes is highly conserved. The zebrafish is a powerful animal model in the study of intestinal development. Moreover, genes and organ functions are also well conserved between zebrafish and higher vertebrates [26–28]. For example, in zebrafish, the internal lining of the intestines forms a ridge (and not villi). This unique characteristic can be observed in cross-sections of mammalian intestines as well. Although zebrafish lack a stomach, crypts, Paneth cells, submucosal glands, and the organization of lymphoid structures, the zebrafish intestine is a simple but unique organ in vertebrate intestinal biology.

The morphological development of zebrafish intestine has been comparatively well studied in embryos and larvae [29–32]. However, zebrafish lack a morphologically and functionally distinct stomach, and do not express genes that encode precise gastric functions. Zebrafish do have an intestinal bulb with a lumen that is larger than the posterior part of the intestine. This intestinal bulb may function as a container that is comparable to the stomach. The digestive enzymes and solute transporters are present in the anterior and mid intestines [33]. A previous report indicated that because the intestinal bulb of zebrafish lacks gastric glands, the pH in the zebrafish intestines never falls below 7.5 [34].

Early research revealed that the zebrafish digestive tract develops in a segmental fashion, and that development begins during the mid-somite stages. Gut tube formation begins during mid- to late-somite stages (~18 somites) in zebrafish; however, in mammals, the gut begins to form during the early-somite stages (1–2 somites). At the 18-somite stage, a continuous thin layer of endoderm becomes distinguishable, which will eventually give rise to the primitive gut endoderm. Although gut formation occurs later in zebrafish, the temporal progression of gut tube formation is similar to that of mammals: the rostral gut of zebrafish develops first, followed by the hindgut and midgut [29].

Zebrafish gut development begins at almost 20 h post fertilization (hpf) and proceeds as follows. Firstly, endodermal precursors form the primitive gut: a thin, rod-like cell layer that lengthens from the future mouth to the future anus of the embryo. Progenitor gut cells then polarize to become columnar epithelium, and junctional complexes form between cells, which are required for lumen inflation and the establishment of the epithelial barrier. These developmental progressions occur in conjunction with cell proliferation along the total length of the intestinal tube. Proliferation is downregulated at approximately 72 hpf, at which time the intestinal epithelial cells are differentiated into the three lineages of mature gut epithelium, including absorptive enterocytes, mucus-producing goblet cells, and hormone-secreting enteroendocrine cells. Around 120 hpf, the yolk is entirely absorbed, and gut development is almost complete. At this time, the embryo is able to feed and digest. Previous studies have described the zebrafish intestine as a tapered tube that begins at the esophageal junction and is folded into three segments: (1), the large diameter rostral intestinal bulb, which is characterized by an expanded lumen and epithelial folding, and is primarily comprised of enterocytes and enteroendocrine cells; (2), the mid-intestine, which is demarcated by the presence of goblet cells and enterocytes with large, supranuclear vacuoles; and (3), the small diameter posterior intestine, which does not possess endocrine and goblet cells. Even though zebrafish do not have five intestinal segments like mammals (i.e., jejunum, duodenum, cecum, ileum, and colon), zebrafish and mammalian intestines do share functional homology. For example, in both zebrafish and mammals, growth factor gradient combinations of bone morphogenetic protein (Bmp), fibroblast growth factor (Fgf), and wingless-type MMTV integration site (Wnt) at the posterior end of the endoderm are able to regulate intestinal development. Additionally, retinoic acid (RA) signaling plays a dose-dependent role in patterning the anterior–posterior (A-P) body axis, including the endoderm [31,32].

Wang et al. [28] previously performed a microarray analysis of adult zebrafish guts, in which guts were separated into seven sections of equal lengths (from anterior 1 to posterior 7). Using metabolic gene data, they were able to confirm the presence of three distinct gut regions. Furthermore, segments 1 to 5 (*S1* to *S5*) showed high expression of intestinal markers that are conserved in humans and mice: fatty acid binding protein 2 (*fabp2*), villin 1 (*vil1*), and apolipoproteins 1 and 4 (*apoa1* and *apoa4*). *Fabp2*, *Apo1*, and *Apo4* all participate in lipid metabolism. Wang et al. [28] also reported that the *Vil1* gene plays a role in regulating anti-apoptosis in small intestinal epithelial cells. Additionally, aquaporin 3 (*aqp3*) and cofilin1 (*cfl1*) (which are biomarkers of the large intestine in mammals) were found to distinguish genes associated with sections *S1* to *S4* from genes associated with *S5* to *S7* in zebrafish. Furthermore, *Cfl1* was reported to regulate the dynamic stabilization of *actin* filaments, and *aqp3* was found to participate in water absorption. Wang et al. [28] also indicated that *S1* to *S5* share molecular characteristics with the small intestine of mammals, and that *S6* and *S7* share similar characteristics with the large intestine of mammals. Finally, *S5* was found to form a transition segment, and was surmised to be the dorsal fraction of the mid-gut that participates in mucosal immunity [28]. However, in order to further investigate the correlation of these genes between diseases, to develop the transgenic zebrafish is quite critical.

3. Developments in Transgenic Zebrafish Technology that Enable the Exploration of Intestinal Tumors Using a Constitutive or Inducible Expression System

Significant progress has been made in the development of transgenic technology, which is an essential technique that is used in research and employed in a variety of model organisms [35,36]. A variety of transgenic expression systems exist, including constitutive and inducible systems [37]. Traditionally, establishing a transgenic fish model involved injecting fish embryos with (1) artificial chromosomes of recombinant bacteria [38], (2) supercoiled [39] or linear DNA [36], and (3) linearized ISce-I meganuclease [40]. Recently, however, the use of Sleeping Beauty (SB) [41], Ac/Ds [42], and Tol2 [43] transposon-based systems has effectively increased transgenic efficiency in zebrafish. The development of SB was based on DNA sequences of Tc1-like elements (TcEs) from teleost fish species [44,45]. When the SB transposon plasmid and SB transposase mRNA are co-injected into fertilized eggs, the SB transposon vector is transposed from the plasmid to the zebrafish genome, and the transposon insertions are transmitted to the next generation of zebrafish germline [46]. The Tol2 transposon element was found in the medaka genome, which can be efficiently excised and integrated into the zebrafish genome. This enables transgenic lines to be generated by co-injecting fish with Tol2 mRNA and vector plasmid [43]. In a plant transposon system, the maize Dissociation (Ds) element is capable of effective Activator (Ac) transposase-mediated transposition in the zebrafish, yielding high transposition frequencies and efficient germline transmission rates [42].

Previous studies noted that the overexpression of oncogenes can lead to serious tumors, early embryonic developmental abnormalities, and death, which prevents oncogene effects from being comprehensively characterized. Controlling gene expression through the use of an induction system can help address this problem. Currently, widely used induction systems include heat shock, Cre-loxP, GAL4-UAS, Tet-On, Tet-Off, and mifepristone. These systems regulate the duration and dosage to achieve spatiotemporal control of transgene expression in fish during both the embryonic and adult stages [37,47].

The important role of intestinal-type fatty acid binding protein (I-FABP; also known as FABP2) has been observed in vertebrates. Specifically, this role involves the intracellular binding and trafficking of long chain fatty acids. Mammalian gene promoters and ubiquitous or endogenous tissue-specific promoters are able to drive the expression of green fluorescent protein (GFP) and red fluorescent protein (RFP) transgenes in zebrafish [48,49]. Zebrafish 4.5-kb *FABP2* gene promoter also drives intestine-specific GFP/RFP expression in the zebrafish. Indeed, previous research noted the ability of the *FABP2* gene promoter to direct GFP/RFP fluorescent expression in the intestinal tube from three days post-fertilization (dpf) (when zebrafish were in the larval stage) until the adult stage [49,50]. The first transgenic fish model of an intestinal tumor was developed through the expression of the *H. pylori* virulence factor *cagA*, which was in turn controlled by the 1.6-kb *FABP2* promoter in *tp53* mutant background zebrafish (tp53^{M214K}) [51]. Heat shock-inducible Cre/Lox expression controlled by the *β-actin* promoter of human *K-RAS*^{G12D} has also been induced in intestinal epithelial tumors alongside several other tumors in zebrafish [52].

4. Zebrafish Models for Intestinal Tumors and Disorders

The zebrafish is a powerful animal model that can be used for the forward and reverse genetic analysis of vertebrate embryogenesis, organ development, disease, tumors, and toxicology. Many zebrafish mutants or transgenic lines have also proven to be excellent animal models for a variety of human diseases and tumors [53]. Experimental carcinogenesis studies have illustrated the development of tumors that can occur in the wild in virtually all organs in zebrafish [54,55]. Furthermore, the histopathology of intestinal neoplasia in zebrafish is similar to the histopathology of intestinal neoplasia in humans [56,57]. One study found that the histological signs of cancer in zebrafish included preneoplastic intestinal changes, such as hyperplasia, dysplasia, adenocarcinoma, small cell carcinoma/carcinoid-like, tubular/tubulovillous adenoma, and enteritis [58]. According to histological diagnosis, the intestinal carcinomas were comprised of neuroendocrine cells. Immunohistochemistry analysis of cytokeratins (that used human epithelial (cytokeratin wide spectrum screening (WSS), AE1/AE3) or neuroendocrines (S100, chromogranin A) markers) confirmed that the majority of intestinal tumors in a cohort of zebrafish were carcinomas [59].

Mutations in the *APC* gene have been identified as being responsible for human familial adenomatous polyposis (FAP) syndrome [60,61]. *APC* gene mutations can also lead to the development of multiple colorectal adenomas following somatic inactivation of the remaining allele via carriers of germline truncating mutation [62]. Similarly, results from a mouse model revealed that multiple tumors developed in the small intestine when the *APC* gene contained a heterozygous truncating mutation [63]. Finally, *APC* was also found to be a key inhibitory gene in the WNT/β-catenin pathway [64].

Zebrafish *apc*-mutants carry a premature stop codon in the putative mutation cluster region (MCR) of *APC*, which mimics the mutations found in FAP patients. Homozygous *apc*-mutant fish embryos die between 72 and 96 hpf. The unusual features that characterize these fish include an aberrantly developed gut, liver, and pancreas. [65]. In one study, 17.6% of adult *apc*-mutant fish (aged >15 months) developed spontaneous liver tumors, and 11.8% of these fish developed spontaneous intestinal tumors. The *apc*-mutant fish appear to have polyps, which is a mammalian resemblance. These intestinal disturbances were observed in the disorganized large structures with ramifications of the villi, which are frequently embedded in fibrovascular stroma. The pathologic lesions were classified as adenomatous polyps. These lesions showed pseudostratification of nuclei, loss of goblet cells, and a high N/C (nuclear-to-cytoplasmic) ratio that is consistent with dysplastic epithelium. In intestinal adenoma tissue of *apc*-mutant fish, high levels of β-catenin accumulated in proliferating cells of both the cytoplasm and nucleus. In addition, 58.3% of *apc*-mutant fish (aged 14 months) treated with 7,12-dimethylbenz[a]anthracene (DMBA) showed intestinal adenomas, whereas only 20.5% of wild-type fish treated with DMBA showed intestinal adenomas. This well-established *apc*-mutant fish is a bona fide tumor suppressor, similar to its mammalian counterpart. Furthermore, the loss of heterozygous *apc*-mutant fish resembles the cancer phenotype in mammals [66]. Recent studies have also used zebrafish to investigate the genetic relationship between mitochondrial pyruvate carrier 1 (*MPC1*) and *APC*. Data from this research has demonstrated that (1) *apc* controls the levels of *mpc1* and (2) the knockdown of *mpc1* recapitulates the phenotypes of impaired *apc* function, such as failed intestinal differentiation. Moreover, exogenous human *MPC1* RNA rescued failed intestinal differentiation in apc-deficient zebrafish [67].

In recent years, zebrafish models have been developed to investigate whether the mutations of human *H-RAS*, *N-RAS*, *K-RAS* or zebrafish *k-ras* caused tumorigenesis, including models that illustrate chordoma [68], melanoma [69], rhabdomyosarcoma [70,71], brain tumors [72], gill tumors [73], liver tumors [74], pancreatic tumors [75], and other tumors that faithfully recapitulate human disease symptoms. The shock-inducible Cre/Lox-mediated $K\text{-}RAS^{G12D}$ transgenic fish approach can be conditionally caused within transgenic fish via heat shock treatment. This heat shock-inducible recombination approach has enabled the generation of multiple types of $K\text{-}RAS^{G12D}$-induced rhabdomyosarcomas (RMS), myeloproliferative disorders, and intestinal epithelial hyperplasia. For example, $K\text{-}RAS^{G12D}$ activation in intestinal epithelial cells triggered intestinal hyperplasia in zebrafish. This is consistent with findings that indicated 50% of human CRC cases have *RAS* gene mutations [76]. In zebrafish, cases of intestinal epithelial hyperplasia were characterized by epithelial cells with severely disorganized intestinal epithelial architecture. Specifically, these cells showed several foci forming large outgrowths in the gastrointestinal cavity of $K\text{-}RAS^{G12D}$ fish. The $K\text{-}RAS^{G12D}$-induced tumor and hyperplasia transgenic models generated here are similar to their related human malignancies [52].

Two *tp53* mutant ($tp53^{N168K}$ and $tp53^{M214K}$) fish that harbor missense mutations in the DNA-binding domain of the *tp53* gene have been mutagenized by N-ethyl-N-nitrosourea (ENU). Both of the mutated *tp53* alleles were dominant-negative, which is orthologous to cancerous mutations in human TP53 cells [77]. Homozygous $tp53^{M214K}$ mutant fish spontaneously formed tumors starting at the age of 8.5 months, and the tumor incidence rate was 28% when fish were 16.5 months old. The most common malignant tumors in *tp53* mutant zebrafish were peripheral nerve sheath tumors [77]. According to the literature, *tp53* zebrafish mutants have been used to study the gastrointestinal tumorigenesis of liver cancer [78] and intestinal tumors [51], as the synergistic interactions between target genes and the *tp53* mutation encourage the formation of these tumors. The allelic loss of TP53 has also been observed in human CRC, and is thought to be a late event that occurs during the transition from adenoma to carcinoma [79]. Data from mouse tumor models have also suggested that TP53 inactivation is an essential event in the progression of pancreatic cancer [80], liver cancer [81], and colorectal cancer [82]. However, assessing the role played by zebrafish *tp53* and *tp53*-related pathways in both wild-type and mutant fish could facilitate a better understanding of the role played by this pleiotropic pathway [79].

Primary risk factors of human gastrointestinal cancer include infection with *Helicobacter pylori* or other bacterial strains that carry the virulence factor *cagA*. To elucidate the mechanism that underlies the *cagA* promotion of cancer formation, the expression of *cagA* by *β-actin* or *FABP2* has been studied in both wild-type and *tp53* mutant zebrafish [77]. The expression of *cagA* led to significantly increased rates of intestinal epithelial cell proliferation in zebrafish by expressing either the wild-type or a phosphorylation-resistant form. Furthermore, the target genes of the WNT pathway, such as *cyclinD1*, *axin2*, and *myca*, were significantly upregulated. Co-expression of *cagA* with the loss-of-function allele *axin1* also increased the proliferation of intestinal cells; however, co-expression of *cagA* with *tcf4* (a null allele of the key β-catenin transcriptional cofactor) restored intestinal proliferation to that of wild-type fish, which showed normal intestinal architecture, with a single layer of epithelial cells lining the mucosal folds, at 18 months. Additionally, overexpression of *cagA* (under the control of ubiquitous *β-actin* or the intestine-specific *FABP2* promoter) induced mucosal fold epithelial hyperplasia, dysplasia within mucosal sulci, and mucosal fold fusion in the intestines of 12-month-old wild-type fish. Intestinal epithelial hyperplasia and definitive neoplasia, such as adenocarcinoma and small cell carcinoma, were also observed in 12-month-old *tp53* and $FABP2\text{-}cagA/tp53^{M214K-/-}$ mutant fish. Finally, a synergistic interaction between *cagA* and the loss-of-function mutation in the tp53 allele were found to facilitate the formation of small cell carcinoma and adenocarcinoma in the intestine of $FABP2\text{-}cagA/tp53^{M214K-/-}$ transgenic fish [51]. This model established that the intestinal tumors transgenic model would be a great advantage in the study of *cagA*-associated gastrointestinal cancers (Table 1).

Table 1. Zebrafish animal models of intestinal disorder and tumors.

Gene Name	System or Mutation Site	Phenotypes	Stage	Refs.
mpc1	Knock down of *mpc1*	Failed intestinal differentiation	96 hpf	[67]
apc	Stop codon in the MCR	Liver and intestine tumors	15 months	[65]
apc+DMBA	Stop codon in the MCR	Intestinal adenomas	14 months	[66]
tp53^{M214}	Point mutations in the DBM	Peripheral nerve sheath tumors, intestinal hyperplasia and adenocarcinoma	12 months	[51,77]
K-RAS^{G12D}	HSP-inducible Cre/Lox	Rhabdomyosarcomas, myeloproliferative disorder and Intestinal hyperplasia	0.8–3.4 months	[52]
cagA	B-*actin*-constitutive expression	Intestinal hyperplasia, dysplasia and mucosal fold fusion	12 months	[52]
cagA^{EPISA}	B-*actin*-constitutive expression	Normal	12 months	[51]
cagA	FABP2-constitutive expression	Intestinal hyperplasia, dysplasia and mucosal fold fusion	12 months	[51]
cagA+tp53^{M214}	FABP2-constitutive expression	Intestinal hyperplasia, adenocarcinoma and small cell carcinoma	12 months	[51]

MCR: Mutation cluster region; DMBA: 7,12-dimethylbenz[a]anthracene; DBM: DNA-binding domain; *cagA*^{EPISA}: A *cagA* mutant lacking ELISA motifs; HSP: Heat shock promoter; FABP2: Intestinal fatty acid-binding protein promoter.

5. The Potential of Zebrafish Xenograft Models to Benefit the Study of CRC Tumor Metastasis and Drug Screening

Pioneering work conducted by several laboratories has indicated that zebrafish embryos have the potential to benefit large-scale drug screening applications [83,84]. Zebrafish can be arrayed in a variety of isolated 12-well, 24-well, and 96-well plates (or even larger plates). For this, fish are bathed in water that contains the small molecules or chemical compounds of interest, a procedure that is ideally suited for high-throughput screening [85]. Over the past decade, the study of these zebrafish models is the most relevant research in clinical relevance [83,84]. Living cells or tissues can be transposed from one species to another using a xenograft method [86].

Casper zebrafish mutants [87] and vascular fluorescent reporter transgenic zebrafish lines (*fli1a:EGFP*) [88] have also previously been generated. Casper zebrafish lack melanocytes and iridophore cells and are therefore transparent from the embryonic stage through to adulthood; the *fli1a:EGFP* reporter line permits the visualization of both blood and lymphatic vessels. Whole-mount alkaline phosphatase vessel staining assays can be used with *fli1a:EGFP* transgenic embryos to investigate angiogenesis, tumor invasion, tumor metastasis, and anti-vascular endothelial growth factor (VEGF) drugs, as well as to disseminate cancer cells [37,89]. In addition, the lymphocyte-deficient *rag2E450fs* (casper) mutant transparent line (ZFIN allele *rag2fb101*) has been engrafted into a wide variety of normal and cancerous zebrafish cells to (1) optimize cell transplantation, (2) improve the visualization of fluorescently-labelled cancer cells at a single-cell resolution, and (3) analyze interactions between tumor cells and other key players in the tumor microenvironment. The tumor cells transplantation method using *rag2E450fs* (casper) mutant also enables cancer processes to be visualized at a single-cell resolution in vivo [90,91]. Indeed, in conjunction with advances in imaging technology, these mutant lines have created new opportunities for zebrafish xenograft models to be employed in the study of tumor cell metastasis and in the screening of novel drugs [37,92].

In another study, researchers labeled two human colorectal cancer cell lines (SW620 and SW480) with 1,1′-dioctadecyl-3,3,3′3′-tetramethylindocarbocyanine (DiI), a lipophilic fluorescent tracking dye. After labeling, cells were collected and injected into the yolk sac or perivitelline space of 2 dpf zebrafish embryos. The colorectal SW620 cells then proliferated, migrated, and formed compact cancer cells. Masses were identified seven days later near the intestinal lining [93]. Conversely, the DiI-labeled non-transfected SW480 cells were irradiated with 0–10 Gy immediately following injection. After 24 h, the number of cells that had disseminated into the tail was determined, wherein a dose-dependent relationship was observed between disseminated cells and radiation intensity (e.g., the number of cancer cells found in the tail of embryos that had received a radiation dose of 10 Gy had significant increased). SW480 cells knocked down for *AEG-1* were also injected into the zebrafish perivitelline cavity and irradiated with 0 Gy or 10 Gy. The number of disseminated cells found in the tail of fish injected with *AEG-1* knockdown cells was significantly lower than that of the control fish. Furthermore, the number of non-transfected SW480 cells (negative control) was significantly higher in the tail of irradiated embryos than in the control embryos that did not receive radiation treatment. Yet, there was not a significant increase upon radiation for the SW480 *AEG-1* knockdown cells compared with the unirradiated control. In summary, this study showed (1) that tumor invasion can be enhanced by radiation, but (2) *AEG-1* knockdown can inhibit this process. This was also the first study to demonstrate that zebrafish comprise an excellent model for the study of early events in radiation-enhanced tumor invasion [94].

In yet another study, stable fluorescent colorectal carcinoma cells expressing GFP protein (HCT-116-GFP) were injected into the yolk sac of 2 dpf embryos. These animals were maintained in 96-well plates at 35 °C for 24 h to facilitate tumor cell proliferation and embryo recovery. Different doses of crambescidine-816 (0.5, 1, and 2 µM) or 5′-fluoracile (500 µM) were then administered for 48 h. This was the first study to demonstrate that crambescidin-816 induces colorectal carcinoma in a zebrafish xenograft model [95]. Recent literature further revealed that CRC zebrafish patient-derived xenografts (zPDX) derived from surgery resected CRC samples and treated with the same treatment administered to the patient provide proof of concept experiments that compare responses to chemotherapy and biological therapies between patients and zPDX [96].

Zebrafish xenograft models can be used for the development and evaluation of anti-cancer drugs. These models enable the response of human tumors to potential anti-cancer drugs to be observed directly. Human tumor material is particularly targeted for primary patient-derived biopsy specimens, and is often hard to maintain in vitro. Therefore, zebrafish models represent an effective way to reduce the time and expense required to conduct cancer treatment research [92]. Additional future advances could allow zebrafish to become an excellent in vivo drug testing model, and may provide an inexpensive and highly scalable platform that can be used in preclinical trials (Figure 1) [97].

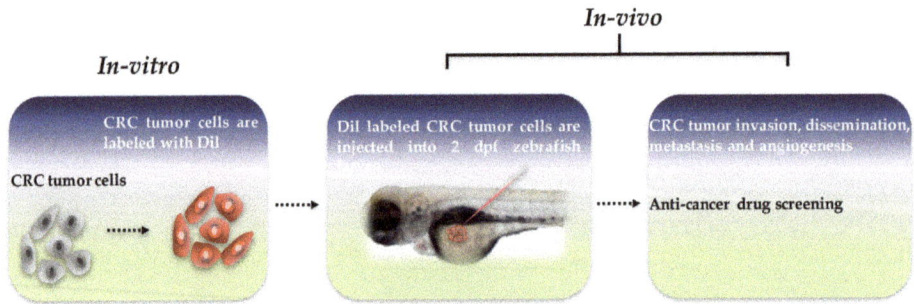

Figure 1. Schematic diagram of zebrafish xenograft model. Colorectal cancer (CRC) tumor cells were labeled with 1,1′-dioctadecyl-3,3,3′3′-tetramethylindocarbocyanine (DiI) dye in vitro, and approximately 300 tumor cells are injected into the yolk sac of each two days post-fertilization zebrafish larvae. Tumor invasion, dissemination, metastasis, and angiogenesis can be visualized, and anti-cancer drug screening can be conducted in vivo in a matter of days.

6. Chemically Induced Enterocolitis in Larvae and Adult Zebrafish

Inflammatory bowel disease (IBD) is a chronic inflammatory disease of the gastrointestinal tract. The symptoms of IBD include diarrhea, abdominal pain, weight loss, ulceration, perforation, and bowel obstruction. IBD is classified into two major forms, Crohn's disease (CD) and ulcerative colitis (UC), both of which can cause high morbidity and mortality. A key feature of CD is the aggregation of macrophages. CD often forms non-caseating granulomas that affect the whole intestine. UC is characterized by an increase in neutrophils and a depletion of goblet cell mucin, and usually affects the mucosal lining of the colon and rectum. Currently, the onset and pathogenic origin of IBD remain unclear; however, zebrafish provide a platform to investigate IBD (Table 2). Specifically, chemically-induced enterocolitis is often used to investigate intestinal inflammation. A variety of zebrafish progeny are suitable for the analysis of chemically induced inflammation [98].

Table 2. The advantages and limitations in the inflammatory bowel disease model of zebrafish.

Items	Larvae	Adult Zebrafish
Advantages	Many individuals Live imaging Germ-free derivation Colonization with specific bacteria High-throughput drug screening Easy operation	Less skin damage Adaptive immune involved
Limitations	Chemically-induced skin damage	With craft Less sample number
Example	TNBS: immersing larvae in 25–75 ug/mL TNBS from 3 dpf DSS: immersing larvae 0.5% (w/v) DSS from 3dpf	OXO: 0.2% oxazolone by intrarectally injection TNBS: 1 uL per 0.1g of body weight by intrarectally injection

TNBS: 2,4,6-trinitrobenzene sulfonic acid; DSS: Dextran sodium sulfate; OXO: oxazolone.

Chemically-induced enterocolitis models have already been established in both zebrafish larvae and adult zebrafish, which could cause intestinal epithelium damage and immune cell recruitment. The first developed an adult fish model for enterocolitis by intrarectally injecting 0.2% oxazolone, a haptenizing agent. Oxazolone caused the architecture of the intestinal wall to become thick and disrupted and also caused the intestine to lose goblet cells and undergo an influx of neutrophils and eosinophils. Furthermore, oxazolone led to an increase in the expression of cytokines, such as interleukin-1 β, tumor necrosis factor-α, and interleukin-10. That research further showed that (1) intestinal microbiota contribute to oxazolone-induced enterocolitis, and (2) vancomycin treatment led to an outgrowth of fusobacteria and reduced the percentage of proteobacteria. Indeed, zebrafish treated with vancomycin showed a reduction in oxazolone-induced enterocolitis score, decreased neutrophil infiltration, and diminished cytokine expression [99].

In research that demonstrated how a zebrafish model can be used in high-throughput chemical screening [100], Fleming et al. established a zebrafish enterocolitis model by immersing 3 dpf larvae in 75 µg/mL of 2,4,6-trinitrobenzene sulfonic acid (TNBS) (which has also been used to induce intestinal inflammation in mice). Fluorescent dye was then used to image live zebrafish larvae and analyze intestinal architecture and peristalsis in vivo. TNBS-induced enterocolitis was found to reduce villus length, enlarge crypts, decrease peristalsis, increase the number of goblet cells, and increase the expression of tumor necrosis factor-α. Moreover, TNBS was found to cause not only intestinal damage, but also skin lesions. However, a separate study by Oehlers et al. noted that larvae did not show skin lesions if they (1) were immersed in lower doses of TNBS or (2) were immersed in the 75 mg/mL dose for less than three days, to influence the analysis of enterocolitis. However, treatment with prednisolone or 5-amino salicylic acid slowed the reduction of the progression of enterocolitis. The data also showed that the number of goblet cells and proliferating cells both increased. Moreover, TNBS induced leukocytosis and reduced the branches of subintestinal vasculature, and a correlation was found between microbiota and TNBS-induced mortality. A potential explanation for this correlation is that microbiota are able to induce the transcription of pro-inflammatory cytokines, such as *il-1beta, tnf-alpha, ccl-20* and *il-8*, which promote inflammation [101].

TNBS has also been directly injected into the rectum of adult zebrafish to induce enterocolitis. Histological analysis revealed that this caused intestinal villi to become thicker and shorter, but did not affect the number of goblet cells. The survival rate of zebrafish with TNBS-induced enterocolitis was found to be related to microbiome diversity. In addition, TNBS caused pro-inflammatory and anti-inflammatory cytokines to be upregulated, and the expression of MCH and its receptor to increase. These findings suggest another potential therapeutic approach to IBD [102]. He et al. posited that TNBS may reduce the diversity of intestinal microbiota, which induces enterocolitis in larvae. Those researchers further showed that the reduction in microbiome diversity was due to an increase in Proteobacteria and a decrease in Firmicutes. It is possible that those chemicals influenced the composition of intestinal microbiota, which may have activated the TLR signaling pathways to initiate mucosal immune-mediated inflammation. However, intestinal damage and TNF-α overexpression was observed before the occurrence of microbiota dysbiosis, which suggests that a feedback loop exists between the interactions of the host and microbiota that perpetuated the inflammatory response [103]. He et al. also conducted additional experiments using germ-free fish, and found that TNBS-induced enterocolitis was not severe, even though toll-like receptor 3, MyD88, TRIF, NF-κB, and TNF-α were expressed. When microbial bacteria colonize, the characters revert to TNBS-treated conventionally-reared zebrafish. In summary, the zebrafish larvae model revealed that gut microbiota play a key role in TNBS-induced enterocolitis [104].

Dextran sodium sulfate (DSS) is a detergent that is also commonly used in animal models of IBD [105]. The highest tolerated dose (i.e., that did not induce significant mortality) had a concentration of 0.5%. Similar to enterocolitis induced by TNBS, DSS-induced enterocolitis caused liver discoloration and increased the number of neutrophils that migrated to the intestine. Moreover, DSS was found to upregulate the transcription of *ccl20*, *il1b*, *il23*, *il8*, *mmp9*, and *tnfa*. However, unlike enterocolitis induced by TNBS, DSS-induced enterocolitis led to the overgrowth of bacteria and reduced the proliferation of cells. Those researchers further observed that DSS induced the accumulation of acidic mucins in the intestinal bulb. This phenotype was associated with microbiota, but was not related to neutrophilic inflammation. Another previous study indicated that increased mucin secretion could prevent TNBS-induced enterocolitis. The mucosecretory phenotype of DSS was used to assess protection against TNBS-induced enterocolitis. DSS was found to reduce mortality and neutrophilic inflammation. In addition, retinoic acid (RA) was a conserved modulator of intestinal epithelial cell differentiation. Other evidence has also suggested that RA is able to suppress mucin secretion, and that co-treatment with RA and TNBS increases the mortality rate associated with TNBS-induced enterocolitis. Furthermore, pre-treatment with DSS in conjunction with RA may reduce the protective ability of DSS. Results of that study emphasized the importance of mucin secretion during enterocolitis progression [106]. In addition, Oehlers et al. wrote an additional technical report that focused on enterocolitis induced by TNBS and DSS that introduced several methods to assess intestinal damage and inflammatory processes. Those researchers reported that, if the proper genetic and imaging tools are employed, a zebrafish model could be useful for (1) high-throughput drug screening and (2) investigations that seek to elucidate the mechanisms that underlie drug efficacy [107]. They also found that most of the anti-inflammatory drugs they studied were able to protect against chemically-induced enterocolitis. For example, cholecystokinin (CCK) and dopamine receptor agonists were found to reduce enterocolitis-associated inflammation, thus providing a new therapeutic target [108]. TNBS and DSS were also used to establish an inflammatory lymphangiogenesis model, because they induced intestinal vascular endothelial growth factor (VEGF) receptor-dependent lymphangiogenesis in zebrafish larvae. This evidence suggests that macrophage recruitment and macrophage expression of intestinal VEGFs are correlated with intestinal inflammatory lymphangiogenesis. Therefore, this study helped to elucidate the mechanism underlying inflammatory lymphangiogenesis during IBD [109].

7. Concluding Comments

In this review paper, we provided an overview of the latest research that employed zebrafish models of intestinal disorders and tumors. Zebrafish have been found to share a substantial number of conserved genes with humans, and zebrafish tissue morphology is also similar to that of humans. Recent reports have used cells or mouse models to elucidate the disease and its pivotal role in cancer initiation. The zebrafish model offers unique advantages and can greatly contribute to the field of cancer research. Therefore, the development of zebrafish models for intestinal disorders and tumors should greatly benefit studies that seek to investigate potential cancer treatments or the mechanisms that underlie tumorigenesis. At present, zebrafish models have been established for several bowel diseases and intestinal tumors, including *apc*-mutant, *K-RAS*^{G12D}, *cagA*, and *cagA*/tp53$^{M214K-/-}$. Zebrafish models have also been used to investigate preclinical and primary tumors, tumor metastasis, cancer biomarkers, targets and small molecule drugs in human digestive organs. Although some understanding of the molecular mechanisms and biological functions associated with intestinal diseases and intestinal neoplasms exists, current knowledge is limited. With the ability to facilitate high-throughput screening for the discovery of novel therapeutic agents, zebrafish could become increasingly important as an in vivo model (Figure 2). Finally, as the utility of zebrafish models in the study of cancer becomes more widely accepted it may promote further drug discovery in the future, thus one day ahead of treatment and prognosis in human patients.

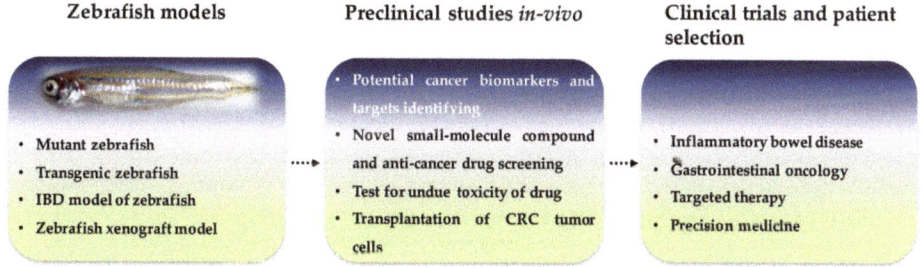

Figure 2. Roles of zebrafish intestinal disorder and tumor models in present and future research. Zebrafish is an ideal genetic and disease model system which is accessible for rapid screening and experimental manipulation for preclinical studies. In the future, zebrafish models could be used for patient selection in clinical trials.

Acknowledgments: This study was supported by grants (R154000667112 and R154000A23112) from Ministry of Education of Singapore.

Conflicts of Interest: The authors declare no conflict of interest.

References

1. Wong, M.C.; Ching, J.Y.; Chan, V.C.; Lam, T.Y.; Luk, A.K.; Wong, S.H.; Ng, S.C.; Ng, S.S.; Wu, J.C.; Chan, F.K.; et al. Colorectal cancer screening based on age and gender: A cost-effectiveness analysis. *Medicine* **2016**, *95*, e2739. [CrossRef] [PubMed]
2. Markowitz, S.D.; Bertagnolli, M.M. Molecular origins of cancer: Molecular basis of colorectal cancer. *N. Eng. J. Med.* **2009**, *361*, 2449–2460. [CrossRef] [PubMed]
3. Vogelstein, B.; Kinzler, K.W. The path to cancer—Three strikes and you're out. *N. Engl. J. Med.* **2015**, *373*, 1895–1898. [CrossRef] [PubMed]
4. Wang, T.L.; Rago, C.; Silliman, N.; Ptak, J.; Markowitz, S.; Willson, J.K.; Parmigiani, G.; Kinzler, K.W.; Vogelstein, B.; Velculescu, V.E. Prevalence of somatic alterations in the colorectal cancer cell genome. *Proc. Natl. Acad. Sci. USA* **2002**, *99*, 3076–3080. [CrossRef] [PubMed]
5. Mann, B.; Gelos, M.; Siedow, A.; Hanski, M.L.; Gratchev, A.; Ilyas, M.; Bodmer, W.F.; Moyer, M.P.; Riecken, E.O.; Buhr, H.J.; et al. Target genes of beta-catenin-t cell-factor/lymphoid-enhancer-factor signaling in human colorectal carcinomas. *Proc. Natl. Acad. Sci. USA* **1999**, *96*, 1603–1608. [CrossRef] [PubMed]
6. Tariq, K.; Ghias, K. Colorectal cancer carcinogenesis: A review of mechanisms. *Cancer Biol. Med.* **2016**, *13*, 120–135. [CrossRef] [PubMed]

7. Christie, M.; Jorissen, R.N.; Mouradov, D.; Sakthianandeswaren, A.; Li, S.; Day, F.; Tsui, C.; Lipton, L.; Desai, J.; Jones, I.T.; et al. Different apc genotypes in proximal and distal sporadic colorectal cancers suggest distinct wnt/beta-catenin signalling thresholds for tumourigenesis. *Oncogene* **2013**, *32*, 4675–4682. [CrossRef] [PubMed]
8. Dow, L.E.; O'Rourke, K.P.; Simon, J.; Tschaharganeh, D.F.; van Es, J.H.; Clevers, H.; Lowe, S.W. Apc restoration promotes cellular differentiation and reestablishes crypt homeostasis in colorectal cancer. *Cell* **2015**, *161*, 1539–1552. [CrossRef] [PubMed]
9. Watanabe, K.; Biesinger, J.; Salmans, M.L.; Roberts, B.S.; Arthur, W.T.; Cleary, M.; Andersen, B.; Xie, X.; Dai, X. Integrative chip-seq/microarray analysis identifies a ctnnb1 target signature enriched in intestinal stem cells and colon cancer. *PLoS ONE* **2014**, *9*. [CrossRef] [PubMed]
10. Vogelstein, B.; Fearon, E.R.; Hamilton, S.R.; Kern, S.E.; Preisinger, A.C.; Leppert, M.; Nakamura, Y.; White, R.; Smits, A.M.; Bos, J.L. Genetic alterations during colorectal-tumor development. *N. Engl. J. Med.* **1988**, *319*, 525–532. [CrossRef] [PubMed]
11. Pretlow, T.P.; Pretlow, T.G. Mutant kras in aberrant crypt foci (acf): Initiation of colorectal cancer? *Biochim. Biophys. Acta* **2005**, *1756*, 83–96. [CrossRef] [PubMed]
12. Rosty, C.; Young, J.P.; Walsh, M.D.; Clendenning, M.; Walters, R.J.; Pearson, S.; Pavluk, E.; Nagler, B.; Pakenas, D.; Jass, J.R.; et al. Colorectal carcinomas with kras mutation are associated with distinctive morphological and molecular features. *Mod. Pathol.* **2013**, *26*, 825–834. [CrossRef] [PubMed]
13. Li, W.; Qiu, T.; Zhi, W.; Shi, S.; Zou, S.; Ling, Y.; Shan, L.; Ying, J.; Lu, N. Colorectal carcinomas with kras codon 12 mutation are associated with more advanced tumor stages. *BMC Cancer* **2015**, *15*. [CrossRef] [PubMed]
14. Pino, M.S.; Chung, D.C. The chromosomal instability pathway in colon cancer. *Gastroenterology* **2010**, *138*, 2059–2072. [CrossRef] [PubMed]
15. Kosmidou, V.; Oikonomou, E.; Vlassi, M.; Avlonitis, S.; Katseli, A.; Tsipras, I.; Mourtzoukou, D.; Kontogeorgos, G.; Zografos, G.; Pintzas, A. Tumor heterogeneity revealed by kras, braf, and pik3ca pyrosequencing: Kras and pik3ca intratumor mutation profile differences and their therapeutic implications. *Hum. Mutat.* **2014**, *35*, 329–340. [CrossRef] [PubMed]
16. Johnson, S.M.; Gulhati, P.; Rampy, B.A.; Han, Y.; Rychahou, P.G.; Doan, H.Q.; Weiss, H.L.; Evers, B.M. Novel expression patterns of pi3k/akt/mtor signaling pathway components in colorectal cancer. *J. Am. Coll. Surg.* **2010**, *210*, 767–776. [CrossRef] [PubMed]
17. Suman, S.; Kurisetty, V.; Das, T.P.; Vadodkar, A.; Ramos, G.; Lakshmanaswamy, R.; Damodaran, C. Activation of akt signaling promotes epithelial-mesenchymal transition and tumor growth in colorectal cancer cells. *Mol. Carcinog.* **2014**, *53* (Suppl. 1), E151–E160. [CrossRef] [PubMed]
18. Chin, Y.R.; Yuan, X.; Balk, S.P.; Toker, A. Pten-deficient tumors depend on akt2 for maintenance and survival. *Cancer Discov.* **2014**, *4*, 942–955. [CrossRef] [PubMed]
19. Ye, Q.; Cai, W.; Zheng, Y.; Evers, B.M.; She, Q.B. Erk and akt signaling cooperate to translationally regulate survivin expression for metastatic progression of colorectal cancer. *Oncogene* **2014**, *33*, 1828–1839. [CrossRef] [PubMed]
20. Cooks, T.; Pateras, I.S.; Tarcic, O.; Solomon, H.; Schetter, A.J.; Wilder, S.; Lozano, G.; Pikarsky, E.; Forshew, T.; Rosenfeld, N.; et al. Mutant p53 prolongs nf-kappab activation and promotes chronic inflammation and inflammation-associated colorectal cancer. *Cancer Cell* **2013**, *23*, 634–646. [CrossRef] [PubMed]
21. Zheng, T.; Wang, J.; Zhao, Y.; Zhang, C.; Lin, M.; Wang, X.; Yu, H.; Liu, L.; Feng, Z.; Hu, W. Spliced mdm2 isoforms promote mutant p53 accumulation and gain-of-function in tumorigenesis. *Nat. Commun.* **2013**, *4*, 2996. [CrossRef] [PubMed]
22. Brighenti, E.; Calabrese, C.; Liguori, G.; Giannone, F.A.; Trere, D.; Montanaro, L.; Derenzini, M. Interleukin 6 downregulates p53 expression and activity by stimulating ribosome biogenesis: A new pathway connecting inflammation to cancer. *Oncogene* **2014**, *33*, 4396–4406. [CrossRef] [PubMed]
23. Aparo, S.; Goel, S. Evolvement of the treatment paradigm for metastatic colon cancer. From chemotherapy to targeted therapy. *Crit. Rev. Oncol. Hematol.* **2012**, *83*, 47–58. [CrossRef] [PubMed]
24. Recondo, G., Jr.; Diaz-Canton, E.; de la Vega, M.; Greco, M.; Recondo, G., Sr.; Valsecchi, M.E. Advances and new perspectives in the treatment of metastatic colon cancer. *World J. Gastrointest. Oncol.* **2014**, *6*, 211–224. [CrossRef] [PubMed]

25. O'Connell, M.J.; Campbell, M.E.; Goldberg, R.M.; Grothey, A.; Seitz, J.F.; Benedetti, J.K.; Andre, T.; Haller, D.G.; Sargent, D.J. Survival following recurrence in stage ii and iii colon cancer: Findings from the accent data set. *J. Clin. Oncol.* **2008**, *26*, 2336–2341. [CrossRef] [PubMed]
26. Heath, J.K. Transcriptional networks and signaling pathways that govern vertebrate intestinal development. *Curr. Top. Dev. Biol.* **2010**, *90*, 159–192. [PubMed]
27. Sander, V.; Davidson, A.J. Kidney injury and regeneration in zebrafish. *Semin. Nephrol.* **2014**, *34*, 437–444. [CrossRef] [PubMed]
28. Wang, Z.; Du, J.; Lam, S.H.; Mathavan, S.; Matsudaira, P.; Gong, Z. Morphological and molecular evidence for functional organization along the rostrocaudal axis of the adult zebrafish intestine. *BMC Genom.* **2010**, *11*, 392. [CrossRef] [PubMed]
29. Wallace, K.N.; Pack, M. Unique and conserved aspects of gut development in zebrafish. *Dev. Biol.* **2003**, *255*, 12–29. [CrossRef]
30. Crosnier, C.; Vargesson, N.; Gschmeissner, S.; Ariza-McNaughton, L.; Morrison, A.; Lewis, J. Delta-notch signalling controls commitment to a secretory fate in the zebrafish intestine. *Development* **2005**, *132*, 1093–1104. [CrossRef] [PubMed]
31. Ng, A.N.; de Jong-Curtain, T.A.; Mawdsley, D.J.; White, S.J.; Shin, J.; Appel, B.; Dong, P.D.; Stainier, D.Y.; Heath, J.K. Formation of the digestive system in zebrafish: Iii. Intestinal epithelium morphogenesis. *Dev. Biol.* **2005**, *286*, 114–135. [CrossRef] [PubMed]
32. Wallace, K.N.; Akhter, S.; Smith, E.M.; Lorent, K.; Pack, M. Intestinal growth and differentiation in zebrafish. *Mech. Dev.* **2005**, *122*, 157–173. [CrossRef] [PubMed]
33. Mudumana, S.P.; Wan, H.; Singh, M.; Korzh, V.; Gong, Z. Expression analyses of zebrafish transferrin, ifabp, and elastaseb mrnas as differentiation markers for the three major endodermal organs: Liver, intestine, and exocrine pancreas. *Dev. Dyn.* **2004**, *230*, 165–173. [CrossRef] [PubMed]
34. Nalbant, P.; Boehmer, C.; Dehmelt, L.; Wehner, F.; Werner, A. Functional characterization of a na$^+$—Phosphate cotransporter (napi-ii) from zebrafish and identification of related transcripts. *J. Physiol.* **1999**, *520*, 79–89. [CrossRef] [PubMed]
35. Stuart, G.W.; McMurray, J.V.; Westerfield, M. Replication, integration and stable germ-line transmission of foreign sequences injected into early zebrafish embryos. *Development* **1988**, *103*, 403–412. [PubMed]
36. Culp, P.; Nusslein-Volhard, C.; Hopkins, N. High-frequency germ-line transmission of plasmid DNA sequences injected into fertilized zebrafish eggs. *Proc. Natl. Acad. Sci. USA* **1991**, *88*, 7953–7957. [CrossRef] [PubMed]
37. Lu, J.W.; Ho, Y.J.; Yang, Y.J.; Liao, H.A.; Ciou, S.C.; Lin, L.I.; Ou, D.L. Zebrafish as a disease model for studying human hepatocellular carcinoma. *World J. Gastroenterol.* **2015**, *21*, 12042–12058. [CrossRef] [PubMed]
38. Park, S.W.; Davison, J.M.; Rhee, J.; Hruban, R.H.; Maitra, A.; Leach, S.D. Oncogenic kras induces progenitor cell expansion and malignant transformation in zebrafish exocrine pancreas. *Gastroenterology* **2008**, *134*, 2080–2090. [CrossRef] [PubMed]
39. Stuart, G.W.; Vielkind, J.R.; McMurray, J.V.; Westerfield, M. Stable lines of transgenic zebrafish exhibit reproducible patterns of transgene expression. *Development* **1990**, *109*, 577–584. [PubMed]
40. Thermes, V.; Grabher, C.; Ristoratore, F.; Bourrat, F.; Choulika, A.; Wittbrodt, J.; Joly, J.S. I-scei meganuclease mediates highly efficient transgenesis in fish. *Mech. Dev.* **2002**, *118*, 91–98. [CrossRef]
41. Ivics, Z.; Hackett, P.B.; Plasterk, R.H.; Izsvak, Z. Molecular reconstruction of sleeping beauty, a tc1-like transposon from fish, and its transposition in human cells. *Cell* **1997**, *91*, 501–510. [CrossRef]
42. Emelyanov, A.; Gao, Y.; Naqvi, N.I.; Parinov, S. Trans-kingdom transposition of the maize dissociation element. *Genetics* **2006**, *174*, 1095–1104. [CrossRef] [PubMed]
43. Kawakami, K.; Shima, A. Identification of the tol2 transposase of the medaka fish oryzias latipes that catalyzes excision of a nonautonomous tol2 element in zebrafish danio rerio. *Gene* **1999**, *240*, 239–244. [CrossRef]
44. Izsvak, Z.; Ivics, Z.; Hackett, P.B. Characterization of a tc1-like transposable element in zebrafish (danio rerio). *Mol. Gen. Genet.* **1995**, *247*, 312–322. [CrossRef] [PubMed]
45. Ivics, Z.; Izsvak, Z.; Minter, A.; Hackett, P.B. Identification of functional domains and evolution of tc1-like transposable elements. *Proc. Natl. Acad. Sci. USA* **1996**, *93*, 5008–5013. [CrossRef] [PubMed]

46. Davidson, A.E.; Balciunas, D.; Mohn, D.; Shaffer, J.; Hermanson, S.; Sivasubbu, S.; Cliff, M.P.; Hackett, P.B.; Ekker, S.C. Efficient gene delivery and gene expression in zebrafish using the sleeping beauty transposon. *Dev. Biol.* **2003**, *263*, 191–202. [CrossRef] [PubMed]
47. Huang, X.; Nguyen, A.T.; Li, Z.; Emelyanov, A.; Parinov, S.; Gong, Z. One step forward: The use of transgenic zebrafish tumor model in drug screens. *Birth Defects Res. C Embryo Today* **2011**, *93*, 173–181. [CrossRef] [PubMed]
48. Deiters, A.; Yoder, J.A. Conditional transgene and gene targeting methodologies in zebrafish. *Zebrafish* **2006**, *3*, 415–429. [CrossRef] [PubMed]
49. Her, G.M.; Chiang, C.C.; Wu, J.L. Zebrafish intestinal fatty acid binding protein (i-fabp) gene promoter drives gut-specific expression in stable transgenic fish. *Genesis* **2004**, *38*, 26–31. [CrossRef] [PubMed]
50. Her, G.M.; Yeh, Y.H.; Wu, J.L. Functional conserved elements mediate intestinal-type fatty acid binding protein (i-fabp) expression in the gut epithelia of zebrafish larvae. *Dev. Dyn.* **2004**, *230*, 734–742. [CrossRef] [PubMed]
51. Neal, J.T.; Peterson, T.S.; Kent, M.L.; Guillemin, K.H. Pylori virulence factor caga increases intestinal cell proliferation by wnt pathway activation in a transgenic zebrafish model. *Dis. Model. Mech.* **2013**, *6*, 802–810. [CrossRef] [PubMed]
52. Le, X.; Langenau, D.M.; Keefe, M.D.; Kutok, J.L.; Neuberg, D.S.; Zon, L.I. Heat shock-inducible cre/lox approaches to induce diverse types of tumors and hyperplasia in transgenic zebrafish. *Proc. Natl. Acad. Sci. USA* **2007**, *104*, 9410–9415. [CrossRef] [PubMed]
53. Dooley, K.; Zon, L.I. Zebrafish: A model system for the study of human disease. *Curr. Opin. Genet. Dev.* **2000**, *10*, 252–256. [CrossRef]
54. Walter, R.B.; Kazianis, S. Xiphophorus interspecies hybrids as genetic models of induced neoplasia. *ILAR J.* **2001**, *42*, 299–321. [CrossRef] [PubMed]
55. Spitsbergen, J.M.; Tsai, H.W.; Reddy, A.; Miller, T.; Arbogast, D.; Hendricks, J.D.; Bailey, G.S. Neoplasia in zebrafish (danio rerio) treated with 7,12-dimethylbenz[a]anthracene by two exposure routes at different developmental stages. *Toxicol. Pathol.* **2000**, *28*, 705–715. [CrossRef] [PubMed]
56. Amatruda, J.F.; Shepard, J.L.; Stern, H.M.; Zon, L.I. Zebrafish as a cancer model system. *Cancer Cell* **2002**, *1*, 229–231. [CrossRef]
57. Stern, H.M.; Zon, L.I. Cancer genetics and drug discovery in the zebrafish. *Nat. Rev. Cancer* **2003**, *3*, 533–539. [CrossRef] [PubMed]
58. Paquette, C.E.; Kent, M.L.; Buchner, C.; Tanguay, R.L.; Guillemin, K.; Mason, T.J.; Peterson, T.S. A retrospective study of the prevalence and classification of intestinal neoplasia in zebrafish (danio rerio). *Zebrafish* **2013**, *10*, 228–236. [CrossRef] [PubMed]
59. Paquette, C.E.; Kent, M.L.; Peterson, T.S.; Wang, R.; Dashwood, R.H.; Lohr, C.V. Immunohistochemical characterization of intestinal neoplasia in zebrafish danio rerio indicates epithelial origin. *Dis. Aquat. Organ.* **2015**, *116*, 191–197. [CrossRef] [PubMed]
60. Groden, J.; Thliveris, A.; Samowitz, W.; Carlson, M.; Gelbert, L.; Albertsen, H.; Joslyn, G.; Stevens, J.; Spirio, L.; Robertson, M.; et al. Identification and characterization of the familial adenomatous polyposis coli gene. *Cell* **1991**, *66*, 589–600. [CrossRef]
61. Kinzler, K.W.; Nilbert, M.C.; Su, L.K.; Vogelstein, B.; Bryan, T.M.; Levy, D.B.; Smith, K.J.; Preisinger, A.C.; Hedge, P.; McKechnie, D.; et al. Identification of fap locus genes from chromosome 5q21. *Science* **1991**, *253*, 661–665. [CrossRef] [PubMed]
62. Kinzler, K.W.; Vogelstein, B. Lessons from hereditary colorectal cancer. *Cell* **1996**, *87*, 159–170. [CrossRef]
63. Su, L.K.; Kinzler, K.W.; Vogelstein, B.; Preisinger, A.C.; Moser, A.R.; Luongo, C.; Gould, K.A.; Dove, W.F. Multiple intestinal neoplasia caused by a mutation in the murine homolog of the apc gene. *Science* **1992**, *256*, 668–670. [CrossRef] [PubMed]
64. Bienz, M.; Clevers, H. Linking colorectal cancer to wnt signaling. *Cell* **2000**, *103*, 311–320. [CrossRef]
65. Hurlstone, A.F.; Haramis, A.P.; Wienholds, E.; Begthel, H.; Korving, J.; Van Eeden, F.; Cuppen, E.; Zivkovic, D.; Plasterk, R.H.; Clevers, H. The wnt/beta-catenin pathway regulates cardiac valve formation. *Nature* **2003**, *425*, 633–637. [CrossRef] [PubMed]
66. Haramis, A.P.; Hurlstone, A.; van der Velden, Y.; Begthel, H.; van den Born, M.; Offerhaus, G.J.; Clevers, H.C. Adenomatous polyposis coli-deficient zebrafish are susceptible to digestive tract neoplasia. *EMBO Rep.* **2006**, *7*, 444–449. [CrossRef] [PubMed]

67. Sandoval, I.T.; Delacruz, R.G.; Miller, B.N.; Hill, S.; Olson, K.A.; Gabriel, A.E.; Boyd, K.; Satterfield, C.; Remmen, H.V.; Rutter, J.; et al. A metabolic switch controls intestinal differentiation downstream of adenomatous polyposis coli (apc). *Elife* **2017**, *6*. [CrossRef] [PubMed]
68. Burger, A.; Vasilyev, A.; Tomar, R.; Selig, M.K.; Nielsen, G.P.; Peterson, R.T.; Drummond, I.A.; Haber, D.A. A zebrafish model of chordoma initiated by notochord-driven expression of hrasv12. *Dis. Model. Mech.* **2014**, *7*, 907–913. [CrossRef] [PubMed]
69. Santoriello, C.; Gennaro, E.; Anelli, V.; Distel, M.; Kelly, A.; Koster, R.W.; Hurlstone, A.; Mione, M. Kita driven expression of oncogenic hras leads to early onset and highly penetrant melanoma in zebrafish. *PLoS ONE* **2010**, *5*, e15170. [CrossRef] [PubMed]
70. Storer, N.Y.; White, R.M.; Uong, A.; Price, E.; Nielsen, G.P.; Langenau, D.M.; Zon, L.I. Zebrafish rhabdomyosarcoma reflects the developmental stage of oncogene expression during myogenesis. *Development* **2013**, *140*, 3040–3050. [CrossRef] [PubMed]
71. Dovey, M.; White, R.M.; Zon, L.I. Oncogenic nras cooperates with p53 loss to generate melanoma in zebrafish. *Zebrafish* **2009**, *6*, 397–404. [CrossRef] [PubMed]
72. Ju, B.; Chen, W.; Orr, B.A.; Spitsbergen, J.M.; Jia, S.; Eden, C.J.; Henson, H.E.; Taylor, M.R. Oncogenic kras promotes malignant brain tumors in zebrafish. *Mol. Cancer* **2015**, *14*, 18. [CrossRef] [PubMed]
73. Shive, H.R.; West, R.R.; Embree, L.J.; Sexton, J.M.; Hickstein, D.D. Expression of krasg12v in zebrafish gills induces hyperplasia and cxcl8-associated inflammation. *Zebrafish* **2015**, *12*, 221–229. [CrossRef] [PubMed]
74. Nguyen, A.T.; Emelyanov, A.; Koh, C.H.; Spitsbergen, J.M.; Lam, S.H.; Mathavan, S.; Parinov, S.; Gong, Z. A high level of liver-specific expression of oncogenic kras(v12) drives robust liver tumorigenesis in transgenic zebrafish. *Dis. Model. Mech.* **2011**, *4*, 801–813. [CrossRef] [PubMed]
75. Provost, E.; Bailey, J.M.; Aldrugh, S.; Liu, S.; Iacobuzio-Donahue, C.; Leach, S.D. The tumor suppressor rpl36 restrains kras(g12v)-induced pancreatic cancer. *Zebrafish* **2014**, *11*, 551–559. [CrossRef] [PubMed]
76. Bos, J.L.; Fearon, E.R.; Hamilton, S.R.; Verlaan-de Vries, M.; van Boom, J.H.; van der Eb, A.J.; Vogelstein, B. Prevalence of ras gene mutations in human colorectal cancers. *Nature* **1987**, *327*, 293–297. [CrossRef] [PubMed]
77. Berghmans, S.; Murphey, R.D.; Wienholds, E.; Neuberg, D.; Kutok, J.L.; Fletcher, C.D.; Morris, J.P.; Liu, T.X.; Schulte-Merker, S.; Kanki, J.P.; et al. Tp53 mutant zebrafish develop malignant peripheral nerve sheath tumors. *Proc. Natl. Acad. Sci. USA* **2005**, *102*, 407–412. [CrossRef] [PubMed]
78. Lu, J.W.; Yang, W.Y.; Tsai, S.M.; Lin, Y.M.; Chang, P.H.; Chen, J.R.; Wang, H.D.; Wu, J.L.; Jin, S.L.; Yuh, C.H. Liver-specific expressions of hbx and src in the p53 mutant trigger hepatocarcinogenesis in zebrafish. *PLoS ONE* **2013**, *8*. [CrossRef] [PubMed]
79. Faro, A.; Boj, S.F.; Clevers, H. Fishing for intestinal cancer models: Unraveling gastrointestinal homeostasis and tumorigenesis in zebrafish. *Zebrafish* **2009**, *6*, 361–376. [CrossRef] [PubMed]
80. Barton, C.M.; Staddon, S.L.; Hughes, C.M.; Hall, P.A.; O'Sullivan, C.; Kloppel, G.; Theis, B.; Russell, R.C.; Neoptolemos, J.; Williamson, R.C.; et al. Abnormalities of the p53 tumour suppressor gene in human pancreatic cancer. *Br. J. Cancer* **1991**, *64*, 1076–1082. [CrossRef] [PubMed]
81. Hsu, I.C.; Metcalf, R.A.; Sun, T.; Welsh, J.A.; Wang, N.J.; Harris, C.C. Mutational hotspot in the p53 gene in human hepatocellular carcinomas. *Nature* **1991**, *350*, 427–428. [CrossRef] [PubMed]
82. Baker, S.J.; Fearon, E.R.; Nigro, J.M.; Hamilton, S.R.; Preisinger, A.C.; Jessup, J.M.; vanTuinen, P.; Ledbetter, D.H.; Barker, D.F.; Nakamura, Y.; et al. Chromosome 17 deletions and p53 gene mutations in colorectal carcinomas. *Science* **1989**, *244*, 217–221. [CrossRef] [PubMed]
83. Zon, L.I.; Peterson, R.T. In vivo drug discovery in the zebrafish. *Nat. Rev. Drug Discov.* **2005**, *4*, 35–44. [CrossRef] [PubMed]
84. Tamplin, O.J.; White, R.M.; Jing, L.; Kaufman, C.K.; Lacadie, S.A.; Li, P.; Taylor, A.M.; Zon, L.I. Small molecule screening in zebrafish: Swimming in potential drug therapies. *Wiley Interdiscip. Rev. Dev. Biol.* **2012**, *1*, 459–468. [CrossRef] [PubMed]
85. Peterson, R.T.; Macrae, C.A. Systematic approaches to toxicology in the zebrafish. *Annu. Rev. Pharmacol. Toxicol.* **2012**, *52*, 433–453. [CrossRef] [PubMed]
86. Cariati, M.; Marlow, R.; Dontu, G. Xenotransplantation of breast cancers. *Methods Mol. Biol.* **2011**, *731*, 471–482. [PubMed]

87. White, R.M.; Sessa, A.; Burke, C.; Bowman, T.; LeBlanc, J.; Ceol, C.; Bourque, C.; Dovey, M.; Goessling, W.; Burns, C.E.; et al. Transparent adult zebrafish as a tool for in vivo transplantation analysis. *Cell Stem Cell* **2008**, *2*, 183–189. [CrossRef] [PubMed]
88. Lawson, N.D.; Weinstein, B.M. In vivo imaging of embryonic vascular development using transgenic zebrafish. *Dev. Biol.* **2002**, *248*, 307–318. [CrossRef] [PubMed]
89. Konantz, M.; Balci, T.B.; Hartwig, U.F.; Dellaire, G.; Andre, M.C.; Berman, J.N.; Lengerke, C. Zebrafish xenografts as a tool for in vivo studies on human cancer. *Ann. N. Y. Acad. Sci.* **2012**, *1266*, 124–137. [CrossRef] [PubMed]
90. Tang, Q.; Abdelfattah, N.S.; Blackburn, J.S.; Moore, J.C.; Martinez, S.A.; Moore, F.E.; Lobbardi, R.; Tenente, I.M.; Ignatius, M.S.; Berman, J.N.; et al. Optimized cell transplantation using adult rag2 mutant zebrafish. *Nat. Methods* **2014**, *11*, 821–824. [CrossRef] [PubMed]
91. Tang, Q.; Moore, J.C.; Ignatius, M.S.; Tenente, I.M.; Hayes, M.N.; Garcia, E.G.; Torres Yordan, N.; Bourque, C.; He, S.; Blackburn, J.S.; et al. Imaging tumour cell heterogeneity following cell transplantation into optically clear immune-deficient zebrafish. *Nat. Commun.* **2016**, *7*, 10358. [CrossRef] [PubMed]
92. Veinotte, C.J.; Dellaire, G.; Berman, J.N. Hooking the big one: The potential of zebrafish xenotransplantation to reform cancer drug screening in the genomic era. *Dis. Model. Mech.* **2014**, *7*, 745–754. [CrossRef] [PubMed]
93. Haldi, M.; Ton, C.; Seng, W.L.; McGrath, P. Human melanoma cells transplanted into zebrafish proliferate, migrate, produce melanin, form masses and stimulate angiogenesis in zebrafish. *Angiogenesis* **2006**, *9*, 139–151. [CrossRef] [PubMed]
94. Gnosa, S.; Capodanno, A.; Murthy, R.V.; Jensen, L.D.; Sun, X.F. Aeg-1 knockdown in colon cancer cell lines inhibits radiation-enhanced migration and invasion in vitro and in a novel in vivo zebrafish model. *Oncotarget* **2016**, *7*, 81634–81644. [CrossRef] [PubMed]
95. Roel, M.; Rubiolo, J.A.; Guerra-Varela, J.; Silva, S.B.; Thomas, O.P.; Cabezas-Sainz, P.; Sanchez, L.; Lopez, R.; Botana, L.M. Marine guanidine alkaloids crambescidins inhibit tumor growth and activate intrinsic apoptotic signaling inducing tumor regression in a colorectal carcinoma zebrafish xenograft model. *Oncotarget* **2016**, *7*, 83071–83087. [CrossRef] [PubMed]
96. Fior, R.; Povoa, V.; Mendes, R.V.; Carvalho, T.; Gomes, A.; Figueiredo, N.; Ferreira, M.G. Single-cell functional and chemosensitive profiling of combinatorial colorectal therapy in zebrafish xenografts. *Proc. Natl. Acad. Sci. USA* **2017**. [CrossRef] [PubMed]
97. Dang, M.; Henderson, R.E.; Garraway, L.A.; Zon, L.I. Long-term drug administration in the adult zebrafish using oral gavage for cancer preclinical studies. *Dis. Model. Mech.* **2016**, *9*, 811–820. [CrossRef] [PubMed]
98. Brugman, S. The zebrafish as a model to study intestinal inflammation. *Dev. Comp. Immunol.* **2016**, *64*, 82–92. [CrossRef] [PubMed]
99. Brugman, S.; Liu, K.Y.; Lindenbergh-Kortleve, D.; Samsom, J.N.; Furuta, G.T.; Renshaw, S.A.; Willemsen, R.; Nieuwenhuis, E.E. Oxazolone-induced enterocolitis in zebrafish depends on the composition of the intestinal microbiota. *Gastroenterology* **2009**, *137*. [CrossRef] [PubMed]
100. Fleming, A.; Jankowski, J.; Goldsmith, P. In vivo analysis of gut function and disease changes in a zebrafish larvae model of inflammatory bowel disease: A feasibility study. *Inflamm. Bowel Dis.* **2010**, *16*, 1162–1172. [CrossRef] [PubMed]
101. Oehlers, S.H.; Flores, M.V.; Okuda, K.S.; Hall, C.J.; Crosier, K.E.; Crosier, P.S. A chemical enterocolitis model in zebrafish larvae that is dependent on microbiota and responsive to pharmacological agents. *Dev. Dyn.* **2011**, *240*, 288–298. [CrossRef] [PubMed]
102. Geiger, B.M.; Gras-Miralles, B.; Ziogas, D.C.; Karagiannis, A.K.; Zhen, A.; Fraenkel, P.; Kokkotou, E. Intestinal upregulation of melanin-concentrating hormone in tnbs-induced enterocolitis in adult zebrafish. *PLoS ONE* **2013**, *8*, e83194. [CrossRef] [PubMed]
103. He, Q.; Wang, L.; Wang, F.; Wang, C.; Tang, C.; Li, Q.; Li, J.; Zhao, Q. Microbial fingerprinting detects intestinal microbiota dysbiosis in zebrafish models with chemically-induced enterocolitis. *BMC Microbiol.* **2013**, *13*, 289. [CrossRef] [PubMed]
104. He, Q.; Wang, L.; Wang, F.; Li, Q. Role of gut microbiota in a zebrafish model with chemically induced enterocolitis involving toll-like receptor signaling pathways. *Zebrafish* **2014**, *11*, 255–264. [CrossRef] [PubMed]
105. Wirtz, S.; Neufert, C.; Weigmann, B.; Neurath, M.F. Chemically induced mouse models of intestinal inflammation. *Nat. Protoc.* **2007**, *2*, 541–546. [CrossRef] [PubMed]

106. Oehlers, S.H.; Flores, M.V.; Hall, C.J.; Crosier, K.E.; Crosier, P.S. Retinoic acid suppresses intestinal mucus production and exacerbates experimental enterocolitis. *Dis. Model. Mech.* **2012**, *5*, 457–467. [CrossRef] [PubMed]
107. Oehlers, S.H.; Flores, M.V.; Hall, C.J.; Okuda, K.S.; Sison, J.O.; Crosier, K.E.; Crosier, P.S. Chemically induced intestinal damage models in zebrafish larvae. *Zebrafish* **2013**, *10*, 184–193. [CrossRef] [PubMed]
108. Oehlers, S.H.; Flores, M.V.; Hall, C.J.; Wang, L.; Ko, D.C.; Crosier, K.E.; Crosier, P.S. A whole animal chemical screen approach to identify modifiers of intestinal neutrophilic inflammation. *FEBS J.* **2017**, *284*, 402–413. [CrossRef] [PubMed]
109. Okuda, K.S.; Misa, J.P.; Oehlers, S.H.; Hall, C.J.; Ellett, F.; Alasmari, S.; Lieschke, G.J.; Crosier, K.E.; Crosier, P.S.; Astin, J.W. A zebrafish model of inflammatory lymphangiogenesis. *Biol. Open* **2015**, *4*, 1270–1280. [CrossRef] [PubMed]

© 2017 by the authors. Licensee MDPI, Basel, Switzerland. This article is an open access article distributed under the terms and conditions of the Creative Commons Attribution (CC BY) license (http://creativecommons.org/licenses/by/4.0/).

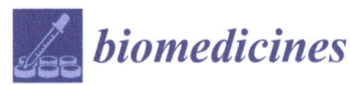

Conference Report

Frontiers in Gastrointestinal Oncology: Advances in Multi-Disciplinary Patient Care

Nelson S. Yee [1,*], Eugene J. Lengerich [2], Kathryn H. Schmitz [2], Jennifer L. Maranki [3], Niraj J. Gusani [4], Leila Tchelebi [5], Heath B. Mackley [6], Karen L. Krok [3], Maria J. Baker [7], Claire de Boer [8] and Julian D. Yee [9]

[1] Division of Hematology-Oncology, Department of Medicine, Penn State Health Milton S. Hershey Medical Center, Experimental Therapeutics Program, Penn State Cancer Institute, The Pennsylvania State University College of Medicine, Hershey, PA 17033, USA

[2] Population Sciences Program, Penn State Cancer Institute, Department of Public Health Sciences, The Pennsylvania State University College of Medicine, Hershey, PA 17033, USA; elengeri@phs.psu.edu (E.J.L.); kschmitz@phs.psu.edu (K.H.S.)

[3] Division of Gastroenterology and Hepatology, Department of Medicine, Penn State Health Milton S. Hershey Medical Center, The Pennsylvania State University College of Medicine, Hershey, PA 17033, USA; jmaranki@pennstatehealth.psu.edu (J.L.M.); kkrok@pennstatehealth.psu.edu (K.L.K.)

[4] Division of General Surgery and Surgical Oncology, Department of Surgery, Penn State Health Milton S. Hershey Medical Center, The Pennsylvania State University College of Medicine, Hershey, PA 17033, USA; ngusani@pennstatehealth.psu.edu

[5] Department of Radiology, Penn State Health Milton S. Hershey Medical Center, The Pennsylvania State University College of Medicine, Hershey, PA 17033, USA; ltchelebi@pennstatehealth.psu.edu

[6] Department of Radiology, Medicine, and Pediatrics, Penn State Health Milton S. Hershey Medical Center, The Pennsylvania State University College of Medicine, Hershey, PA 17033, USA; hmackley@pennstatehealth.psu.edu

[7] Department of Medicine, Penn State Health Milton S. Hershey Medical Center, Penn State Cancer Institute, The Pennsylvania State University College of Medicine, Hershey, PA 17033, USA; mbaker@pennstatehealth.psu.edu

[8] Center Stage Arts in Health, Penn State Health Milton S. Hershey Medical Center, Department of Humanities, The Pennsylvania State University College of Medicine, Hershey, PA 17033, USA; cdeboer@pennstatehealth.psu.edu

[9] College of Liberal Arts, The Pennsylvania State University, State College, PA 16801, USA; jdy133@psu.edu

* Correspondence: nyee@pennstatehealth.psu.edu; Tel.: +1-717-531-0003

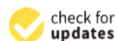

Received: 25 April 2018; Accepted: 11 May 2018; Published: 1 June 2018

Abstract: Cancers of the digestive system remain highly lethal; therefore, the care of patients with malignant diseases of the digestive tract requires the expertise of providers from multiple health disciplines. Progress has been made to advance the understanding of epidemiology and genetics, diagnostic and screening evaluation, treatment modalities, and supportive care for patients with gastrointestinal cancers. At the Multi-Disciplinary Patient Care in Gastrointestinal Oncology conference at the Hershey Country Club in Hershey, Pennsylvania on 29 September 2017, the faculty members of the Penn State Health Milton S. Hershey Medical Center presented a variety of topics that focused on this oncological specialty. In this continuing medical education-certified conference, updates on the population sciences including health disparities and resistance training were presented. Progress made in various diagnostic evaluation and screening procedures was outlined. New developments in therapeutic modalities in surgical, radiation, and medical oncology were discussed. Cancer genetic testing and counseling and the supportive roles of music and arts in health and cancer were demonstrated. In summary, this disease-focused medical conference highlighted the new frontiers in gastrointestinal oncology, and showcase the multi-disciplinary care provided at the Penn State Cancer Institute.

Keywords: gastrointestinal oncology; pancreatic carcinoma; hepatocellular carcinoma; biliary tract carcinoma; gastric carcinoma; colorectal carcinoma; stereotactic body radiation therapy; liver transplant; targeted therapy; psychosocial support

1. Introduction

The Multi-Disciplinary Patient Care in Gastrointestinal Oncology conference was held on September 29, 2017 at the Hershey Country Club in Hershey, Pennsylvania, U.S. This conference's target audience included primary care physicians, gastroenterologists, medical oncologists, surgical oncologists, radiation oncologists, nurse practitioners, physician assistants, and nurses. The faculty members of the Penn State Cancer Institute and Penn State Health Milton S. Hershey Medical Center presented a variety of topics that focused on the frontiers in caring for patients with various gastrointestinal cancers. The purpose of this conference was to provide updates on new developments and emerging trends in caring for patients with various malignant diseases of the digestive system. The objectives of this program were to (1) recognize the risk factors and genetic mutations of cancers in the digestive system for prevention and early detection, (2) discuss diagnostic modalities and multi-disciplinary treatment of patients with digestive organ cancers, and (3) explore supportive interventions for patients with malignant diseases of the digestive system.

2. Population Sciences in Cancers of the Digestive System

2.1. Epidemiology of Cancers in the Digestive System

In 2018, the estimated number of new cases of cancer of the digestive system was the highest among all cancer sites in the United States [1]. Among the cancers of the digestive organs, colon cancer was the most prevalent. From 2007 to 2013, the five-year relative survival rates by all tumor stages at diagnosis for pancreatic cancer was the lowest among all cancer sites. The next lowest five-year relative survival rate was attributed to cancers in the liver, intrahepatic bile duct, esophagus, stomach, and lung. Lengerich, V.M.D., M.S., Associate Director of Health Disparities and Engagement, provided an overview of the epidemiology of digestive system cancer in the United States.

2.1.1. Health Disparities in Appalachia

Lengerich presented public health data on various cancers of the digestive system in Appalachia, in which certain counties of central Pennsylvania are located. Compared with the general population in the United States, the Appalachian residents tend to have less contact with physicians, lower levels of preventive care, and less health insurance coverage for non-elderly people. Lengerich reported epidemiological data on health disparities in the Appalachian communities. In particular, the incidence and mortality rates of colon cancer and rectal cancer in the Appalachia were greater than of the U.S. population [2–4]. These data suggest relatively little use of screening interventions for colorectal cancer in rural Appalachia. This may be related to the low level of awareness of regular screening for colorectal cancer among the general population in Appalachia. Other contributing factors may include low availability of screening centers, long distances to health care facilities, high rates of unemployment and poverty, and inability to afford travel to screening facilities [5].

Various strategies attempted to reduce health disparities in cancer in the Appalachian communities were presented. An active area of investigation is the use of screening interventions for prevention and early detection of colorectal cancer, including a national, multimedia campaign called Screen for Life, which aims to educate people aged 50 or older about the importance of regular screening tests for colorectal cancer [6]. The effectiveness and methods for dissemination of Screen for Life materials in rural Appalachia were examined by a network of investigators working in medically under-served regions. These reports indicated a substantial potential for the Screen for Life materials and campaign, though limited at the local level, in rural Appalachia [7–9]. However, these observations led to the hypothesis that the number of individuals in rural Appalachia seeking colorectal cancer screening could be increased by disseminating Screen for Life materials at state, regional, and community levels through health care practices and organizations [5]. Additionally, primary care physicians may help engage patients in screening for colorectal cancer by encouraging the use of fecal occult blood testing when colonoscopy is not possible and systems-based reminders that provide electronic resources that are not visit-dependent [10].

Limited access to healthcare services is challenging for those who live in rural communities, and strategies to involve Appalachian populations as participants in research and overcome that disparity were discussed. These include community-based participatory research in rural communities with the goals of increasing awareness of community assets and enhancing treatment-related care and psychosocial care [11]. Through collaboration with community physicians, these initiatives may help improve patients' access to tertiary care and clinical studies at academic cancer centers, and facilitate education of patients and the general population. Other strategies include raising funding support for research on health disparities, increasing availability of screening interventions for early detection of cancer, and development of community plans to enhance survivorship by improving the long-term health and well-being of cancer survivors in rural locations.

2.1.2. Key Points and Recommendations

Despite advances in screening, early detection, diagnosis, and treatment of various malignant diseases, digestive system cancer incidence and mortality rates remain among the highest. The disparity in cancer care for people in Appalachia is a longstanding problem, which is partly a socioeconomic issue. Malignant diseases in the digestive organs besides colorectal cancer are largely unexplored in the Appalachian population. Special emphasis of research efforts, judicial allocation of funding support for research, and prudent distribution of resources will hopefully make a meaningful impact on health by lessening the burden of cancers of the digestive system.

2.2. Exercise in Cancer Patients and Survivors

Growing evidence suggests the roles of exercise in improving treatment response and reducing treatment-related toxicities in cancer patients, as well as preventing disease recurrence in cancer survivors. The report of a recent survey demonstrates that oncologists have little knowledge regarding exercise counseling, and they are not routinely discussing exercise with their patients [12]. Schmitz, Associate Director of Population Sciences, described the benefits of exercise in patients diagnosed with various malignant diseases with an emphasis on colon cancer.

2.2.1. Clinical Studies of Exercise in Cancer Patients and Survivors

Schmitz provided the existing and emerging evidence for the safety and efficacy of exercise training during and following systemic treatment of cancer. A large number of studies demonstrated that exercise is safe in patients with breast cancer, including those who had exercise training during chemotherapy or radiation therapy, as well as those who had exercise training following completion of chemotherapy or radiation therapy [13]. The adverse events reported in those studies, such as plantar fasciitis and other musculoskeletal injuries, were mild and rare. Notably, for women who have had surgical resection of their axillary lymph nodes and/or radiation therapy to the axilla, aerobic, and/or resistance training did not cause or worsen lymphedema. Additionally, studies of exercise interventions in survivors of prostate cancer showed that exercise is safe in this population [13]. Importantly, a significant association between high levels of exercise and low risks of cancer-specific mortality and cancer recurrence were observed in patients with breast cancer or prostate cancer as well as other malignant diseases [14].

Colon cancer is the third most common cancer, which is associated with a fairly good prognosis. Yet, few clinical studies have evaluated the potential benefits of exercise for reducing chemotherapy-related toxicities and improving treatment efficacy. None of the trials addressed safety or adverse events except one report, which indicated that there was no significant abnormality in electrocardiograms during maximal aerobic fitness testing [15]. However, one study reported a statistically significant association between high exercise levels and a low risk of recurrence and all-cause mortality of colorectal cancer [16]. A clinical study to investigate the effects of aerobic exercise on tumor recurrence and as the molecular and cellular pathways associated with physical activity among patients with stage II and III colon cancer was completed (www.clinicaltrials.govNCT02250053). Analysis of the results of this important study pends.

2.2.2. Clinical Studies of Exercise in Cancer Patients at Penn State Cancer Institute

Currently, a clinical study is ongoing at the Penn State Cancer Institute and regional facilities to further investigate the safety and efficacy of resistance training in patients receiving chemotherapy for treatment of colorectal cancer (www.clinicaltrials.govNCT03291951). This is a randomized, open-label, controlled trial of resistance training intervention in patients with newly-diagnosed stage II or III colon cancer receiving chemotherapy. The primary goal of this study is to examine the effects of resistance training on chemotherapy-related outcomes, including dose delays, dose reductions, early stoppage, and grade 3 and 4 toxicities. This clinical trial consists of two aspects: an in-person and telephone-based intervention to promote home-based resistance training, and a wait-list, control group. In the resistance training group, the subjects will work with an exercise professional on the same day as a chemotherapy infusion session, and the subjects will complete a series of exercises at home twice weekly throughout the intervention. For the control group, the subjects will be told to continue whatever exercise program they have been undertaking up to enrolling in the study, but to not increase exercise or begin weight-lifting over the period of study participation.

Another study is currently open for enrollment at Penn State Cancer Institute for patients who receive chemotherapy for treatment of any solid tumor including cancers in the digestive system (www.clinicaltrials.govNCT03461471). The primary objective of this study is to assess the safety, feasibility, and acceptability of an exercise program within the course of chemotherapy. This is an open-label, single group study for patients diagnosed with a solid tumor malignancy at stages I to IV. Feasibility will be accomplished if one-third of the patients receiving chemotherapy actually perform the prescribed exercise (one exercise session per week for four weeks). Other outcome measures include changes in pain, physical function, nausea, emesis, and arthralgia as well as alterations of chemotherapy (dose delays and changes).

2.2.3. Key Points and Recommendations

Numerous clinical studies have demonstrated the benefits of exercise training in terms of physical functions and quality of life for patients with cancer. Significant association has been reported between high exercise levels and reduced risks of cancer recurrence and cancer-specific mortality. The evidence to date supports the recommendation of regular exercise for people with cancer as well as those who have completed cancer treatment. Ongoing studies are being designed and conducted to test the hypothesis that exercise is safe and improves treatment response, quality of life, and survival in patients, and reduces toxicities for various malignant diseases including those in the digestive system.

3. Diagnostic Evaluation of Esophageal, Pancreatic, Biliary Tract, and Hepatocellular Carcinoma

Technological advances have been made in the diagnostic evaluation of cancers of the digestive system. Improved accuracy of diagnosis and staging of malignant diseases in the upper gastrointestinal organs has been enabled by endoscopy along with various imaging modalities. Surveillance of hepatocellular carcinoma (HCC) and liver transplantation have become increasingly important for early detection and treatment of this disease.

3.1. Diagnostic Evaluation and Staging for Cancers of Esophagus, Pancreas, and Biliary System

Endoscopy plays a central role in the diagnosis of cancer in both the upper and lower gastrointestinal tracts. Maranki, Medical Director of Endoscopy, discussed the diagnostic evaluation and staging for cancers of the esophagus, pancreas, and biliary system. In particular, endoscopic ultrasonography (EUS) is an important diagnostic modality for patients with esophageal and pancreatic carcinoma by evaluating the extent of tumor invasion and any involvement of the regional lymph nodes, and by enabling tumor biopsy through fine needle aspiration. The use of a new technique via SpyGlass^{TM} cholangioscopy has improved the diagnostic yield of biliary tract carcinoma through high-resolution direct visualization with biopsy of the bile ducts.

3.1.1. Diagnosis and Staging of Esophageal Cancer

Esophageal carcinoma, either squamous cell carcinoma or adenocarcinoma, is typically diagnosed by esophagogastroduodenoscopy with tissue biopsy. Computed tomography (CT) of the chest and abdomen and positron emission tomography (PET) in combination with CT scans are indicated to evaluate any metastatic disease. EUS plays an important role in staging the disease based on depth of invasion of the esophageal wall and involvement of any regional lymph nodes if there is no evidence of metastatic disease. Endoscopic mucosal resection of early stage tumors (T1a, T1b) can be therapeutic and curative.

3.1.2. Diagnosis and Staging of Pancreatic Cancer

Imaging studies for diagnosis of pancreatic carcinoma include dual-phase helical CT scans, transabdominal ultrasonography (US), EUS-guided fine needle aspiration (FNA), endoscopic retrograde cholangiopancreatography (ERCP), magnetic resonance cholangiopancreatography (MRCP), and PET scans. The accuracy of these imaging studies for diagnosis of pancreatic carcinoma (PC) was compared [17]. In particular, the sensitivity and specificity of EUS-guided FNA are 92% and 100%, respectively; those of ERCP are 70% and 94%, respectively. Moreover, the performance of EUS for pancreatic adenocarcinoma was compared to CT and MRI scans with regard to nodal staging, vascular invasion, and resectability.

As shown in Table 1, EUS appears less sensitive but more specific than CT scans for staging of lymph node involvement, detecting vascular invasion, and determining resectability of tumors. For nodal staging, EUS is more sensitive and less specific than MRI scans; for detecting vascular invasion, EUS is less sensitive and more specific than MRI scans. Notably, the performance of EUS is dependent on the operator, and EUS should be considered complementary to either CT or MRI scans for the staging of pancreatic adenocarcinoma.

Table 1. Comparison of endoscopic ultrasonography (EUS) and either computed tomography (CT) or magnetic resonance imaging (MRI) scans for pancreatic adenocarcinoma.

	EUS vs. CT		EUS vs. MRI	
	Sensitivity	Specificity	Sensitivity	Specificity
Nodal staging	24% vs. 58%	88% vs. 85%	36% vs. 15%	87% vs. 97%
Vascular invasion	58% vs. 86%	95% vs. 93%	42% vs. 59%	97% vs. 84%
Resectability	87% vs. 90%	89% vs. 69%	NA	NA

NA: not available. This table is modified from reference [17].

3.1.3. Diagnosis and Staging of Cholangiocarcinoma

If a lesion in the biliary tract is identified on imaging studies, such as US, CT, MRI, or MRCP, EUS-guided FNA or ERCP with biliary brushings are indicated for establishing the diagnosis. CT-guided biopsy of the tissue is considered if necessary. All lesions suspicious of cholangiocarcinoma should be further evaluated with MRI or MRCP. However, diagnosis of cholangiocarcinoma by tissue biopsy can be challenging, and tissue may be obtained via several techniques. Of note, EUS-guided FNA is not advisable for hilar and intrahepatic lesions if the tumor is considered resectable. This is due to concerns of tumor seeding the needle tract. A new technique via SpyGlass™ cholangioscopy has been shown to improve diagnostic yield for cholangiocarcinoma.

SpyGlass™ cholangioscopy uses fiberoptic technology for high-resolution direct visualization of the bile ducts. Since the launch of the Spyglass™ Direct Visualization System, the sensitivity for detecting cholangiocarcinoma has been improved [18,19]. ERCP with Spyglass™ Direct Visualization System enables the direct visualization of the bile ducts, thus facilitating tissue biopsy and therapeutic intervention. With the implementation of a new digital system, the SpyGlass™ cholangioscopy provides a sensitivity and specificity of 90% and 95.8%, respectively, for diagnosis of malignant disease in the bile ducts [20].

3.1.4. Key Points and Recommendations

For diagnostic and staging evaluation of esophageal carcinoma, PET and CT scans and EUS are the standard of care. Besides CT scans, the role of EUS is particularly valuable for evaluating patients with localized pancreatic carcinoma that appears resectable on the initial imaging study. A new technique using ERCP with Spyglass™ Direct Visualization System has improved the sensitivity and specificity for the diagnosis of cholangiocarcinoma.

3.2. Hepatocellular Carcinoma

HCC is a major cause of cancer-related mortality worldwide. The incidence, disease burden, and mortality of HCC have been rising in the United States. Krok, Medical Director of Liver Transplantation, provided a hepatologist's perspective on HCC. Krok's presentation focused on the risk factors of HCC, screening modalities of HCC, and liver transplant for treatment of selected patients.

3.2.1. Risk Factors for HCC

An update on the risk factors for HCC in the United States was provided. For persons above 65 years old, diabetes and obesity represent the major risk factors for HCC, and they are followed by hepatitis C virus (HCV), alcoholism, smoking, hepatitis B virus (HBV), and rare genetic disorders [21]. In obese men, liver cancer is associated with the highest relative risk of death among all types of cancer [22]. For patients with hepatitis C viral (HCV) infection, HCC is generally developed in the setting of advanced hepatic cirrhosis [23]. HBV DNA is considered a key risk for the development of HCC, and the baseline serum level of HBV DNA is correlated with the incidence of HCC over time.

3.2.2. Screening of HCC

Surveillance of HCC has been shown to improve outcomes by early tumor detection, reduction of total mortality, and improved survival [24]. Surveillance guidelines for high-risk patients by ultrasonography (US), with or without serum alpha-fetoprotein (AFP) or prothrombin induced by vitamin K absence-II (PIVKA-II), have been recommended by various cancer organizations in the United States, Europe, Japan, and other Asian-Pacific countries. These screening tests are indicated at various time intervals, from every 3 months or 6 months to 12 months. Besides the U.S., other imaging modalities for surveillance of HCC, including CT and MRI scans, were described. Their advantages and disadvantages were compared, with MRI scans showing the highest sensitivity of detecting HCC [25]. Special emphasis was placed on contrast-enhanced ultrasonography (CEUS), which demonstrates higher sensitivity, negative predictive value, and overall accuracy that standard US [26]. Furthermore, a meta-analysis indicated that CEUS and gadoxetate-enhanced MRI scans show the highest sensitivity and positive predictive value for detecting HCC [27].

3.2.3. Liver Transplantation for Treatment of HCC

Liver transplant is a viable treatment option for many patients with HCC. Liver transplant can be a curative intervention of choice for HCC, especially for patients with cirrhosis that cannot easily have a surgical resection. The five-year survival rate is about 75%, which is comparable to patients without HCC who undergo liver transplant. Both cadaverous and living donor liver transplant can be offered. In the United States, there have been more than 1,000 liver transplants per year for patients with HCC since 2008. A total of 15,045 liver transplants have been performed for patients with HCC. Currently, there are 14,104 patients waiting for a liver transplant with a diagnosis of HCC. Currently, the Milan criteria are the most commonly used for evaluating candidates for liver transplant [28]. Once a patient is considered to be within the Milan criteria and meets all criteria for listing for liver transplant, they will be listed for transplant. Various modalities, including transcatheter arterial chemoembolization (TACE), radiofrequency ablation, and Yttrium-90, may be used for bridge treatment prior to liver transplantation. For HCC with vascular invasion, tumor recurrence following liver transplant progressively increases with time [29].

3.2.4. Key Points and Recommendations

The major risk factors for HCC in the United States include obesity, hepatitis C viral infection, and alcoholism. Interventions and research efforts should be focused on developing strategies, especially behavioral modification for preventing HCC. Imaging studies using US, CT, and MRI scans along with serum tumor markers, including AFP and PIVKA-II, facilitate early detection of HCC. For individuals at risk of developing HCC, active surveillance is indicated with the hope of detecting small tumors at a localized stage, so that they can be cured by liver transplantation or surgical resection. Whereas liver transplantation is a curative intervention for both HCC and the underlying hepatic cirrhosis, organ donation remains a limiting factor and requires continued public support.

4. Therapeutic Interventions by Surgical Resection, Radiation Therapy, and Systemic Treatment

A number of advances have been made in the localized, systemic, and targeted treatment of cancers of the digestive organs. New developments in surgical management as well as pre-operative and post-operative interventions have been applied for improved clinical outcomes. Refinement of criteria for radiation therapy continues, and new technologies for precise radiotherapy while minimizing toxicity has been investigated. Constant new developments have occurred in systemic therapies for improving the treatment response for patients with advanced or metastatic diseases.

4.1. Surgical Gastrointestinal Oncology

Surgical interventions have been playing a crucial role in the treatment of various malignant diseases in the digestive system. Gusani, Group Leader of Liver, Pancreas, and Foregut Program and Surgical Oncologist, presented new paradigms in the surgical management of gastrointestinal cancer. Gusani discussed the importance of treatment of the whole patient involving prehabilitation and survivorship, and treatment of advanced tumors by considering the whole range of treatment options. These include multi-visceral and extended resections and the use of neoadjuvant therapy. Improved surgical outcomes through better understanding of anatomy, surgical techniques, and peri-operative medicine, and minimally invasive surgery were also discussed.

Gusani presented a surgeon's perspective on various aspects of gastrointestinal oncology. The surgical techniques for resection of gastric and gastroesophageal junction adenocarcinoma, hepatocellular carcinoma, metastatic colon adenocarcinoma in liver, and pancreatic tumors (adenocarcinoma, cysts, and neuroendocrine tumor) were described. Highlights of their presentation include the role and goal of physical activity in survivorship of patients who have undergone surgical resection of gastrointestinal carcinoma, and minimally invasive surgery that offers benefits in peri-operative outcomes while preserving oncologic outcomes.

4.2. Radiation Gastrointestinal Oncology

Technological advances have been made and applied in radiation oncology, and increasing evidence has indicated the clinical efficacy of stereotactic body radiation therapy (SBRT) in cancers of the digestive system. Mackley, Attending and Consultant Radiation Oncologist, provided an update on the general indications of radiation therapy for upper gastrointestinal malignancies based on the National Cancer Consortium Network (NCCN) treatment guidelines. This included current recommendations that support SBRT as an option in the treatment of unresectable PC and HCC. Tchelebi, Attending and Consultant Radiation Oncologist, further discussed the technical delivery of SBRT and the clinical evidence that supports this emerging treatment modality.

4.2.1. SBRT in Pancreatic Carcinoma

SBRT involves very high dose radiation delivered to a highly conformal treatment volume over a short treatment course (about one to five fractions over one to two weeks). As compared to three-dimensional conformal radiation therapy, SBRT may achieve superior tumor control by delivering a higher biological effective dose over a shorter overall treatment time with increased sparing of adjacent of critical organs. Moreover, Tchelebi presented data from recent clinical studies about using SBRT in the neoadjuvant setting for patients with borderline resectable pancreatic carcinoma (BRPC) and unresectable locally advanced pancreatic carcinoma (LAPC) [30]. Clinical data from an earlier study and recent studies on the use of SBRT as definitive treatment of locally advanced unresectable pancreatic carcinoma were also presented. Tchelebi concluded that SBRT improves resectability of BRPC and enables 5–10% of patients with unresectable LAPC to undergo resection. Additionally, clinical trials are ongoing to investigate chemotherapy (modified FOLFIRINOX) with or without SBRT in LAPC (www.clinicaltrials.govNCT01926197), and using adjuvant SBRT for patients following radical resection of pancreatic carcinoma with advanced tumor stages or lymph node involvement (www.clinicaltrials.govNCT02461836).

4.2.2. SBRT in Hepatocellular Carcinoma

External beam radiation therapy (EBRT) has been used for treatment of patients with HCC in various settings. EBRT may be considered for definitive treatment of HCC unsuitable for resection, liver transplant, or radiofrequency ablation; as a bridge to liver transplant; as definitive therapy for HCC unsuitable/refractory to TACE; or when there is tumor invasion of the portal vein. EBRT may be used at low doses for symptomatic HCC. Tchelebi reviewed the data from multiple clinical studies that investigated SBRT for HCC [30]. They discussed the advantages of SBRT for HCC including the effectiveness for large tumors (>10 cm), HCC with thrombosis in the portal vein, or when other local therapeutic modalities are contraindicated or less effective; sparing of adjacent un-involved liver; and producing complete pathological responses in patients who undergo liver transplant. Tchelebi concluded that SBRT can be used in HCC when other local therapies are not feasible (such as for large tumors or thrombosis in the portal vein), or in conjunction with TACE, or as a bridge to liver transplant.

4.3. Medical Gastrointestinal Oncology

Systemic therapies play important roles in various gastrointestinal malignancies at different tumor stages. Progressive advances have been made in improving the therapeutic efficacy of systemic treatment using chemotherapy, targeted therapy, and immunotherapy [31–41]. Results of recent clinical studies suggested new treatment options for patients with various malignant disease in the digestive system. Yee, Team Leader of Gastrointestinal Oncology and Attending and Consultant Medical Oncologist, provided an overview of the standard treatment of pancreatic, gastroesophageal, hepatobiliary, and colorectal carcinoma. Yee presented and discussed the most recent evidence from international medical conferences and medical literature on chemotherapy, targeted therapy, and immunotherapy in gastrointestinal oncology.

4.3.1. Systemic Treatment of Pancreatic Carcinoma

Systemic chemotherapy is an essential component of standard treatment for patients with PC diagnosed at all stages. New developments have been focusing on targeted agents directed against the tumor microenvironment and cancer stem cells. In a phase II clinical study of 246 patients, PEGylated hyaluronidase (PEGPH20), that degrades hyaluronan in the tumor-associated stroma, in combination with *nab*-paclitaxel and gemcitabine, significantly prolonged progression-free survival (PFS) and overall survival (OS), as compared to *nab*-paclitaxel and gemcitabine [42]. Moreover, this study suggested that hyaluronic acid is a potential predictive biomarker of tumor response to PEGPH20.

Results of a first-in-human clinical trial using napabucasin that targets cancer stem cells by inhibiting the activation of the signaling molecule STAT3 have been reported. In a phase 1b/II study of 66 patients with metastatic PC, the STAT3 inhibitor napabucasin that targets cancer stem cells, in combination with *nab*-paclitaxel and gemcitabine, produced anti-tumor response, with an overall response rate of 55%, disease control rate 93%, and progression-free survival 7.1 months [43]. A phase III study to investigate napabucasin in combination with nab-paclitaxel and gemcitabine versus nab-paclitaxel and gemcitabine is currently recruiting worldwide including at the Penn State Cancer Institute (www.clinicaltrials.govNCT02993731).

4.3.2. Systemic Treatment of Gastric and Gastroesophageal Carcinoma

For localized gastric carcinoma (GC) and gastroesophageal junction carcinoma (GEJC), peri-operative systemic chemotherapy using a combination regimen consisting of cisplatin and 5-fluorouracil is the standard of care. In a phase III study of 716 patients, a group of patients received peri-operative FLOT (docetaxel, oxaliplatin, 5-fluorouracil), and another group received peri-operative ECF (epirubicin, cisplatin, 5-fluorouracil) or ECX (epirubicin, cisplatin, capecitabine) [44]. Peri-operative FLOT improved clinical outcomes with a significant prolongation of progression-free and overall survival, reduction in the progression of disease during or following pre-operative chemotherapy, and an increase in pT0, pT1, and R0 resection. Results of this study support peri-operative FLOT as the new standard of systemic treatment for patients with resectable GC or GEJC.

The anti-PD-1 antibodies pembrolizumab significantly improved the response rate and overall survival beyond second line treatment of patients with advanced GC or GEJC expressing PD-L1. Results of this study led to approval of pembrolizumab by the Food and Drug Administration (FDA) in this patient population [45].

4.3.3. Systemic Treatment of Hepatocellular and Biliary Tract Carcinoma

The anti-PD-1 antibody nivolumab was investigated in a study of 262 sorafenib naïve or sorafenib-treated patients with advanced HCC. Nivolumab produced tumor responses regardless of etiology of HCC or tumor expression of PD-L1 [46]. Results of this study led to FDA approval of nivolumab for treatment of patients with HCC following prior sorafenib regardless of PD-L1 status.

In a phase III trial, the clinical efficacy of adjuvant capecitabine was evaluated in resected biliary tract carcinoma (BTC). In this study, 447 patients were randomized to receive adjuvant capecitabine versus observation. Intrahepatic (19%), hilar (28%), extra-hepatic (35%), gallbladder (18%). Capecitabine 1250 mg/m^2 on day 1 through day 14 of every 21-day cycle for a total of 8 cycles. The results of this study indicated that adjuvant capecitabine significantly prolonged overall survival in resected biliary tract carcinoma [47].

4.3.4. Systemic Treatment of Colorectal Carcinoma

Nivolumab, an anti-PD-1 antibody, has been recently FDA-approved for treatment of patients with metastatic colorectal carcinoma (CRC) with microsatellite instability-high (MSI-H) or mismatch repair-deficiency (dMMR) that has progressed following fluoropyrimidime, oxaliplatin, and irinotecan.

This indication is based on the data from a multicenter, open-label, single-arm, phase 2 clinical trial (CheckMate 142) [48].

The benefits of three months vs. six months of adjuvant chemotherapy using FOLFOX (5-fluorouracil, leucovorin, and oxaliplatin) or CAPOX (capecitabine and oxaliplatin) in stage III or high-risk stage II CRC were investigated [49,50]. Results of these studies indicated that three months of adjuvant chemotherapy is not inferior to six months of treatment. As a result, three months of adjuvant chemotherapy is recommended for low-risk disease (T1-3, N1). However, the use of three months of adjuvant chemotherapy for high-risk disease (T4 or N2 tumors) should be tailored to the individual patient.

4.4. Key Points and Recommendations

Surgical interventions continue to play crucial roles in the treatment of various malignant diseases in the digestive system. Besides the importance of surgical techniques for resection, treatment of the whole patient involving prehabilitation, survivorship, and physical activity, as well as minimally invasive surgery, offer benefits in both peri-operative and oncological outcomes. While three-dimensional conformal radiation remains the conventional therapeutic modality in gastrointestinal oncology, SBRT that involves a highly conformal treatment volume over a short treatment course has emerged as a treatment option that provides benefits in efficacy and safety, particularly in PC and HCC. Results of the recent clinical trials that investigated chemotherapy, targeted therapy, and immunotherapy have led to U.S. FDA approval of nivolumab in HCC and CRC with dMMR or MSI-H, and pembrolizumab in GC or GEJC expressing PD-L1, as well as solid tumors that display dMMR. Peri-operative FLOT for resectable GC and GEJC, adjuvant capecitabine for resected (R0) BTC, and three months of adjuvant FOLFOX or CAPOX for low-risk CRC are expected to become the new standard of care.

5. Gastrointestinal Cancer Genetics

Convincing evidence indicated that the development of cancer typically involves genetic disposition and behavioral and environmental factors. Although certain risk factors are potentially modifiable [51], genetic testing of hereditary gastrointestinal cancer syndromes has become an integral part of patient care in oncology [52]. Technological advances in the next generation sequencing of human genomes have improved genetic testing for the screening of various malignant diseases, particularly cancers of the digestive system. Baker, Director of Cancer Genetics, provided an overview of the genetic syndromes that predispose a person to GC, CRC, and PC. They discussed the practical aspects and clinical application of next generation sequencing (NGS) panels for hereditary gastrointestinal cancer.

5.1. Cancer Genetic Testing and Counseling

The genetics of gastric, colorectal, and pancreatic carcinoma were presented. For GC, approximately 3–5% of patients have a hereditary risk, and three heritable syndromes are known to predispose primarily to GC: hereditary diffuse gastric cancer (HDGC), familial intestinal gastric cancer (FIGC), and gastric adenocarcinoma and proximal polyposis of the stomach (GAPPS). Specific genes and types of mutations were identified in HDGC (*E-cadherin* and *α-E-catenin* genes), and GAPPS (promoter 1B mutations the *APC* gene), whereas no known genetic variants have been identified in FIGC. The diagnostic criteria for both FIGC, and GAPPS were described, as was the testing criteria for HDGC [53]. Other cancer syndromes and the associated genes that predispose a person to GC were also presented. These include familial adenomatous polyposis (*APC*), hereditary breast and ovarian cancer syndrome (*BRCA1, BRCA2*), juvenile polyposis syndrome (*SMAD4, BMPR1A*), Li-Fraumeni syndrome (*TP53*), Lynch syndrome (*MLH1, MSH2, MSH6, PMS2, EPCAM*), and Peutz-Jeghers syndrome (*STK11*).

In addition to GC, the genetic syndromes associated with hereditary CRC [52] and PC [52,54] were presented. Other hereditary cancer syndromes with gastrointestinal involvement [55] and the standards for informed consent for genetic testing in gastrointestinal practice [52] were also described.

5.2. Next-Generation Sequencing Panels

The traditional approach to cancer genetic testing that entails analysis of one gene per condition at a time using Sanger sequencing was compared to the contemporary approach using NGS panels. Given the increased number of genes analyzed with NGS panels, the process of informed consent, out of necessity, had to change dramatically. No longer was each gene discussed independently, but rather genes were categorized into groups of high, moderate, or low susceptibility regarding their impact on cancer risk. Risks, benefits, and limitations of NGS panels were also discussed, using case examples for illustration. Potential benefits include the ability to simultaneously analyze multiple cancer susceptibility genes in a more cost-efficient manner, thus increasing the likelihood of identifying one or more cancer predisposition syndromes within a family. Potential risks and limitations, though, include the higher likelihood of identifying one or more variants of uncertain significance and the likelihood that a mutation may be identified in a gene for which our knowledge base is still evolving with regards to the spectrum of associated cancers, the estimated lifetime risks of these cancers, as well as appropriate management guidelines. In addition, unexpected findings may be identified such as a gene mutation that is not consistent with the family history of cancer or a mutation in a recessive gene that has reproductive implications.

Lastly, choosing a laboratory for NGS panels is a practical aspect of cancer genetic testing and a number of questions will need to be considered and addressed [56]. Evaluation of the technology being used involves consideration of the testing platform, depth of coverage, and presence of a deletion/duplication assay. Analysis of the genes involves considering the number of genes examined, whether a cancer site-specific panel or a pan-cancer panel would be more appropriate, looking at the proportion of genes that are "medically actionable", and whether the option exists to modify the panel or create a custom panel. Other pertinent factors for consideration include the cost of testing and insurance coverage, the turn-around time, the rate of variants of uncertain significance (VUS), the reliability of the laboratory, and the ease of laboratory use.

5.3. Key Points and Recommendations

The genetic syndromes and the associated genetic mutations for GC, CRC, and PC have been identified. Clinicians should be vigilant about individuals with cancer and their family history of cancer, and should be prompt to refer patients to cancer geneticists for genetic testing and counseling. Patients with germline mutations that predispose to various malignant diseases will likely benefit from screening tests for early detection of tumors and taking appropriate measures for preventive and therapeutic interventions. Cancer genetic testing using NGS panels is expected to produce potential benefits by concurrent analysis of multiple cancer susceptibility genes in a cost-efficient manner, thus increasing the likelihood of identifying cancer predisposition syndromes within a family.

6. Supportive Care in Oncology

Complementary to the treatment of cancer, emotional, psychological, and social support are essential for the well-being of patients, particularly those with gastrointestinal cancers. In clinical practice, patients with advanced cancer are recommended to receive palliative care early in the disease course and concurrent with anti-cancer treatment [57]. At the Penn State Cancer Institute, supportive care services are provided by healthcare providers from multiple disciplines to patients with malignant diseases. They include palliative care physicians and nurses, clinical psychologists, kinesiologists, nutritionists, physical therapists, artists and music therapists, acupuncturists, and population scientists for smoking cessation. A support group that focuses on gastrointestinal cancer patients and survivors is underway at the Penn State Cancer Institute. The goals include improving the quality of life for cancer patients and survivors as well as the well-being of their caretakers.

6.1. Music and Arts in Health and Oncology

A program that integrates music, arts, and creative writing has been established at the Milton S. Hershey Medical Center through the Center for Humanistic Medicine and Center Stage Arts in Health. The goal of this program is to provide supportive care by psychological and cognitive improvement. This program is particularly needed for patients with gastrointestinal malignancies that are associated with high levels of psychosocial distress, disease burden, and mortality rate. de Boer, Director of Center Stage Arts in Health, provided an overview of the music and arts programs at Penn State Health including the Cancer Institute.

6.2. Center Stage Arts in Health

Center Stage Arts in Health is a multi-faceted program that aims to nourish well-being through the arts. At Center Stage, professional musicians play cheerful and reflective music with a variety of genres and instruments in the lobby and numerous clinical and family areas. The staff of Center Stage visit patients upon their admission to the hospital, and patients have the opportunity to choose artwork created by regional artists to hang in their room during their hospital stay [58]. Murals are created in the clinical and family waiting areas (https://sites.psu.edu/centerstage/murals/), and original art is commissioned for display throughout the hospital. A summer lunchtime concert series is conducted in the outdoor courtyard, featuring local professional ensembles including jazz, classical, and soft rock music. At Center Stage and the Penn State Cancer Institute, a set of arts workshops of multiple modalities, including an expressive workshop program, is offered to cancer patients and their caregivers. A brief video introduction of the Center Stage program can be watched at https://www.youtube.com/watch?time_continue=8&v=HT3wJn8OoF4.

Faculty-led investigations are ongoing to observe, explore, and quantify the impact of the arts on the experience of patients and caregivers. During the summer of 2017, a Pennsylvania State University undergraduate student, Julian Yee, who majors in psychology, participated in research as a Center Stage Intern. During the internship, Yee assisted the Center Stage Team to promote music and arts in health. First of all, Yee observed the pertinence of the social interactions between musical artists and visitors, staff, and patients. From there, Yee recorded the data of musical acts against the audience's reactions. Then, they transported art supplies to guide cancer survivors and their families to make art crafts on Survivorship Day. Finally, they helped paint a mural in a hallway so when children pass by, they are reminded that the hospital can be a colorful environment.

6.3. Key Points and Recommendations

Emotional, psychological, and social support is an essential component of the multi-disciplinary care of patients, and particularly those with cancers in the digestive system. For patients with advanced gastrointestinal cancer, palliative care is recommended concurrent with anti-cancer treatment early in the disease course. The Center Stage Arts in Health integrates music, arts, and creative writing with the aim to nurture the well-being of patients through psychological and cognitive improvement.

7. Conclusions

Cancers of the digestive system continue to represent a major cause of physical and psychosocial burden. Healthcare practitioners and scientists with expertise in multiple disciplines play critical roles in providing optimal care for patients with these malignant diseases. Recent advances have been made in gastrointestinal cancer epidemiology and genetics, diagnostic evaluation, treatment modalities, and supportive care. This conference paper summarizes the presentations by the faculty members of the Penn State Health Milton S. Hershey Medical Center with a focus on gastrointestinal oncology. These specialists provided updates on new developments in (1) health disparities and resistance training, (2) diagnostic evaluation and screening procedures, (3) conventional and novel therapeutic modalities, (4) cancer genetic testing and counseling, and (5) music and arts in health and cancer. In summary, this medical conference highlighted the new frontiers in the multi-disciplinary care for patients with gastrointestinal cancers.

Author Contributions: N.S.Y., E.J.L., K.H.S., J.L.M., N.J.G., L.T., H.B.M., K.L.K., M.J.B., C.d.B., and J.D.Y. wrote the paper.

Acknowledgments: No grant has been received in support of this research work. No fund has been received for covering the costs to publish in open access.

Conflicts of Interest: The authors declare no conflict of interest.

References

1. Siegel, R.L.; Miller, K.D.; Jemal, A. Cancer statistics, 2018. *CA Cancer J. Clin.* **2017**, *68*, 7–30. [CrossRef] [PubMed]
2. Lengerich, E.J.; Tucker, T.C.; Powell, R.K.; Colsher, P.; Lehman, E.; Ward, A.J.; Siedlecki, J.C.; Wyatt, S.W. Cancer incidence in Kentucky, Pennsylvania, and West Virginia: Disparities in Appalachia. *J. Rural Health* **2005**, *21*, 39–47. [CrossRef] [PubMed]
3. Centers for Disease Control and Prevention (CDC). Cancer Death Rates—Appalachia, 1994–1998. In *MMWR Morb Mortal Wkly Rep*; Centers for Disease Control and Prevention: Atlanta, GA, USA, 2002; Volume 51, pp. 527–529.
4. Armstrong, L.R.; Thompson, T.; Hall, H.I.; Coughlin, S.S.; Steel, B.; Rogers, J.D. Colorectal carcinoma mortality among Appalachian men and women, 1969–1999. *Cancer* **2004**, *101*, 2851–2858. [CrossRef] [PubMed]
5. Lengerich, E.J.; Rubio, A.; Brown, P.; Knight, E.A.; Wyatt, S.W. Results of Coordinated Investigations of a National Colorectal Cancer Education Campaign in Appalachia. *Prev. Chronic Dis.* **2006**, *3*, A32. [PubMed]
6. Jorgensen, C.M.; Gelb, C.A.; Merritt, T.L.; Seeff, L.C. Observations from the CDC: CDC's Screen for Life: A National Colorectal Cancer Action Campaign. *J. Womens Health Gend. Based Med.* **2001**, *10*, 417–422. [CrossRef] [PubMed]
7. Vanderpool, R.C.; Coyne, C.A. Qualitative assessment of local distribution of Screen for Life mass media materials in Appalachia. *Prev. Chronic. Dis.* **2006**, *3*, A54. [PubMed]
8. Davis, R.E.; Armstrong, D.K.; Dignan, M.; Norling, G.R.; Redmond, J. Evaluation of educational materials on colorectal cancer screening in Appalachian Kentucky. *Prev. Chronic. Dis.* **2006**, *3*, A54.
9. Ward, A.J.; Kluhsman, B.C.; Lengerich, E.J.; Piccinin, A.M. The impact of cancer coalitions on the dissemination of colorectal cancer materials to community organizations in rural Appalachia. *Prev. Chronic Dis.* **2006**, *3*, A55. [PubMed]
10. Rosenwasser, L.A.; McCall-Hosenfeld, J.S.; Weisman, C.S.; Hillemeier, M.M.; Perry, A.N.; Chuang, C.H. Barriers to colorectal cancer screening among women in rural central Pennsylvania: Primary care physicians' perspective. *Rural Remote Health* **2013**, *13*, 2504. [PubMed]
11. Lengerich, E.J.; Kluhsman, B.C.; Bencivenga, M.; Allen, R.; Miele, M.B.; Farace, E. Development of community plans to enhance survivorship from colorectal cancer: Community-based participatory research in rural communities. *J. Cancer Surviv.* **2007**, *1*, 205–211. [CrossRef] [PubMed]
12. Nadler, M.; Bainbridge, D.; Tomasone, J.; Cheifetz, O.; Juergens, R.A.; Sussman, J. Oncology care provider perspectives on exercise promotion in people with cancer: An examination of knowledge, practices, barriers, and facilitators. *Support. Care Cancer* **2017**, *25*, 2297–2304. [CrossRef] [PubMed]
13. Schmitz, K.H.; Courneya, K.S.; Matthews, C.; Demark-Wahnefried, W.; Galvão, D.A.; Pinto, B.M.; Irwin, M.L.; Wolin, K.Y.; Segal, R.J.; Lucia, A.; et al. American College of Sports Medicine Roundtable on exercise guidelines for cancer survivors. *Med. Sci. Sport Exerc.* **2010**, *42*, 1409–1426. [CrossRef] [PubMed]
14. Cromie, P.; Zopf, E.M.; Zhang, X.; Schmitz, K.H. The impact of exercise on cancer mortality, recurrence, and treatment-related adverse effects. *Epidemiol. Rev.* **2017**, *39*, 71–92. [CrossRef] [PubMed]
15. Allgayer, H.; Nicolaus, S.; Schreiber, S. Decreased interleukin-1 receptor antagonist response following moderate exercise in patients with colorectal carcinoma after primary treatment. *Cancer Detect. Prev.* **2004**, *28*, 208–213. [CrossRef] [PubMed]

16. Meyerhardt, J.A.; Heseltine, D.; Niedzwiecki, D.; Hollis, D.; Saltz, L.B.; Mayer, R.J.; Thomas, J.; Nelson, H.; Whittom, R.; Hantel, A.; et al. Impact of physical activity on cancer recurrence and survival in patients with stage III colon cancer: Findings from CALGB 89803. *J. Clin. Oncol.* **2006**, *24*, 3535–3541. [CrossRef] [PubMed]
17. Goncalves, B.; Soares, J.B.; Bastos, P. Endoscopic ultrasound in the diagnosis and staging of pancreatic cancer. *GE Port. J. Gastroenterol.* **2015**, *22*, 161–171. [CrossRef] [PubMed]
18. Chen, Y.K.; Pleskow, D.K. SpyGlass single-operator peroral cholangiopancreatoscopy system for the diagnosis and therapy of bile-duct disorders: A clinical feasibility study (with video). *Gastrointest. Endosc.* **2007**, *65*, 832–841. [CrossRef] [PubMed]
19. Theodoropoulou, A.; Vardas, E.; Voudoukis, E.; Tavernaraki, A.; Tribonias, G.; Konstantinidis, K.; Paspatis, G.A. SpyGlass direct visualization system facilitated management of iatrogenic biliary stricture: A novel approach in difficult cannulation. *Endoscopy* **2012**, *44* (Suppl. 2), E433–E434. [CrossRef] [PubMed]
20. Navaneethan, U.; Hasan, M.K.; Kommaraju, K.; Zhu, X.; Hebert-Magee, S.; Hawes, R.H.; Vargo, J.J.; Varadarajulu, S.; Parsi, M.A. Digital, single-operator cholangiopancreatiscopy in the diagnosis and management of pancreatobiliary disorders: A multicenter clinical experience (with video). *Gastrointest. Endosc.* **2016**, *84*, 649–655. [CrossRef] [PubMed]
21. Makarova-Rusher, O.V.; Altekruse, S.F.; McNeel, T.S.; Ulahannan, S.; Duffy, A.G.; Graubard, B.I.; Greten, T.F.; McGlynn, K.A. Population attributable fractions of risk factors for hepatocellular carcinoma in the Unites States. *Cancer* **2016**, *122*, 1757–1765. [CrossRef] [PubMed]
22. Calle, E.E.; Rodriguez, C.; Walker-Thurmond, K.; Thun, M.J. Overweight, obesity, and mortality from cancer in a prospectively studied cohort of U.S. adults. *New. Engl. J. Med.* **2003**, *348*, 1625–1638. [CrossRef] [PubMed]
23. El Serag, H.B.; Kanwal, F.; Richardson, P.; Kramer, J. Risk of hepatocellular carcinoma after sustained virological response in Veterans with hepatitis C virus infection. *Hepatology* **2016**, *64*, 130–137. [CrossRef] [PubMed]
24. Singal, A.G.; Pillai, A.; Tiro, J. Early detection, curative treatment, and survival rates for hepatocellular carcinoma surveillance in patients with cirrhosis: A meta-analysis. *PLoS Med.* **2014**, *11*, e1001624. [CrossRef] [PubMed]
25. Yu, N.C.; Chaudhari, V.; Raman, S.S.; Lassman, C.; Tong, M.J.; Busuttil, R.W.; Lu, D.S. CT and MRI improve detection of hepatocellular carcinoma, compared with ultrasound alone, in patients with cirrhosis. *Clin. Gastroenterol. Hepatol.* **2011**, *9*, 161–167. [CrossRef] [PubMed]
26. Xu, H.X.; Xie, X.Y.; Lu, M.D.; Liu, G.J.; Xu, Z.F.; Zheng, Y.L.; Liang, J.-Y.; Chen, L.D. Contrast-enhanced sonography in the diagnosis of small hepatocellular carcinoma < or = 2 cm. *J. Clin. Ultrasound* **2008**, *36*, 257–266. [PubMed]
27. Hanna, R.F.; Miloushev, V.Z.; Tang, A.; Finklestone, L.A.; Brejt, S.Z.; Sandhu, R.S.; Santillan, C.S.; Wolfson, T.; Gamst, A.; Sirlin, C.B. Comparative 13-year meta-analysis of the sensitivity and positive predictive value of ultrasound, CT, and MRI for detecting hepatocellular carcinoma. *Abdom. Radiol.* **2016**, *41*, 71–90. [CrossRef] [PubMed]
28. Mazzaferro, V.; Regalia, E.; Doci, R.; Andreola, S.; Pulvirenti, A.; Bozzetti, F.; Montalto, F.; Ammatuna, M.; Morabito, A.; Gennari, L. Liver transplantation for the treatment of small hepatocellular carcinomas in patients with cirrhosis. *N. Engl. J. Med.* **1996**, *334*, 693–699. [CrossRef] [PubMed]
29. Hemming, A.W.; Langham, M.R.; Reed, A.I.; van der Werf, W.J.; Howard, R.J. Resection of the inferior vena cava for hepatic malignancy. *Am. Surg.* **2001**, *67*, 1081–1087. [CrossRef] [PubMed]
30. Tchelebi, L.; Zaorsky, N.; Mackley, H. Stereotactic body radiation therapy in the management of upper GI malignancies. *Biomedicines* **2018**, *6*, 7–doi10. [CrossRef] [PubMed]
31. Yee, N.S. Toward the goal of personalized therapy in pancreatic cancer by targeting the molecular phenotype. *Adv. Exp. Med. Biol.* **2013**, *779*, 91–143. [PubMed]
32. Joshi, M.; Yang, Z.; Harvey, H.; Belani, C.; Yee, N.S. Current and emerging therapies in neuro-endocrine tumors: Impact of genetic targets on clinical outcomes. *Clin. Cancer Drugs* **2014**, *1*, 28–39. [CrossRef]
33. Yee, N.S.; Kazi, A.A.; Yee, R.K. Current systemic treatment and emerging therapeutic strategies in pancreatic adenocarcinoma. *Curr. Clin. Pharmcol.* **2015**, *10*, 256–266. [CrossRef]
34. Marks, E.I.; Yee, N.S. Immunotherapy in biliary tract carcinoma: Current status and emerging approaches. *World J. Gastro. Oncol.* **2015**, *7*, 338–346. [CrossRef] [PubMed]

35. Wyluda, E.; Yee, N.S. Systemic treatment of advanced biliary tract cancer: Emerging roles of targeted therapy and molecular profiling. *Clin. Cancer Drug* **2015**, *2*, 80–86. [CrossRef]
36. Kankeu Fonkoua, L.; Yee, N.S. Immunotherapy in gastric carcinoma: Current status and emerging strategies. *Clin. Cancer Drug* **2015**, *2*, 91–99. [CrossRef]
37. Marks, E.I.; Yee, N.S. Molecular genetics and targeted therapy in hepatocellular carcinoma. *Curr. Cancer Drug Target* **2015**, *16*, 53–70. [CrossRef]
38. Yee, N.S. Immunotherapeutic approaches in pancreatic adenocarcinoma: Current status and future perspectives. *Curr. Mol. Pharmacol.* **2016**, *9*, 231–241. [CrossRef] [PubMed]
39. Marks, E.I.; Yee, N.S. Molecular genetics and targeted therapeutics in biliary tract carcinoma. *World J. Gastro.* **2016**, *22*, 1335–1347. [CrossRef] [PubMed]
40. Balaban, E.P.; Mangu, P.B.; Khorana, A.A.; Shah, M.A.; Mukherjee, S.; Crane, C.H.; Javle, M.M.; Eads, J.R.; Allen, P.; Ko, A.H.; et al. Locally advanced, unresectable pancreatic cancer: American Society of Clinical Oncology clinical practice guideline. *J. Clin. Oncol.* **2016**, *34*, 2654–2658. [CrossRef] [PubMed]
41. Chen, Y.; Yee, N.S. Pharmacokinetics-guided dosing of 5-fluorouracil for precision cancer treatment: A focus on colorectal carcinoma. *Appl. Clin. Res. Clin. Trials Regul. Aff.* **2016**, *3*, 159–163. [CrossRef]
42. Hingorani, S.R.; Bullock, A.J.; Seery, T.E.; Zheng, L.; Sigal, D.; Ritch, P.S.; Braiteh, F.S.; Zalupski, M.; Bahary, N.; Harris, W.P.; et al. Randomized phase II study of PEGPH20 plus nab-paclitaxel/gemcitabine vs. nab-paclitaxel plus gemcitabine in patients with untreated, metastatic pancreatic ductal adenocarcinoma. *J. Clin. Oncol.* **2017**, *35*. [CrossRef]
43. Bekaii-Saab, T.S.; Starodub, A.; El-Rayes, B.F.; O'Neil, B.H.; Shahda, S.; Ciombor, K.K.; Noonan, A.M.; Hanna, W.T.; Sehdev, A.; Shaib, W.L.; et al. A phase Ib/II study of cancer stemness inhibitor napabucasin in combination with gemcitabine (gem) & nab-paclitaxel (nabPTX) in metastatic pancreatic adenocarcinoma (mPDAC) patients (pts). *Ann. Oncol.* **2017**, *28* (Suppl. 3), 4106.
44. Al-Batran, S.E.; Homann, N.; Schmalenberg, H.; Kopp, H.G.; Haag, G.M.; Luley, K.B.; Schmiegel, W.H.; Folprecht, G.; Probst, S.; Prasnikar, N.; et al. Perioperative chemotherapy with docetaxel, oxaliplatin, and fluorouracil/leucovorin (FLOT) versus epirubicin, cisplatin, and fluorouracil or capecitabine (ECF/ECX) for resectable gastric or gastroesophageal junction (GEJ) adenocarcinoma (FLOT4-AIO): A multicenter, randomized phase 3 trial. *J. Clin. Oncol.* **2017**, *35*. [CrossRef]
45. Fuchs, C.S.; Doi, T.; Jang, R.W.; Muro, K.; Satoh, T.; Machado, M.; Sun, W.; Jalal, S.I.; Shah, M.A.; Metges, J.P.; et al. KEYNOTE-059 cohort 1: Efficacy and safety of pembrolizumab (pembro) monotherapy in patients with previously treated advanced gastric cancer. *J. Clin. Oncol.* **2017**, *35*. [CrossRef]
46. Todd, S.C.; El-Khoueiry, A.B.; Yau, T.; Melero, I.; Sangro, B.; Kudo, M. Nivolumab in sorafenib-naïve and -experienced patients with advanced hepatocellular carcinoma: CheckMate040 Study. *J. Clin. Oncol.* **2017**, *35* (Suppl. 15), 4013.
47. Primrose, J.N.; Fox, R.; Palmer, D.H.; Prasad, R.; Mirza, D.; Anthoney, D.A.; Corrie, P.; Falk, S.; Wasan, H.S.; Ross, P.J.; et al. Adjuvant capecitabine for biliary tract cancer: The BILCAP randomized study. *J. Clin. Oncol.* **2017**, *35*. [CrossRef]
48. Overman, M.J.; McDermott, R.; Leach, J.L.; Lonardi, S.; Lenz, H.-J.; Morse, M.A.; Desai, J.; Hill, A.; Axelson, M.; Moss, R.A.; et al. Nivolumab in patients with metastatic DNA mismatch repair-deficient or microsatellite instability-high colorectal cancer (CheckMate 142): an open-label, multicenter, phase 2 study. *Lancet Oncol.* **2017**, *18*, 1182–1191. [CrossRef]
49. Shi, Q.; Sobrero, A.F.; Shields, A.F.; Yoshino, T.; Paul, J.; Taieb, J.; Sougklakos, I.; Kerr, R.; Labianca, R.; Meyerhardt, J.A.; et al. Prospective pooled analysis of six phase III trials investigating duration of adjuvant (adjuv) oxaliplatin-based therapy (3 vs. 6 months) for patients (pts) with stage III colon cancer (CC): The IDEA (International Duration Evaluation of Adjuvant chemotherapy) collaboration. *J. Clin. Oncol.* **2017**, *35*. [CrossRef]
50. Iveson, T.; Kerr, R.; Saunders, M.P.; Hollander, N.H.; Tabernero, J.; Haydon, A.M.; Glimelius, B.; Harkin, A.; Scudder, C.; Boyd, K.; et al. Final DFS results of the SCOT study: An international phase III randomized (1:1) non-inferiority trial comparing 3 versus 6 months of oxaliplatin based adjuvant chemotherapy for colorectal cancer. *J. Clin. Oncol.* **2017**, *35*. [CrossRef]
51. Islami, F.; Sauer, A.G.; Miller, K.D.; Siegel, R.L.; Fedewa, S.A.; Jacobs, E.J.; McCullough, M.L.; Patel, A.V.; Ma, J.; Soerjomataram, I.; et al. Proportion and number of cancer cases and death attributable to potentially modifiable risk factors in the United States. *CA Cancer J. Clin.* **2018**, *68*, 31–54. [CrossRef] [PubMed]

52. Syngal, S.; Brand, R.E.; Church, J.M.; Giardiello, F.M.; Hampel, H.L.; Burt, R.W. ACG Clinical guideline: Genetic testing and management of hereditary gastrointestinal cancer syndromes. *Am. J. Gastroenterol.* **2015**, *110*, 223–263. [CrossRef] [PubMed]
53. Colvin, H.; Yamamoto, K.; Wada, N.; Mori, M. Hereditary gastric cancer syndromes. *Surg. Oncol. Clin. N. Am.* **2015**, *24*, 765–777. [CrossRef] [PubMed]
54. Connor, A.A.; Gallinger, S. Hereditary pancreatic cancer syndromes. *Surg. Oncol. Clin. N. Am.* **2015**, *24*, 733–764. [CrossRef] [PubMed]
55. Rubinstein, W.S.; Weissman, S.M. Managing hereditary gastrointestinal cancer syndromes: The partnership between genetic counselors and gastroenterologists. *Nat. Clin. Pract. Gastroenterol. Hepatol.* **2008**, *5*, 569–582. [CrossRef] [PubMed]
56. Fecteau, H.; Vogel, K.J.; Hanson, K.; Morrill-Cornelius, S. The evoluation of cancer risk assessment in the era of next generation sequencing. *J. Genet. Couns.* **2014**, *23*, 633–639. [CrossRef] [PubMed]
57. Ferrell, B.R.; Temel, J.S.; Temin, S.; Alesi, E.R.; Balboni, T.A.; Basch, E.M.; Firn, J.I.; Paice, J.A.; Peppercorn, J.M.; Phillips, T.; et al. Integration of palliative care into standard oncology care: American Society of Clinical Oncology Clinical Practice Guideline Update. *J. Clin. Oncol.* **2017**, *35*, 96–112. [CrossRef] [PubMed]
58. George, D.R.; de Boer, C.; Green, M.J. "That landscape is where I'd like to be ... " Offering patients with cancer a choice of artwork. *JAMA* **2017**, *317*, 890–892. [CrossRef] [PubMed]

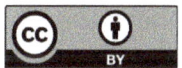

© 2018 by the authors. Licensee MDPI, Basel, Switzerland. This article is an open access article distributed under the terms and conditions of the Creative Commons Attribution (CC BY) license (http://creativecommons.org/licenses/by/4.0/).

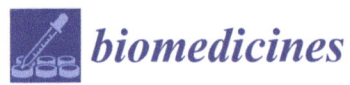

Case Report

Tumor Molecular Profiling for an Individualized Approach to the Treatment of Hepatocellular Carcinoma: A Patient Case Study

Kristine Posadas [1], Anita Ankola [2], Zhaohai Yang [3] and Nelson S. Yee [4,*]

1. Pennsylvania State University College of Medicine, Hershey, PA 17033, USA; kposadas@pennstatehealth.psu.edu
2. Department of Radiology, Penn State Health Milton S. Hershey Medical Center, Hershey, PA 17033, USA; aankola@pennstatehealth.psu.edu
3. Department of Pathology, Penn State Health Milton S. Hershey Medical Center, Hershey, PA 17033, USA; zyang2@pennstatehealth.psu.edu
4. Division of Hematology-Oncology, Department of Medicine, Penn State Health Milton S. Hershey Medical Center; Experimental Therapeutics Program, Penn State Cancer Institute, Pennsylvania State University College of Medicine, Hershey, PA 17033, USA
* Correspondence: nyee@pennstatehealth.psu.edu; Tel.: +1-717-531-0003

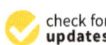

Received: 13 March 2018; Accepted: 9 April 2018; Published: 17 April 2018

Abstract: Hepatocellular carcinoma (HCC) is increasing in incidence, and the associated mortality rate remains among the highest. For advanced HCC, sorafenib has been shown to slightly prolong survival, and regorafenib and nivolumab, both recently approved by the United States Food and Drug Administration (FDA), may produce clinical benefits to a limited extent. Systemic chemotherapy has been shown to produce a modest response, but there is no clinically valid biomarker that can be used to predict which patients may benefit. In this case study, we present two patients with metastatic HCC, they received systemic treatment using capecitabine, oxaliplatin, and either bevacizumab or sorafenib. The tumor response to treatment was determined by the progression-free survival (PFS). Molecular profiling of the tumors showed differential expression of biochemical markers and different mutational status of the *TP53* and β-catenin (*CTNNB1*) genes. We hypothesize that the PFS correlates with the tumor molecular profiles, which may be predictive of the therapeutic response to systemic chemotherapy. Further investigation is indicated to correlate tumor biomarkers and treatment responses, with the objective of personalizing the therapies for patients with advanced HCC.

Keywords: hepatocellular carcinoma; immunohistochemistry; molecular profiling; next-generation sequencing; precision medicine; predictive biomarkers

1. Introduction

Hepatocellular carcinoma (HCC) is increasing in incidence, and the associated mortality rate remains among the highest [1]. For patients with localized HCC, surgical resection and liver transplantation may be offered with curative intent. Palliative local therapy, such as chemoembolization, radiofrequency ablation, and stereotactic body radiation therapy, are options for treatment [2]. However, for patients with advanced or metastatic HCC, palliative systemic treatment is the only option, and the associated survival benefit is limited [3].

For select patients with advanced HCC, sorafenib is the standard first-line systemic treatment [4]. In the second-line setting, regorafenib (a small molecule inhibitor targeting tyrosine kinases and angiogenesis receptors) and nivolumab (an anti-PD-1 monoclonal antibody) have been recently approved by the United States Food and Drug Administration (FDA) for patients with advanced HCC, which have failed to respond to sorafenib [5,6]. According to the National Comprehensive Cancer Network (NCCN), patients with unresectable HCC should receive systemic chemotherapy preferably in a clinical trial setting [7]. HCC is resistant to conventional chemotherapeutic agents possibly related to pathogenic mutations in certain genes such as *TP53* and *CTNNB1* (coding for β-catenin), which are commonly mutated in HCC [3]. This is supported by evidence that mutated TP53 and CTNNB1 contribute to increased cell proliferation and reduced apoptosis in HCC [8,9]. Multiple studies have indicated that patients with HCC that carry mutations in *TP53* have a relatively poor prognosis [10]. Molecular profiling of HCC has been performed to characterize this type of malignancy with the hope of identifying predictive biomarkers and therapeutic targets.

A retrospective study showed considerable molecular heterogeneity among 350 specimens of HCC [11]. An immunohistochemical analysis indicated various frequencies of change in the expression of protein biomarkers and the associated potential therapeutic agents. For instance, a decreased expression of thymidine synthetase (TS) and excision repair cross-complementation group 1 (ERCC1) was found in 79.8% and 66.1% of specimens, respectively. Reduced expression of these biochemical markers suggests potential benefits from fluoropyrimidines and platinum agents, respectively [12,13]. Furthermore, genetic mutations were most frequently identified in the *TP53* and *CTNNB1* genes in 30% and 20% of the tested specimens, respectively. While there was no standard effective chemotherapy for advanced HCC, early phase studies suggested capecitabine and oxaliplatin (CAPOX) to be effective in patients with HCC. This was demonstrated in a phase II study that showed modest anti-tumor activity when using CAPOX as a first-line therapy, with a median progression-free survival (PFS) of 4.1 months [14]. Furthermore, a clinical trial to investigate a combination of capecitabine, oxaliplatin, and bevacizumab (CAPOX-B) as a first-line regimen in patients with advanced/metastatic HCC showed a median PFS of 6.8 months [15].

In this case study, we present two patients who were diagnosed with metastatic HCC, analyzed for tumor molecular profiles, and treated with CAPOX in combination with either bevacizumab or sorafenib. These two patients had different clinical features regarding the etiology of HCC and treatment responses, and the molecular profiles of their tumors were distinct in the expression of biochemical markers and genomic DNA mutations. The correlation of the therapeutic response with the tumor molecular profiling suggests the potential for developing predictive biomarkers using a large data set, and evaluating the use of individualized treatment for patients with HCC in future prospective studies.

2. Case Reports

2.1. Patient #1

This is a 65-year-old Caucasian man who presented with progressive weakness and paresthesia in the bilateral lower extremities. He also complained about urinary retention lasting two days. His past medical problems included hypertension, psoriatic arthritis, lymphedema in the right lower extremity, a cardiac murmur, and osteoarthritis in bilateral knees status post left knee replacement. He had no history of hepatic cirrhosis, diabetes mellitus, steatohepatitis, viral hepatitis, alcoholism, hemochromatosis, or Wilson's disease. His family history showed significant "liver cancer" and hemochromatosis in his father and "cancer in a digestive organ" in his paternal grandmother. He had worked in the navy as a maintenance supervisor and a shuttle bus driver. He had previously smoked one pack of cigarettes per day for 20 years and quit smoking 20 years ago; he had previously consumed alcohol and he last drank in December 2015. The physical examination was remarkable for chronic edema in the bilateral lower extremities, the spine was non-tender, and no peritoneal ascites was noted. Laboratory tests showed elevated serum alpha-fetoprotein (AFP) level in the liver, corresponding to 60.9 ng/mL (reference range: 0–15 ng/mL), and normal AFP-L3 (3.6%, reference range: 0–9.9%), while his carbohydrate antigen 19–9, carcinoembryonic antigen, prostate-specific antigen, and β-human chorionic gonadotropin were all within normal limits. Viral hepatitis serology was non-reactive for both the hepatitis B viral envelope antigen and the hepatitis C virus.

The initial evaluation conducted using computed tomography (CT) scans (December 2015) revealed multiple lesions in the liver and bones (T6 spine, sacrum, bilateral ribs) (Figure 1). He underwent a T5–T7 laminectomy, an open biopsy of the thoracic intraspinal (extradural) lesion, and excision of the thoracic epidural neoplasm. The pathology of the biopsied T6 epidural mass showed metastatic carcinoma, and the histopathology and immunohistochemical staining for Hep-Par-1 were consistent with a hepatic primary tumor (Figure 2). Thus, this patient had stage IV B (T3a N0 M1) HCC. Starting in February 2016, he was started on sorafenib (200 mg orally every 12 h daily) as a first-line therapy. Two months later, CT scans showed enlarged tumors in the liver, with omental and mesenteric carcinomatosis, stable osseous metastases, and the serum AFP-liver level increased to 71 ng/mL, consistent with tumor progression.

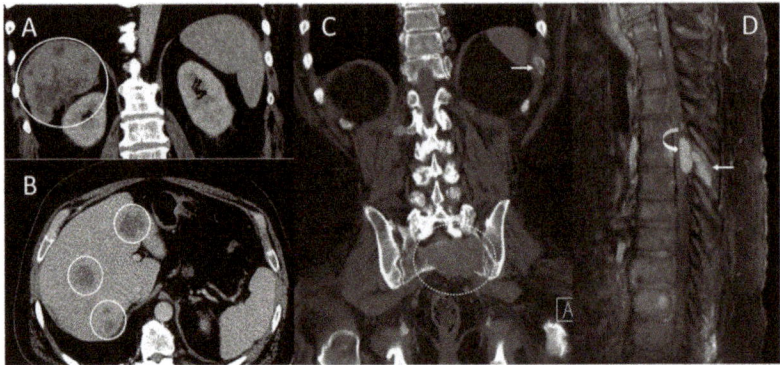

Figure 1. Computed tomography (CT) scans and magnetic resonance imaging (MRI) scans at initial diagnosis showed metastatic lesions in the liver, left 11th rib, 6th thoracic spine (T6), and sacrum. (**A**) Coronal and (**B**) axial contrast-enhanced CT scans demonstrate multifocal heterogeneous irregular hepatic tumors of varying sizes throughout the liver (solid circles) primarily in the right hepatic lobe. (**C**) Coronal CT scans in bone window demonstrate a lytic bone metastasis involving the left eleventh rib (arrow) and a large, destructive upper sacral metastasis (dashed circle). (**D**) Sagittal contrast-enhanced MRI scans demonstrate an enhancing mid-thoracic spine epidural metastasis (curved arrow) with an adjacent bone metastasis involving the T6 spinous process (arrow).

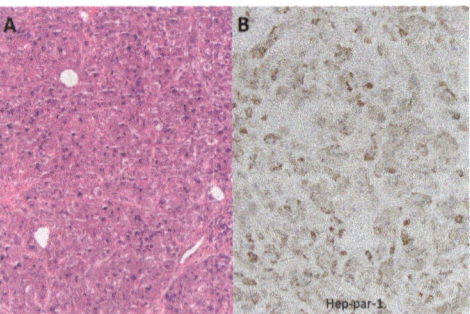

Figure 2. Histopathological and immunohistochemical analysis of the biopsied T6 epidural mass. (**A**) The hematoxylin- and eosin-stained section shows infiltration by nests of polygonal cells with enlarged atypical nuclei and abundant eosinophilic cytoplasm. Nuclear pseudo-inclusion and mitotic figures are apparent. (**B**) Immunohistochemical analysis for Hep-Par-1 shows granular cytoplasmic staining, supporting a diagnosis of metastatic hepatocellular carcinoma (original magnification ×200).

In May 2016, he started immunotherapy on a clinical trial using an investigative anti-PD-1 monoclonal antibody. The patient received four cycles of this treatment (a total of eight weeks), and then the tumor progressed. This was evidenced by CT scans (July 2016) showing an increase in both size and number of omental, peritoneal, mesenteric metastases, a stable disease in liver, bones, and lymph nodes, and the serum AFP-liver level increased further to 102.3 ng/mL.

Molecular profiling of the epidural metastatic tumor was performed by the Caris® Life Sciences (https://www.carislifesciences.com/cmi-overview/). The materials and methods for the tumor molecular profiling were previously described in detail [11]. Briefly, using formalin-fixed paraffin-embedded tumor tissues, successive 4 μm sections were generated until sufficient material for testing was obtained. For the molecular analysis, tumor cells were excised by microdissection, until a total area of at least 50 mm^2 was obtained. The expression of a panel of protein and RNA biomarkers predictive of the response to cytotoxic chemotherapy and molecularly targeted agents was determined by immunohistochemistry (IHC), chromogenic in-situ hybridization (CISH), and RNA sequencing (RNA-Seq). The expression levels of various biochemical markers and the associated therapeutic agents with potential benefits are listed in Table 1. Notably, the immunohistochemical analysis of tumor tissues showed a lack of expression for thymidine synthetase (TS) and a diminished expression of excision repair cross-complementation group 1 (ERCC1), suggesting a potential benefit from capecitabine and oxaliplatin, respectively. Moreover, next-generation sequencing (NGS) of tumor genomic DNA showed no pathogenic mutation in the tested genes. In particular, no pathogenic mutation was detected in the genes *TP53*, *CTNNB1*, *BRCA1*, *BRCA2*, *BRAF*, *KRAS*, *EGFR*, and *PIK3CA* (Table 2).

Table 1. Biomarker analysis and associated therapies.

Test	Method	Result	Value	Conditions for a Positive Results	Potential Benefit	Therapies
TS	IHC	Negative	0 + 100%	≥1 + ≥10%	Yes	capecitabine, fluorouracil, pemetrexed
ERCC1	IHC	Negative	2 + 5%	≥3 + ≥10% or ≥2 + ≥50%	Yes	carboplatin, cisplatin, oxaliplatin
TUBB3	IHC	Negative	0 + 100%	≥2 + ≥30%	Yes	docetaxel, *nab*-paclitaxel, paclitaxel
TOP2A	IHC	Negative	2 + 3%	≥1 + ≥10%	No	doxorubicin, epirubicin, liposomal doxorubicin
TOPO1	IHC	Positive	2 + 50%	≥2 + ≥30%	Yes	irinotecan, topotecan
HER2/Neu	CISH, IHC, NGS	Not amplified, Negative			No	adotrastuzumab emtansine (T-DM1), pertuzumab, trastuzumab, lapatinib
ALK	RNA-Seq	Fusion not detected			No	ceritinib, crizotinib
ROS1	RNA-Seq	Fusion not detected			No	crizotinib

The immunohistochemical analyses were developed by Caris MPI, Inc. d/b/a Caris Life Sciences®, which also determine their performance characteristics. The therapies with potential benefits are based on the body of evidence, overall clinical utility, competing biomarker interactions, and tumor type from which the evidence was gathered, as listed in www.carislifesciences.com. The value represents the staining intensity and the percent of cells showing staining. ALK: anaplastic lymphoma kinase. CISH: chromogenic in-situ hybridization. ERCC1: excision repair cross-complementation group 1. HER2/Neu: human epidermal growth factor receptor 2. IHC: immunohistochemistry. RNA-Seq: RNA sequencing. ROS1: avian UR2 sarcoma virus oncogene. TOP2A: DNA topoisomerase II alpha. TOPO1: DNA topoisomerase I. TS: thymidine synthetase. TUBB3: tubulin beta 3 class III.

Table 2. Tumor genomic DNA analysis by next-generation sequencing for genetic mutations.

ABL1	BRCA2	EGFR	HRAS	NF1	RET
AKT1	c-KIT	HER2/Neu (ERBB2)	IDH1	NOTCH1	ROS1
ALK	CDK4	ERBB3	IDH2	NRAS	SMO
Androgen Receptor	CDKN2A	FGFR1	JAK2	NTRK1	SRC
APC	CHEK1	FGFR2	KDR (VEGFR2)	PDGFRA	TP53
ARAF	CHEK2	FGFR3	KRAS	PDGFRB	VHL
ATM	cMET	FLT3	MEK1	PIK3CA	WT1
BAP1	CSF1R	GNA11	MEK2	PTCH1	
BRAF	CTNNB1	GNAQ	MLH1	PTEN	
BRCA1	DDR2	GNAS	MPL	RAF1	

Using the Illumina NextSeq platform, a direct sequence analysis was performed on the genomic DNA isolated from a formalin-fixed paraffin-embedded tumor sample. This analysis can detect all variants with >99% confidence based on the mutational frequency present as well as the amplicon coverage. This test is sensitive enough to detect as little as a 10% population of cells containing a genomic mutation. The details can be found at www.carislifesciences.com.

On the basis of the tumor molecular profile, treatment with capecitabine, oxaliplatin, and bevacizumab (CAPOX-B) was initiated. The selection of this regimen (CAPOX-B) was based on results of the phase II study in patients with advanced HCC. The combination appeared efficacious and tolerable. This study demonstrated a median PFS of 6.8 months, a median overall survival (OS) of 9.8 months, a partial response rate of 20%, and a disease control rate of 77.5% [15]. For every 21-day cycle of the CAPOX-B regimen, capecitabine (825 mg/m^2) was administered orally twice daily on day 1 through to day 14, oxaliplatin (130 mg/m^2) was administered intravenously on day 1, and bevacizumab (5 mg/kg) was administered intravenously on day 1. Following treatment with three cycles of CAPOX-B, CT scans revealed a decrease in the size of the hepatic and omental lesions with stable osseous and peri-portal lymphadenopathy (Figure 3A). After another three cycles of therapy, CT scans showed a continued decrease in the size of the hepatic, lymph nodal, and omental lesions (Figure 3B).

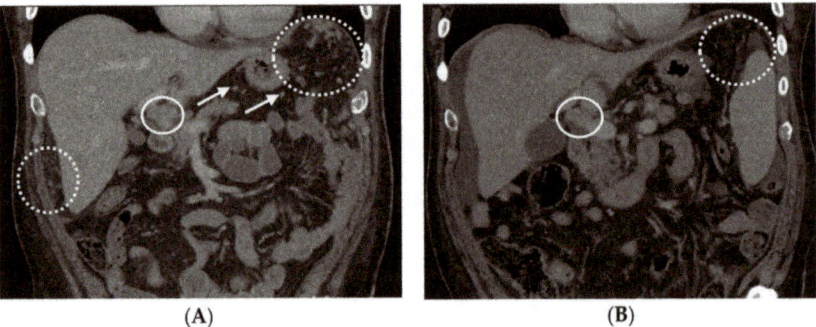

Figure 3. Following cycle 3 and cycle 6 with capecitabine, oxaliplatin, and bevacizumab (CAPOX-B), the CT scans showed tumor response. (**A**) Following cycle 3 with CAPOX-B, the coronal contrast-enhanced CT scans demonstrate innumerable left sub-diaphragmatic and peri-hepatic omental nodules (dashed circles) along with peri-gastric nodules (several annotated by arrows) consistent with omental carcinomatosis and mesenteric metastases. Peri-portal lymphadenopathy can be observed in the solid circle. (**B**) Following cycle 6 with CAPOX-B, the coronal contrast-enhanced CT scans demonstrate a decrease in omental metastases (dashed circle) and peri-portal lymphadenopathy (solid circle), and a small amount of peri-hepatic ascites.

Following cycle 9 with CAPOX-B, the CT scans showed stable hepatic and metastatic lesions (Figure 4A). The hepatic and metastatic lesions remained unchanged following cycle 15 with CAPOX-B, as shown in the CT scans (Figure 4B). The patient went on to receive a total of 18 cycles of CAPOX-B; the disease eventually progressed as evidenced by new and enlarged hepatic masses in the CT scans based on Response Evaluation Criteria in Solid Tumors (RECIST) guideline version 1.1 (Figure 5). Clinically, the patient experienced fatigue, ascites, and edema in the bilateral lower extremities, all grade 3 according to the Common Terminology Criteria for Adverse Events (CTCAE Version 4.0). At that time, the patient decided to pursue the option of home hospice and he subsequently expired at home.

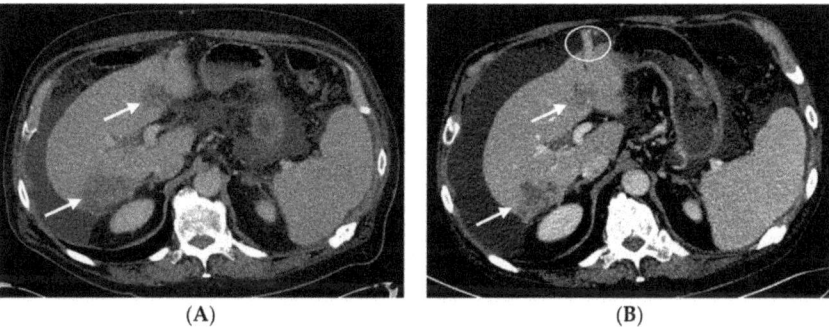

Figure 4. The tumors remained stable following cycle 9 and cycle 15 with CAPOX-B. (**A**) Following cycle 9 with CAPOX-B, the axial contrast-enhanced CT scans demonstrate stable heterogeneous hepatic tumors (arrows) compatible with a diagnosis of hepatocellular carcinoma. The right hepatic lobe tumor is subcapsular in location. There are small peri-hepatic and peri-gastric ascites. (**B**) Following cycle 15 with CAPOX-B, the axial contrast-enhanced CT scans demonstrate persistent heterogeneously enhanced hepatic tumors of a stable size (arrows). Progressive peri-hepatic and peri-gastric ascites with recanalized para-umbilical vein (circle) and splenomegaly can be seen.

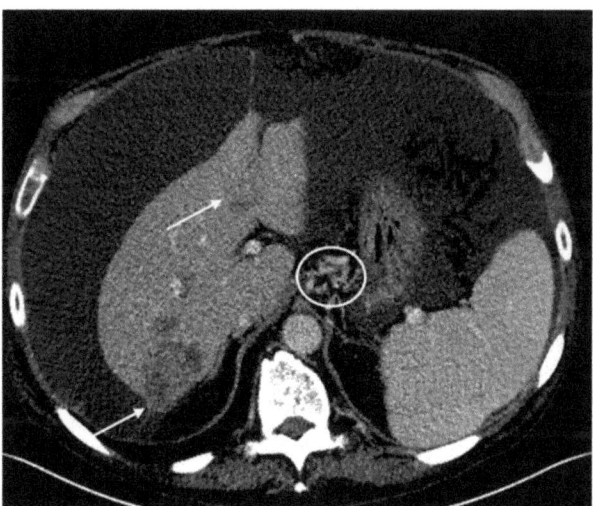

Figure 5. Following cycle 18 with CAPOX-B, there was evidence of tumor progression in the CT scans on the basis of the Response Evaluation Criteria in Solid Tumors (RECIST) guideline version 1.1. Axial contrast-enhanced CT scans demonstrate enlarging heterogeneous hepatic tumors (arrows). The larger right hepatic tumor now measures 6.3 cm with an exophytic component. There is a large-volume abdominal ascites that has progressively increased in size, with gastrohepatic varices (circle).

2.2. Patient #2

In contrast to patient #1, another patient with recurrent metastatic HCC was treated using a similar regimen of chemotherapy; he had a relatively short PFS and a distinct tumor molecular profile. Patient #2 is a 57-year-old Caucasian man who underwent an orthotopic liver transplantation (in April 2015) because of HCC, in the setting of a hepatitis C viral infection and hepatic cirrhosis. A pathological examination of the native liver revealed multiple foci of moderately differentiated HCC, stage pT3b, pN1, and the portal vein margin was also affected by invasive carcinoma. The past medical history was significant for hepatitis C viral infection (genotype 1; previously treated with sofosbuvir and ribavirin), hepatic cirrhosis, hypertension, aortic stenosis, and insulin-dependent diabetes mellitus. The family history was significant for "liver cancer" in his brother, colon cancer in his brother, thyroid cancer in his sister, and "cancer of type unknown to patient" in his brother. He had worked as a machine operator. He had previously smoked one pack of cigarettes daily for 30 years and he admitted to previous consumption of alcohol and intravenous drug use. At clinical presentation, he complained of fatigue and incisional pain, but denied suffering from nausea, vomiting, and diarrhea. The physical examination was remarkable for a mildly distended abdomen and chronic 1+ pitting edema in the bilateral lower extremities; there was no scleral icterus or jaundice. The serum AFP-liver level was normal at 2.1 ng/mL, and AFP-L3 was elevated at 39.1%. Surveillance CT scans (in January 2015) showed a new small thrombus within the right portal vein.

Between May and December 2015, this patient received eight cycles of adjuvant doxorubicin and sorafenib. For every 21-day cycle, doxorubicin (60 mg/m^2) was administered intravenously on day 1, and two tablets of sorafenib (200 mg) were administered orally every 12 h continuously [16]. In December 2015, surveillance CT scans showed a new 2 cm × 1.4 cm mass in the lower lobe of the left lung and an enlarged and enhanced (tumor) thrombus within the portal vein. The biopsy of the pulmonary mass revealed metastatic carcinoma. He received stereotactic body radiation therapy (SBRT) to the tumor thrombus in the portal vein (in February 2016) and to the tumor in the left lung lobe (in March 2016). CT scans in April 2016 showed an enlarged left lower lung mass and new bilateral adrenal nodules corresponding to metastases. The serum AFP-liver level and AFP-L3 were both elevated at 20.4 ng/mL and 67.4%, respectively.

A tumor molecular profiling of the metastatic carcinoma biopsied from the left lower lobe of the lung was performed using formalin-fixed paraffin-embedded tumor tissues by Caris® Life Sciences (https://www.carislifesciences.com/cmi-overview/). The results of the analyses by IHC, CISH, and RNA-Seq revealed the expression levels of biomarkers and the associated chemotherapy agents with potential benefits (Table 3). There was a decreased expression of ERCC1, suggesting the potential benefits of oxaliplatin. However, TS levels were increased, predicting a potential lack of benefits of capecitabine. The mutational analysis of genomic DNA by NGS was significant for pathogenic mutations in both *TP53* (exon 6, Y220C) and *CTNNB1* (exon 3, S37Y); there was no detected pathogenic mutation in the other genes tested.

In April 2016, the patient was started on a treatment plan using a combination of sorafenib, oxaliplatin, and capecitabine (SECOX) [17]. This regimen was previously shown to produce anti-tumor activity and was tolerable, with no treatment-related death being reported. In this single-arm, multi-center, phase II study, 51 patients with advanced HCC were enrolled and treated with the SECOX regimen. The best response rate was 16% (all partial response), the median PFS was 5.26 months, and the median OS was 11.73 months [18]. For every 14-day cycle of the SECOX regimen, two tablets of sorafenib (200 mg) were administered orally every 12 h continuously, two tablets of capecitabine (500 mg) were administered orally every 12 h on day 1 through to day 7, and 85 mg/m^2 of oxaliplatin was administered intravenously on day 1.

Following cycle 4 of SECOX, the patient tolerated the treatment well without specific complaints. CT scans in June 2016 showed a mixed response including an interval progression of the infiltrative disease within the liver, slightly enlarged bilateral adrenals nodules, an enlarged small right upper lung lobe, and a reduction in size of the left lower lung lobe. The serum AFP-liver level and AFP-L3 were both increased, being 55 ng/mL and 55.2%, respectively. The patient received a further four cycles of SECOX with a slightly increased dosage of oxaliplatin (having been previously reduced because of thrombocytopenia). In August 2016, CT scans showed progression of the disease in the right upper lung lobe, liver, adrenals, and peritoneum on the basis of the RECIST guideline v1.1. The serum AFP-liver level and AFP-L3 both rose further to 78.3 ng/mL and 60.9%, respectively. SECOX was subsequently discontinued. PFS was 3.7 months. At that time, the patient experienced grade 1 nausea/emesis/diarrhea and transient grade 1 oxaliplatin-induced cold hypersensitivity (CTCAE v4.0). Prior to starting regorafenib for treatment, he expired at home.

Table 3. Biomarker analysis and associated therapies.

Test	Method	Result	Value	Potential Benefit	Therapies
TS	IHC	Positive	1 + 10%	No	capecitabine, fluorouracil, pemetrexed
ERCC1	IHC	Negative	2 + 35%	Yes	carboplatin, cisplatin, oxaliplatin
TUBB3	IHC	Negative	1 + 90%	Yes	docetaxel, nab-paclitaxel, paclitaxel
TOP2A	IHC	Positive	2 + 20%	Yes	doxorubicin, epirubicin, liposomal doxorubicin
TOPO1	IHC	Positive	2 + 80%	Yes	irinotecan, topotecan

Value represents staining intensity and percent of cells showing staining. ERCC1: excision repair cross-complementation group 1. IHC: immunohistochemistry. TOPO1: DNA topoisomerase I. TOP2A: DNA topoisomerase II alpha. TS: thymidine synthase. TUBB3: tubulin beta class III.

2.3. Timeline

The clinical data of both patients #1 and #2, including diagnosis, treatment, the key result of tumor molecular profiles, and responses to treatment, are summarized as a timeline as illustrated in Figure 6.

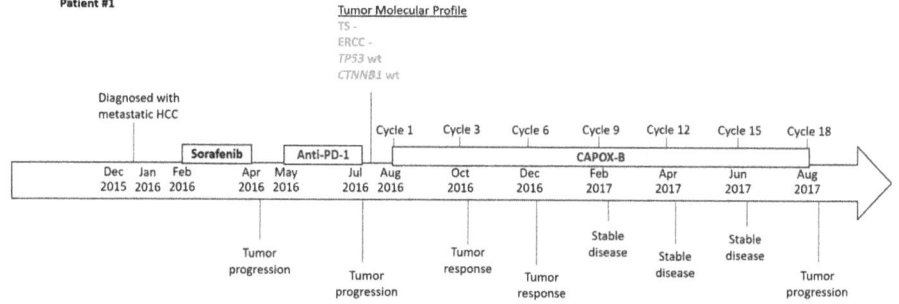

Figure 6. Cont.

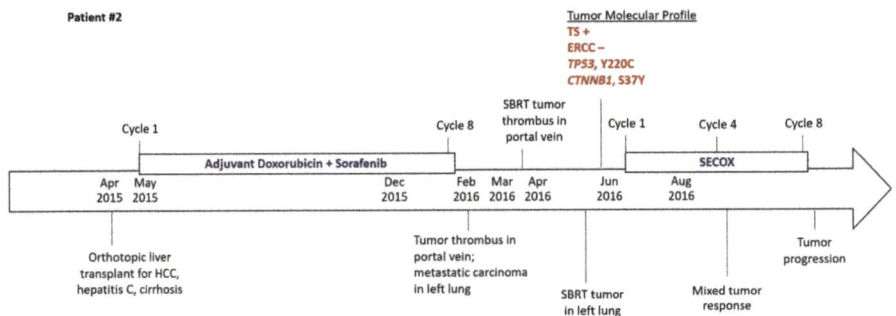

Figure 6. Timeline to illustrate the chronology of treatment and responses to treatment for patients #1 and #2 and the key data of their tumor molecular profiles.

3. Discussion

In this case study, we present two patients who had different clinical features regarding the etiology of HCC and treatment responses. The molecular profiling of their tumors were distinct in the expression of biochemical markers and genomic DNA mutations. In particular, patient #1 showed an unusually good tumor response with CAPOX-B, and his tumor molecular profiling indicated a negative expression of TS and ERCC1, as well as a lack of pathogenic mutations in the *TP53* and *CTNNB1* genes. In contrast, patient #2 received eight cycles of SECOX with a PFS of 3.7 months, and his tumor molecular profiling showed negative expression of ERCC1, but increased expression of TS, and also pathogenic mutations in both the *TP53* and the *CTNNB1* genes. It is known that *TP53* and *CTNNB1* are the two most common mutations in HCC and they contribute to tumor resistance to chemotherapeutic agents. These data suggest that the tumor molecular profile of HCC may correlate with the treatment efficacy as determined by PFS.

HCC is generally considered resistant to cytotoxic chemotherapeutic drugs, but treatment responses of tumors are variable among patients. Currently, there is no predictive biomarker of treatment response for patients with HCC. These cases highlight the value of molecular profiling in HCC, especially in patients with advanced and/or metastatic HCC that has progressed following standard therapies. Patient #1 had a PFS of 12.3 months; this is well beyond the median PFS of 6.8 months as reported in the phase II trials using CAPOX or nivolumab [6,14], and almost twice as long as the median PFS in the study evaluating CAPOX-B as a first-line treatment [15]. Given the patient's negative IHC analysis for TS and ERCC1 and the lack of pathogenic mutations in the tested genes, we hypothesize that his robust response to CAPOX-B was related to a favorable molecular profile. His response to CAPOX-B was particularly impressive, considering his PFS in response to CAPOX-B as a third-line treatment. On the other hand, patient #2 had a relatively short PFS of 3.7 months, less than the median PFS of 5.26 months as reported in the phase II study evaluating the efficacy of SECOX in advanced HCC [18]. Similarly, we hypothesize that patient #2's low response to SECOX was related to his molecular profile which showed a potential lack of benefit from capecitabine and exhibited pathogenic mutations in two key genes, *TP53* and *CTNNB1*. No data on tumor molecular profiling were available from the previous phase II studies that investigated CAPOX-B and SECOX.

How the etiology of HCC contributes to therapeutic responsiveness or resistance is unclear, though the various modalities of treatment for patients with HCC have been the same in clinical practice regardless of their etiology. While the etiology of patient #1's HCC is unclear, patient #2 undoubtedly had developed HCC as a consequence of a hepatitis C viral infection and hepatic cirrhosis. It is noteworthy that the tumor profile of patient #1 showed negative TS expression and no pathogenic mutation in *TP53*, and that of patient #2 showed positive TS expression with pathogenic mutation in *TP53*; such an association is consistent with the data of a previous study [11]. Nevertheless, it will be important to determine any association between the etiology of HCC and the tumor molecular profiles, as well as the clinical efficacy of systemic treatments including chemotherapy.

4. Conclusions and Future Perspectives

This case study sheds new light on the potential value of molecular profiling of advanced/metastatic HCC in terms of guiding treatment. However, definitive conclusions on the clinical utility of the tumor molecular profiles of HCC as predictive biomarkers cannot be drawn based on the limited scope of the data from these case reports. Retrospective studies using data from a large patient population are indicated to correlate biomarkers with treatment responses. Ultimately, a prospective clinical study will be needed to test the hypothesis that molecular profile-based biomarkers can predict clinical outcomes. Our goal is to identify and develop predictive biomarkers for treatment response in order to help guide the selection of personalized therapy for patients with HCC.

Acknowledgments: We wish to express our sincere gratitude for the two patients described in this case study. Informed consent by the two patients could not be obtained since they expired at home prior to the preparation of this manuscript. Moreover, the Human Subjects Protection Office of the Penn State Health Milton S. Hershey Medical Center determined that this case study (Study ID: STUDY00008982, Version Date: 15 January 2018) does not meet the definition of human subject research as defined in 45 CFR 46.102(d) and/or (f); Institutional Review Board (IRB) review and approval is not required. No grant has been received in support of this research work. No fund was received for covering the costs to publish in open access.

Author Contributions: Nelson S. Yee provided patient history. Kristine Posadas and Nelson S. Yee analyzed the molecular profiling data and reviewed the literature. Anita Ankola evaluated the radiographical images and provided the figures with CT and MRI scans. Zhaohai Yang examined the biopsied epidural metastatic tumor and provided the figure with histopathology and immunohistochemical analysis. Kristine Posadas, Anita Ankola, Zhaohai Yang, and Nelson S. Yee wrote the paper.

Conflicts of Interest: The authors declare no conflict of interest.

References

1. Siegel, R.L.; Miller, K.D.; Jemal, A. Cancer statistics, 2018. *CA Cancer J. Clin.* **2018**, *68*, 7–30. [CrossRef] [PubMed]
2. Benson, A.B.; D'Angelica, M.I.; Abbott, D.E.; Abrams, T.A.; Alberts, S.R.; Anaya, D.A.; Are, C.; Brown, D.B.; Chang, D.T.; Covey, A.M.; et al. NCCN Guidelines Insights Hepatobiliary cancers, Version 1.2017. Featured updates to the NCCN Guidelines. *J. Natl. Compr. Cancer Netw.* **2017**, *15*, 563–573. [CrossRef]
3. Marks, E.I.; Yee, N.S. Molecular genetics and targeted therapy in hepatocellular carcinoma. *Curr. Cancer Drug Target* **2015**, *16*, 53–70. [CrossRef]
4. Forner, A.; Reig, M.; Bruix, J. Hepatocellular carcinoma. *Lancet* **2018**, *391*, 1301–1314. [CrossRef]
5. Bruix, J.; Qin, S.; Merle, P.; Granito, A.; Huang, Y.H.; Bodoky, G.; Pracht, M.; Yokosuka, O.; Rosmorduc, O.; Breder, V.; et al. Regorafenib for patients with hepatocellular carcinoma who progressed on sorafenib treatment (RESORCE): A randomized, double-blind, placebo-controlled, phase 3 trial. *Lancet* **2017**, *389*, 56–66. [CrossRef]
6. El-Khoueiry, A.B.; Sangro, B.; Yau, T.; Crocenzi, T.S.; Kudo, M.; Hsu, C.; Kim, T.Y.; Choo, S.P.; Trojan, J.; Welling, T.H., 3rd; et al. Nivolumab in patients with advanced hepatocellular carcinoma (CheckMate 040): An open-label, non-comparative, phase 1/2 dose escalation and expansion trial. *Lancet* **2017**, *389*, 2492–2502. [CrossRef]
7. Benson, A.B.; Abrams, T.A.; Ben-Josef, E.; Bloomston, P.M.; Botha, J.F.; Clary, B.M.; Covey, A.; Curley, S.A.; D'Angelica, M.I.; Davila, R.; et al. The NCCN Hepatobiliary Cancers Clinical Practice Guidelines in Oncology. *J. Natl. Compr. Cancer Netw.* **2009**, *7*, 350–391. [CrossRef]
8. Nhieu, J.T.; Renard, C.A.; Wei, Y.; Cherqui, D.; Zafrani, E.S.; Buendia, M.A. Nuclear accumulation of mutated β-catenin in hepatocellular carcinoma is associated with increased cell proliferation. *Am. J. Pathol.* **1999**, *155*, 703–710. [CrossRef]
9. Lai, P.B.; Chi, T.Y.; Chen, G.G. Different levels of p53 induced either apoptosis or cell cycle arrest in a doxycycline-regulated hepatocellular carcinoma cell line in vitro. *Apoptosis* **2007**, *12*, 387–393. [CrossRef] [PubMed]

10. Zhan, P.; Ji, Y.-N.; Yu, L.-K. TP53 mutation is associated with a poor outcome for patients with hepatocellular carcinoma: Evidence from a meta-analysis. *Hepatobiliary Surg. Nutr.* **2013**, *2*, 260–265. [CrossRef] [PubMed]
11. Ang, C.; Miura, J.T.; Gamblin, T.C.; He, R.; Xiu, J.; Millis, S.Z.; Gatalica, Z.; Reddy, S.K.; Yee, N.S.; Abou-Alfa, G.K. Comprehensive multiplatform biomarker analysis of 350 hepatocellular carcinomas identifies potential novel therapeutic options. *J. Surg. Oncol.* **2016**, *113*, 55–61. [CrossRef] [PubMed]
12. Qiu, L.X.; Tang, Q.Y.; Bai, J.L.; Qian, X.P.; Li, R.T.; Liu, B.R.; Zheng, M.H. Predictive value of thymidylate synthase expression in advanced colorectal cancer patients receiving fluoropyrimidine-based chemotherapy: Evidence from 24 studies. *Int. J. Cancer* **2008**, *123*, 2384–2389. [CrossRef] [PubMed]
13. Li, P.; Fang, Y.-J.; Li, F.; Ou, Q.J.; Chen, G.; Ma, G. ERCC1, defective mismatch repair status as predictive biomarkers of survival for stage III colon cancer patients receiving oxaliplatin-based adjuvant chemotherapy. *Br. J. Cancer* **2013**, *108*, 1238–1244. [CrossRef] [PubMed]
14. Boige, V.; Raoul, J.-L.; Pignon, J.-P.; Bouche, O.; Blanc, J.F.; Dahan, L.; Jouve, J.L.; Dupouy, N.; Ducreux, M. Multicentre phase II trial of capecitabine plus oxaliplatin (XELOX) in patients with advanced hepatocellular carcinoma: FFCD 03-03 trial. *Br. J. Cancer* **2007**, *97*, 862–867. [CrossRef] [PubMed]
15. Sun, W.; Sohal, D.; Haller, D.G.; Mykulowycz, K.; Rosen, M.; Soulen, M.C.; Caparro, M.; Teitelbaum, U.R.; Giantonio, B.; O'dwyer, P.J.; et al. Phase 2 trial of bevacizumab, capecitabine, and oxaliplatin in treatment of advanced hepatocellular carcinoma. *Cancer* **2011**, *117*, 3187–3192. [CrossRef] [PubMed]
16. Abou-Alfa, G.K.; Johnson, P.; Knox, J.J.; Capanu, M.; Davidenko, I.; Lacava, J.; Leung, T.; Gansukh, B.; Saltz, L.B. Doxorubicin plus sorafenib vs doxorubicin alone in patients with advanced hepatocellular carcinoma: A randomized trial. *JAMA* **2010**, *304*, 2154–2160. [CrossRef] [PubMed]
17. Chiu, J.; Tang, V.; Chan, P.; Leung, R.; Wong, H.; Poon, R.T.P.; Fan, S.T.; Yau, T. The use of SECOX (sorafenib, oxaliplatin, capecitabine) as the treatment of advanced hepatocellular carcinoma (HCC)—A single center retrospective study. In Proceedings of the European Society for Medical Oncology, Vienna, Austria, 28 September–2 October 2012.
18. Yau, T.C.; Cheung, F.Y.; Lee, F.; Choo, S.P.; Wong, H.; Toh, H.C.; Leung, A.K.; Chan, P.; Yau, T.K.; Wong, J.; et al. A multicenter phase II study of sorafenib, capecitabine, and oxaliplatin (SECOX) in patients with advanced hepatocellular carcinoma: Final results of Hong Kong-Singapore Hepatocellular Carcinoma Research Collaborative Group Study. *J. Clin. Oncol.* **2017**. [CrossRef]

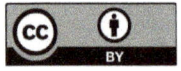

© 2018 by the authors. Licensee MDPI, Basel, Switzerland. This article is an open access article distributed under the terms and conditions of the Creative Commons Attribution (CC BY) license (http://creativecommons.org/licenses/by/4.0/).

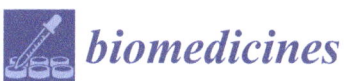

Conference Report

Update in Systemic and Targeted Therapies in Gastrointestinal Oncology

Nelson S. Yee

Division of Hematology-Oncology, Department of Medicine, Penn State Health Milton S. Hershey Medical Center, Experimental Therapeutics Program, Penn State Cancer Institute, The Pennsylvania State University College of Medicine, Hershey, PA 17033, USA; nyee@pennstatehealth.psu.edu; Tel.: +1-717-531-0003

Received: 1 January 2018; Accepted: 6 March 2018; Published: 16 March 2018

Abstract: Progress has been made in the treatment of gastrointestinal cancers through advances in systemic therapies, surgical interventions, and radiation therapy. At the Multi-Disciplinary Patient Care in Gastrointestinal Oncology conference, the faculty members of the Penn State Health Milton S. Hershey Medical Center presented a variety of topics that focused on this sub-specialty. This conference paper highlights the new development in systemic treatment of various malignant diseases in the digestive system. Results of the recent clinical trials that investigated the clinical efficacy of pegylated hyaluronidase, napabucasin, and L-asparaginase in pancreatic carcinoma are presented. The use of peri-operative chemotherapy comprised of 5-fluorouracil or capecitabine, leucovorin, oxaliplatin, and docetaxel (FLOT), and immunotherapy including pembrolizumab, nivolumab, and ipilimumab in gastroesophageal carcinoma are discussed. Data from clinical trials that investigated the targeted therapeutics including nivolumab, ramucirumab, lenvatinib, and BLU-554 are reported. The role of adjuvant capecitabine in resected biliary tract carcinoma (BTC) and nab-paclitaxel in combination with gemcitabine and cisplatin in advanced BTC are presented. In colorectal carcinoma, the efficacy of nivolumab, adjuvant FOLFOX or CAPOX, irinotecan/cetuximab/vemurafenib, and trifluridine/tipiracil/bevacizumab, is examined. In summary, some of the above systemic therapies have become or are expected to become new standard of care, while the others demonstrate the potential of becoming new treatment options.

Keywords: biliary tract carcinoma; chemotherapy; clinical trial; colorectal carcinoma; gastric carcinoma; gastrointestinal oncology; hepatocellular carcinoma; immunotherapy; pancreatic carcinoma; targeted therapy

---

1. Introduction

Cancers in the digestive system are among the most common malignant diseases worldwide, and are associated with relatively high mortality rates. Optimal caring of patients with malignant diseases of digestive organs requires the expertise of providers from multiple health disciplines. At the Multi-Disciplinary Patient Care in Gastrointestinal Oncology conference held on 29 September 2017 in Hershey, Pennsylvania, the faculty members of the Penn State Cancer Institute and Penn State Health Milton S. Hershey Medical Center presented a variety of topics that focused on this sub-specialty. These included presentations regarding the new frontiers in diagnostic and staging evaluation, surgical interventions, and radiation therapy. In particular, important advances in systemic chemotherapy, as well as the discovery of molecular biomarkers and therapeutic targets in those cancers, were discussed. This article focuses on the presentations about new development of systemic and targeted therapies in various malignancies of the digestive system.

2. Update of Systemic and Targeted Therapies

A number of advances have been made in the systemic and targeted treatment of cancers of the digestive organs. These include cancers in the pancreas, stomach and gastroesophageal junction, liver, biliary tract, colon, and rectum. Here is a summary of the most recent evidence on chemotherapy and targeted therapy in gastrointestinal oncology as presented at the international medical conferences and in the published medical literature. Those conferences were held in 2017, including Annual Conference of the American Society of Clinical Oncology, Annual Conference of the European Society of Medical Oncology World Gastrointestinal Congress, and the Annual Conference of the International Liver Cancer Association in Seoul, South Korea.

3. Pancreatic Carcinoma

Systemic chemotherapy plays important roles in the treatment of pancreatic carcinoma diagnosed at all stages [1]. New development has been focusing on targeted agents directed against the tumor microenvironment, cancer stem cells, and cellular metabolism [2]. In this section, highlights of the recent clinical trials investigating the clinical efficacy of (i) hyaluronidase that degrades tumor-associated stroma, (ii) napabucasin that targets cancer stem cells, and (iii) L-asparaginase that inhibits cellular metabolism, are reported.

3.1. Targeting Tumor-Associated Stroma Using Pegylated Hyaluronidase

A unique feature of pancreatic carcinoma is desmoplastic reaction, resulting in formation of a dense stroma that hinders delivery of therapeutic agents to the cancer cells. Hyaluronan is a component of the tumor-associated stroma, and pegylated hyaluronidase (PEGPH20) has been developed to degrade hyaluronan in order to facilitate delivery of chemotherapeutic agents to the cancer cells. In a phase II, open-label clinical study of 246 patients with metastatic pancreatic adenocarcinoma, nab-paclitaxel (125 mg/m^2 iv weekly for 3 weeks) + gemcitabine (1000 mg/m^2 iv weekly for 3 weeks) with or without PEGPH20 (3 µg/kg iv twice a week for cycle 1 and weekly for cycle 2 and beyond) were administered for every 4-weeks cycle (ClinicalTrials.gov identifier: NCT01839487). PEGPH20 in combination with nab-paclitaxel and gemcitabine significantly prolongs progression-free survival (PFS), as compared to nab-paclitaxel and gemcitabine (Table 1). The improvement of PFS is even greater for patients with tumors expressing high levels of HA, and this is also seen with overall survival (OS). Moreover, this study suggested that hyaluronic acid is a potential predictive biomarker of tumor response to PEGPH20 [3]. A phase III, randomized, double-blind, placebo-controlled, multicenter clinical study is ongoing to confirm the clinical efficacy of PEGPH20 in combination with nab-paclitaxel and gemcitabine (NCT02715804).

Table 1. Results of a phase II clinical study to investigate pegylated hyaluronidase in combination with nab-paclitaxel and gemcitabine in metastatic pancreatic carcinoma.

Outcomes	PEGPH20 + nab-Paclitaxel + Gemcitabine	nab-Paclitaxel + Gemcitabine
PFS (months) All patients	6.0 HR 0.73, * $P < 0.05$	5.3
PFS (months) HA-High (35%)	9.2 HR 0.51, * $P < 0.048$	5.2
OS (months) HA-High (35%)	11.5	8.5

HA: hyaluronan. HR: hazard ratio. OS: overall survival. PEGPH20: pegylated hyaluronidase. PFS: progression-free survival. * P indicates statistical significance.

3.2. Targeting Cancer Stem Cells by a STAT3 Inhibitor

Tumor metastasis and therapeutic resistance have been attributed to cancer stem cells. Targeting the cancer stem cells is expected to improve survival through improving anti-tumor response to treatment. A first-in-human clinical trial was conducted to investigate the clinical efficacy of napabucasin that targets cancer stem cells by inhibiting the activation of signal transducer and activator of transcription 3 (STAT3). In a phase 1b/II study of 66 patients (55 evaluable) with metastatic pancreatic adenocarcinoma, napabucasin 240 mg orally twice daily in combination with nab-paclitaxel (125 mg/m^2 iv) and gemcitabine (1000 mg/m^2 iv) was administered weekly for 3 weeks of every 4-week cycle until disease progression (NCT02231723). Results of this study indicate that the combination of napabucasin with nab-paclitaxel and gemcitabine produced anti-tumor response (Table 2) [4]. A phase III, open-label clinical study to confirm the efficacy of napabucasin in combination with nab-paclitaxel and gemcitabine in patients with metastatic pancreatic adenocarcinoma is ongoing (NCT02993731).

Table 2. Results of a phase I/II clinical study to investigate napabucasin in combination with *nab*-paclitaxel and gemcitabine in metastatic pancreatic adenocarcinoma.

Efficacy Endpoints	Outcome
Complete Response	1 (1.8%)
Partial Response	26 (47.3%)
Stable Disease	24 (43.6%)
Overall Response Rate	55%
Disease Control Rate	93%
Disease Progression	3 (on treatment), 1 after off treatment due to toxicity
Progression-Free Survival	7.1 months
1-Year Overall Survival Rate	56%

3.3. Targeting Asparagine by Enzymatic Degradation

Asparagine is an essential amino acid required for survival of pancreatic cancer cells, which have no or little asparagine synthetase to produce endogenous asparagine. Asparagine promotes proliferation of cancer cells through regulating serine uptake, influencing serine metabolism and thus synthesis of protein and nucleotides [5]. Eryaspase consists of L-asparaginase encapsulated within erythrocytes, and it hydrolyzes and depletes asparagine from the circulating blood plasma (http://erytech.com/ery-asp.html). In a phase IIb study, 140 patients with metastatic pancreatic carcinoma were randomized to receive eryaspase (100 IU/kg on day 3 and day 17 of every 4-weeks cycle) in combination with either gemcitabine or FOLFOX (5-fluorouracil, leucovorin, and oxaliplatin); versus chemotherapy alone (NCT02195180). Expression of asparagine synthetase was either none (0) or low (1) as determined by immunohistochemistry. Eryaspase in combination with either gemcitabine or FOLFOX significantly prolonged overall survival as compared to either gemcitabine or FOLFOX (26.1 weeks vs 19 weeks, HR 0.57, * P = 0.03) [6].

While some of the above clinical trials are ongoing, the evidence suggests that subsets of patients whose tumors with expression of certain molecular biomarkers likely benefit from the targeted therapeutic agents. Conceivably, patients with pancreatic carcinoma with high expression level of HA may benefit from addition of PEGPH20 to either nab-paclitaxel/gemcitabine or FOLFIRINOX. Those with pancreatic cancer cells with constitutively activated STAT3 may benefit from addition of napabucasin to nab-paclitaxel/gemcitabine. Pancreatic carcinoma with no or low level of expression of asparagine synthetase will likely be sensitive to treatment with eryaspase in combination with either gemcitabine or FOLFOX.

4. Gastric, Gastroesophageal Junction, and Esophageal Carcinoma

Systemic chemotherapy is the standard of care for patients with advanced or metastatic gastric carcinoma (GC), gastroesophageal junction carcinoma (GEJC), and esophageal carcinoma (EC). Monoclonal antibodies including trastuzumab directed against human epidermal growth factor receptor 2 (HER2) and ramucirumab that targets vascular endothelial growth factor receptor 2 (VEGFR2), either as single agents or in combination with chemotherapy, have become part of the standard of care for treatment of advanced GC and GEJC. For resectable GC or GEJC, chemotherapy improves the surgical outcome; whereas chemotherapy concurrent with radiation therapy with or without surgery can be potentially curable for localized EC. Immunotherapy has emerged as a new treatment option for patients with gastroesophageal carcinoma [7]. In this section, highlights of the clinical studies that investigated peri-operative chemotherapy and immunotherapy are discussed.

4.1. Peri-Operative FLOT in Resectable Tumors

For resectable GC or GEJC, peri-operative chemotherapy using epirubicin, cisplatin and either 5-fluorouracil or capecitabine (ECF and ECX, respectively) has been the standard of care. However, the survival benefit of this regimen remains limited. The combination of docetaxel, oxaliplatin, and either 5-fluorouracil or capecitabine (FLOT) produced survival benefit in advanced gastroesophageal carcinoma, but its clinical efficacy in resectable tumors had not been determined. In a phase III trial (FLOT4) of 716 patients with resectable GC or GEJC, peri-operative FLOT was compared with ECF or ECX. In the treatment group receiving FLOT, 4 pre-operative and 4 post-operative 2-week cycles of docetaxel 50 mg/m^2 iv, oxaliplatin 85 mg/m^2 iv, leucovorin 200 mg/m^2 iv, and 5-fluorouracil 2600 mg/m^2 as 24h iv infusion, all were administered on day 1. For the ECF or ECX treatment group, the patients received 3 pre-operative and 3 post-operative 3-week cycles of epirubicin 50 mg/m^2 iv and cisplatin 60 mg/m^2 iv both on day 1, and either 5-fluorouracil 200 mg/m^2/24 h continuous iv infusion or capecitabine 1250 mg/m^2 orally on day 1 through day 21 (NCT01216644). Results of this study showed that, as compared to either ECF or ECX, FLOT significantly prolonged PFS and OS, associated with lower rate of disease progression, and increased rate of complete resection of tumors (Table 3). ECF or ECX was associated with more grade 3 or 4 nausea and emesis than FLOT, which was associated with more grade 3 or 4 neutropenia [8]. This study supports peri-operative FLOT as the new standard of systemic treatment for patients with resectable GC or GEJC.

Table 3. Results of peri-operative FLOT in patients with resectable gastric or gastroesophageal junction carcinoma.

Regimens	PFS (Months)	OS (Months)	PD during or after Pre-Op	pT0/T1	R0 Resection
FLOT	30 HR 0.75, * P = 0.004	50 HR 0.77, * P = 0.012	1% * P = 0.001	25% * P = 0.001	84% * P = 0.001
ECF or ECX	18	35	5%	15%	77%

ECF: epirubicin, cisplatin, 5-fluorouracil. ECX: epirubicin, cisplatin, capecitabine. FLOT: 5-fluorouracil, leucovorin, oxaliplatin, docetaxel. OS: overall survival. PD: progression of disease. PFS: progression-free survival. * P indicates statistical significance.

4.2. Pembrolizumab in PD-L1-Expressing Gastric and Gastroesophageal Carcinoma

In a phase I clinical study, the anti-programmed death-1 (anti-PD-1) antibody pembrolizumab exhibited anti-tumor activity in patients with previously treated advanced GC. In a phase II clinical study, 259 patients with recurrent or metastatic GC or GCJC that have progressed on 2 or more prior chemotherapy received pembrolizumab (200 mg iv every 21 days) (KEYNOTE-059, NCT02335411). Pembrolizumab significantly improved response rate and overall survival beyond 2nd line treatment in patients with advanced GC or GEJC expressing PD-L1 ($\geq$1% expression of PD-L1). The overall response rate (ORR) is 16.4% in all patients. Among patients with $\geq$1% expression of PD-L1, ORR 22.7%, vs. 8.6%

if PD-L1 negative [9]. Results of this study has led to US FDA approval of pembrolizumab for treatment of patients with advanced, PD-L1-positive ($\geq$1%) GC or GEJC that have progressed following 2 or more lines of therapy.

4.3. Nivolumab and Ipilimumab in Gastric, Gastroesophageal Junction, and Esophageal Carcinoma

A combination of immune checkpoint inhibitors was investigated in advanced GC, GEJC, and EC. In a previous phase III clinical study (ONO-12), the anti-PD-1 antibody nivolumab has been shown to prolong overall survival (OS), as compared to placebo, as a 3rd-line or beyond treatment in Asian patients with advanced GC or GEJC [10]. In a phase I/II study, nivolumab in combination with or without the anti-CTLA4 antibody, ipilimumab, produced anti-tumor activity in Western patients with advanced GC, GEJC, and EC (CheckMate 032, NCT01928394). The data of a long-term follow-up of the CheckMate 032 study were reported [11]. In the phase II study, nivolumab either alone or in combination with ipilimumab showed durable anti-tumor responses in metastatic GC or GEJC, particularly in tumors expressing PD-L1 ($\geq$1%), and also long-term OS in those Western patients with previously treated GC, GEJC, and EC (Table 4).

Table 4. Results of a phase II clinical study to investigate nivolumab and ipilimumab in metastatic gastric or gastroesophageal junction carcinoma.

Outcomes	Nivolumab (3 mg/kg) Every 2 Weeks	Nivolumab (1 mg/kg) + Ipilimumab (3 mg/kg) every 3 Weeks	Nivolumab (3 mg/kg) + Ipilimumab (1 mg/kg) Every 3 Weeks
ORR (%)	12	24	8
ORR (%) PD-L1 $\geq$ 1%	19	40	23
ORR (%) PD-L1 $\leq$ 1%	12	22	0
OS (months)	6.2	6.9	4.8

ORR: overall response rate. OS: overall survival.

4.4. Pembrolizumab in PD-L1-Expressing Esophageal Carcinoma

For patients with advanced or metastatic EC, the conventionally used systemic chemotherapy has been extrapolated from evidence of clinical studies in GC or GEJC. In a phase IB study, pembrolizumab was investigated in patients with PD-L1-positive advanced esophageal carcinoma (KEYNOTE-028, NCT02054806). Among the 83 patients being evaluated, 37 (45%) had PD-L1-positive tumors and 23 patients were enrolled. ORR was 30% (95% CI, 13% to 53%), and median duration of response 15 months (6 to 26 months). Treatment-related adverse events were reported in 9 patients, and those most commonly include anorexia, lymphocytopenia, and skin rash. There were no grade 4 pembrolizumab-related adverse events or deaths. Increased tumor response and delayed tumor progression were associated with relatively high interferon-γ composite scores. It was concluded that pembrolizumab produced durable anti-tumor activity and manageable toxicity in patients with pretreated, PD-L1-positive advanced esophageal carcinoma [12].

The promising data of the above mentioned clinical studies are expected to create new opportunities of effective treatment for patients with GC, GEJC, and EC. While pembrolizumab has been FDA-approved as a 3rd-line or beyond treatment of advanced GC and GEJC expressing PD-L1, the potential use of pembrolizumab either alone or in combination with cytotoxic chemotherapy is being explored as 1st-line treatment. Meanwhile, nivolumab, either as a single agent or in combination with ipilimumab, may provide additional treatment options for patients with GC, GEJC, and EC. The use of peri-operative FLOT is expected to be the new standard of care for patients with resectable GC and GEJC. However, this regimen tends to be associated with severe

5. Hepatocellular Carcinoma

For patients with advanced or metastatic hepatocellular carcinoma (HCC), sorafenib is the standard first-line treatment. For HCC that has progressed following treatment with sorafenib, regorafenib as a second-line treatment provides survival benefit. However, treatment using sorafenib or regorafenib is palliative, and the clinical benefits of these targeted agents are somewhat limited [13]. Results of clinical trials that investigated the clinical efficacy of targeted therapeutic agents including nivolumab, ramucirumab, lenvatinib, and BLU-554 have recently been reported.

5.1. Nivolumab

The efficacy of nivolumab, an anti-PD-1 antibody, was investigated in sorafenib naïve or sorafenib-treated patients with advanced HCC. In this clinical study (CheckMate 040), 262 patients were enrolled and 98% of them had hepatic cirrhosis of Child-Pugh scores 5–6. In both groups of subjects, those who had never received sorafenib and those who had previously been treated with sorafenib, nivolumab showed anti-tumor response to varying extent (Table 5). Importantly, nivolumab produced tumor responses regardless of the etiology of HCC or tumor expression of PD-L1. Based on results of this study, FDA approved nivolumab for treatment of patients with HCC following prior sorafenib regardless of PD-L1 status [14].

Table 5. Results of a clinical study to investigate nivolumab in advanced hepatocellular carcinoma.

Outcomes	Sorafenib-Naïve ($n = 80$)	Sorafenib-Treated ($n = 182$)
Overall response rate	24%	19%
Complete response	1%	1%
Partial response	19%	13%
Stable disease	34%	41%
Disease control rate	63%	56%

In the CheckMate-040 study, the efficacy of nivolumab was further evaluated in a subgroup of 154 patients with HCC who progressed on sorafenib or who were intolerant to sorafenib with additional eligibility criteria (NCT01658878). By assessment using RECIST v1.1, the overall response rate (ORR) was 14.3%, complete response (CR) 1.9%, and partial response (PR) 12.3%. Among those who responded to nivolumab, 91% of the patients had a response duration ≥ 6 months, and 55% with duration ≥ 12 months. Assessment using modified RECIST criteria, the efficacy of nivolumab is even greater, with ORR 18.2%, CR 3.2%, and PR 14.9%.

However, nivolumab is associated with the risk of various immune-related adverse reactions. Skin rash is relatively common. Other reactions include pneumonitis, colitis, hepatitis, endocrinopathies (in hypophysis, adrenal, thyroid, endocrine pancreas), nephritis, encephalitis, and infusion-related. These reactions may require treatment with corticosteroids. Depending on the severity of the reactions, nivolumab may need to be withheld or discontinued.

5.2. Ramucirumab

Hepatocellular carcinogenesis is promoted by tumor-associated neo-angiogenesis, and vascular endothelial growth factor (VEGF) and receptor-induced signaling plays an important role [13]. The anti-VEGF antibody bevacizumab was previously investigated in advanced HCC without proven clinical benefit. Ramucirumab is a monoclonal antibody directed against VEGFR2 and it produced anti-tumor response in colon, gastric and gastroesophageal junction, and pulmonary carcinoma. The anti-tumor effect of ramucirumab in HCC was previously known.

In a phase III trial (REACH), the clinical efficacy of ramucirumab was investigated in patients with advanced HCC. In this study, 643 patients with advanced HCC who had previously been treated with sorafenib, were randomized to receive ramucirumab or placebo. Results of this study showed that ramucirumab produced statistically significant improvement of the hazard ratio of HCC in patients with hepatic cirrhosis of Child-Pugh 5. The efficacy is further increased in patients with hepatic cirrhosis of Child-Pugh 5 and serum AFP $\geq$ 400 ng/mL (Table 6). Thus, ramucirumab produced survival benefit in patients with advanced HCC, particularly those with hepatic cirrhosis of Child-Pugh Class A (score 5 or 6) and serum AFP $\geq$ 400 ng/mL [15].

Table 6. Results of a phase III clinical study to investigate ramucirumab in advanced hepatocellular carcinoma.

Outcomes	Ramucirumab vs. Placebo	Ramucirumab vs. Placebo (AFP $\geq$ 400 ng/mL)
HR (Child-Pugh 5)	0.80 (P = 0.06)	0.61 (* P = 0.01)
HR (Child-Pugh 6)	0.96 (P = 0.76)	0.64 (* P = 0.04)
HR (Child-Pugh 7 or 8)	1.00 (P > 0.99)	0.67 (P = 0.28)

AFP: Alpha fetoprotein; HR: Hazard Ratio. * P indicates statistical significance.

5.3. Lenvatinib

Lenvatinib is a small molecule inhibitor of receptor tyrosine kinases (RTKs) involved in neo-angiogenesis by inhibiting the kinase activities of VEGFR1, 2, and 3. Lenvatinib also inhibits RTKs implicated in tumor growth and metastasis, including fibroblast growth factor receptors (FGFR1, 2, 3, and 4); platelet-derived growth factor receptor (PDGFRα), KIT, and RET. Currently, lenvatinib is FDA-approved for treatment of patients with locally recurrent or metastatic, progressive, radioactive iodine-refractory differentiated thyroid cancer (available online: https://www.accessdata.fda.gov/drugsatfda_docs/label/2015/206947s000lbl.pdf). In a phase III trial, the clinical efficacy of lenvatinib versus sorafenib was investigated as 1st-line treatment of unresectable HCC. In this open-label study, 954 subjects with advanced HCC and hepatic cirrhosis of Child-Pugh A were randomized to receive either lenvatinib or sorafenib as first-line therapy [16]. Results of this study show that lenvatinib produced significant improvements in PFS, TTP, and ORR (Table 7). The investigators concluded that lenvatinib is non-inferior to sorafenib in overall survival.

Table 7. Results of a phase III clinical trial to investigate lenvatinib vs sorafenib in unresectable hepatocellular carcinoma.

Outcomes	Lenvatinib	Sorafenib
Median OS (months)	13.6 HR 0.92; NS	12.3
Median PFS (months)	7.4 HR 0.66; * P < 0.00001	3.7
Median TTP (months)	8.9 HR 0.63; * P < 0.00001	3.7
ORR (%)	24 * P < 0.00001	9

HR: hazard ratio. NS, not statistically significant. ORR: overall response rate. OS: overall survival. PFS: progression-free survival. TTP: time to tumor progression. * P indicates statistical significance.

5.4. BLU-554

FGF19 stimulates proliferation of hepatocytes and induces hepatocellular carcinoma through activation of FGFR4 [17]. BLU-554 is a highly selective small molecular inhibitor of FGFR4, and FGF19 has been identified as a potential predictive biomarker of treatment response to BLU-554. A phase I clinical trial was conducted to investigate the safety and efficacy of BLU-554 in patients with advanced HCC that had been pre-treated (Table 8). This trial includes a dose-escalation phase and an expansion portion. Of the first 77 enrolled subjects being analyzed, 44 of them had FGF19-expressing (at least 1% expression) HCC. In the dose-escalation phase, the maximum-tolerated dose of 600 mg of BLU-554 daily was established. BLU-554 produced anti-tumor response in FGF19+ HCC. Patients with HCC without expression of FGF19 did not demonstrate anti-tumor response to BLU-554. [18]. This study suggests the potential use of BLU-544 as a new treatment of patients with HCC that express FGF19.

Table 8. Results of a phase I clinical trial to investigate BLU-544 in pretreated advanced hepatocellular carcinoma.

Outcomes	Result
Complete Response	1 patient
Partial Response	5 patients
Stable Disease	20 patients
Overall Response Rate	16%
Disease Control Rate	68%

While nivolumab produces efficacy in a subset of patients with advanced HCC previously treated with sorafenib, future investigation is indicated to improve the response rate conceivably by combination of nivolumab with other interventions. These may include radiation therapy, other immune checkpoint inhibitors, or chemotherapy. The clinical data showing the efficacy of ramucirumab in patients with HCC and elevated serum AFP levels appear promising. It will be worthy to determine if a combination of ramucirumab with other therapeutics active in HCC such as sorafenib or nivolumab produces enhanced therapeutic response. Considering the inhibitory activity of lenvatinib in multiple RTKs including VEGFR2 and FGFR4, it is possible that subsets of patients may particularly benefit from lenvatinib, such as those with elevated serum AFP and FGF19 + HCC (as demonstrated in the study using ramucirumab and BLU-554, respectively).

6. Biliary Tract Carcinoma

The prognosis of patients with biliary tract carcinoma (BTC) is generally poor, and effective treatment is desperately needed to improve treatment response and survival [19]. For patients who have localized BTC being surgically resected, tumors tend to recur both locally and as distant metastasis. Even when BTC is completely surgically removed (R0 resection), tumor recurrence may occur and the current standard of care is observation [20]. However, a meta-analysis indicated that adjuvant chemotherapy provides a benefit of overall survival in patients with resected BTC [21]. Moreover, for patients with radically resected extrahepatic cholangiocarcinoma and gallbladder carcinoma, adjuvant capecitabine and gemcitabine followed by capecitabine concurrent with radiation therapy was efficacious and well tolerated [22]. Recently, the results of a clinical trial that investigated the role of adjuvant capecitabine in resected BTC have been reported. Besides, for advanced or metastatic BTC, gemcitabine and cisplatin are the standard first-line treatment though with limited survival benefit [20]. The potential value of combining *nab*-paclitaxel with gemcitabine and cisplatin as first-line treatment of advanced BTC has been examined in a clinical study.

6.1. Adjuvant Capecitabine in Resected BTC

In a phase III clinical trial, the survival benefit of adjuvant capecitabine versus observation in resected BTC was investigated. In this study, 447 patients with surgical removed BTC (R0 resection) were enrolled. BTC in these patients include intrahepatic (19%), hilar (28%), extra-hepatic (35%) cholangiocarcinoma, and gallbladder carcinoma (18%) [23]. In the treatment arm, the subjects received adjuvant capecitabine 1250 mg/m^2 on day 1 through day 14 of every 21-day cycle for a total of 8 cycles. The subjects in the control arm were observed with no treatment following surgery.

Adjuvant capecitabine significantly prolonged overall survival and recurrence-free survival in resected BTC (Table 9). Results of this study suggest adjuvant capecitabine as the new standard of care for resected (R0) BTC.

Table 9. Results of a phase III clinical trial to investigate adjuvant capecitabine in resected (R0) biliary tract carcinoma.

Regimen	Capecitabine	Observation
Overall survival	51 months HR 0.75; * P = 0.028	36 months
Recurrence-free survival	25 months	18 months

HR: Hazard ratio. * P indicates statistical significance.

6.2. Combination of nab-Paclitaxel, Gemcitabine, and Cisplatin in Advanced BTC

For patients with locally advanced unresectable or metastatic BTC, palliative systemic chemotherapy using gemcitabine and cisplatin is the standard of care [20]. The clinical efficacy of the combination of nab-paclitaxel, gemcitabine, and cisplatin as 1st-line treatment of advanced BTC was investigated. In a phase II trial, a single arm of 51 patients were enrolled for treatment using nab-paclitaxel in combination with gemcitabine and cisplatin [24]. Results of this study suggest that the combination of nab-paclitaxel with gemcitabine and cisplatin may provide additional survival benefit as compared with historical control using gemcitabine and cisplatin (Table 10). A phase III clinical trial is indicated to test this hypothesis.

Table 10. Results of a phase II clinical trial to investigate nab-paclitaxel in combination with gemcitabine and cisplatin in advanced biliary tract carcinoma.

Regimen	Progression-Free Survival	Overall Survival	1-Year Survival Rate
nab-Paclitaxel + Gemcitabine + Cisplatin	11.4 months	>20 months (estimated)	66.7%
Gemcitabine + Cisplatin	8.0 months (Historical control)	11.7 months (Historical control)	-

While the phase III study results support the use of adjuvant capecitabine as the new standard of care for resected (R0) BTC, the optimal adjuvant therapy for patients with R1 or R2 resected BTC, as well as tumors with lymph nodes and/or resection margins involved by invasive carcinoma, remains to be determined. Whether the combination of nab-paclitaxel with gemcitabine and cisplatin provides superior survival benefit as compared to gemcitabine/cisplatin will need to be directly compared in a randomized, placebo-controlled clinical study. While the combination of gemcitabine and cisplatin is the current standard treatment for advanced or metastatic BTC, the roles of targeted therapy and immunotherapy in BTC remain to be explored.

7. Colorectal Carcinoma

Systemic chemotherapy and targeted therapy have been used as the standard of care for patients with colorectal carcinoma (CRC), as neoadjuvant therapy, adjuvant therapy, and palliative treatment. In this section, results of recent clinical studies investigating (i) immunotherapy (nivolumab), (ii) duration of adjuvant chemotherapy (oxaliplatin and either 5-fluorouracil or capecitabine), (iii) targeted therapy (irinotecan and cetuximab ± vemurafinib), and (iv) palliative chemotherapy (trifluridine/tipiracil and bevacizumab) are presented and discussed.

7.1. Nivolumab

Metastatic CRC with DNA mismatch repair-deficient (dMMR) or microsatellite instability-high (MSI-H) displays high levels of tumor-associated neoantigens and tumor-infiltrating lymphocytes. These pathological features suggest anti-tumor response as observed with anti-PD-1 antibodies in other types of tumors. In a multicenter, open-label, single-arm, phase II clinical trial, the therapeutic efficacy of nivolumab was investigated in patients with metastatic CRC who had progressed or been intolerant of ≥ 1 line of treatment (CheckMate 142, NCT02060188). Patients received nivolumab 3 mg/kg iv every 2 weeks until tumor progression, intolerable toxicity, death, or withdrawal from study. At a median follow-up of 12 months, 23 of 74 enrolled patients showed objective tumor response, and 51 patients had disease control for ≥ 12 weeks [25]. Results of this clinical study have led to U.S. FDA approval of nivolumab for treatment of patients with metastatic CRC with MSI-H or dMMR previously treated with chemotherapy (fluoropyrimidine and either oxaliplatin or irinotecan).

7.2. Adjuvant FOLFOX or CAPOX: 3 Months vs. 6 Months

Adjuvant chemotherapy using oxaliplatin in combination with either 5-fluorouracil or capecitabine (FOLFOX and CAPOX, respectively) for 6 months has been the standard of care for patients following surgical resection of stage III or high-risk stage II CRC. A major drawback of this treatment is that, oxaliplatin-induced neurotoxicity tends to accumulate over time and possibly become permanent.

To determine if adjuvant chemotherapy (either FOLFOX or CAPOX) for 3 months was as effective as 6 months, a global prospective study known as the International Duration Evaluation of Adjuvant therapy (IDEA) was planned. The IDEA study combined data from six concurrent, phase III clinical trials conducted in twelve countries in North America, Europe, and Asia. More than 12,800 patients were enrolled and followed for a median time of 39 months [26]. Results of the IDEA study showed that the rate of disease-free survival with a 3-month course of adjuvant chemotherapy was slightly lower as compared to the standard 6-month course, 74.6% vs. 75.5%, respectively. Moreover, in a subset of patients with low-risk colon cancer (60% of patients in the IDEA study, pT1-T3, pN1), the rates of recurrence-free survival in patients receiving a 3-month course vs a 6-month course were 83.1% and 83.3%, respectively. Besides, patients who received a 6-month course of chemotherapy experienced more side effects including fatigue, diarrhea, and neuropathy than those receiving a 3-month course. In particular, the rates of grade ≥ 2 chemotherapy-induced neuropathy for patients who received 6 months vs. 3 months of chemotherapy were 45% vs. 15% with FOLFOX, and 48% vs. 17% with CAPOX.

One of those trials in the IDEA collaboration is a non-inferiority, randomized (1:1) clinical study aimed to evaluate if 3 months of adjuvant FOLFOX or CAPOX as effective as 6 months' adjuvant chemotherapy in stage III or high-risk stage II CRC (SCOT study). In this phase III, open-label, multi-center study, 6088 patients with either stage III or high-risk stage II CRC were enrolled, 32.5% of patients received FOLFOX and 67.5% CAPOX [27]. Results of this study show that 3 months of adjuvant chemotherapy is not inferior to 6 months of treatment (Table 11).

Table 11. Results of a phase III clinical study to investigate the efficacy of 3 months vs. 6 months of adjuvant chemotherapy in surgically resected stage III or high-risk stage II colorectal carcinoma.

Outcome	3 Months of CAPOX or FOLFOX	6 Months of CAPOX or FOLFOX
DFS Events	734	735
3-Year DFS Rate (%)	76.8 HR 1.008 (95% CI 0.910–1.117) Non-inferiority, * $P = 0.014$	77.4

CAPOX: capecitabine and oxaliplatin. CI: confidence interval. DFS: disease-free survival. FOLFOX: 5-fluorouracil, leucovorin, and oxaliplatin. HR: hazard ratio. * P indicates statistical significance.

Based on these data, for low-risk disease (T1-3, N1), the recommendation for the duration of adjuvant chemotherapy is 3 months; for high-risk disease (T4 or N2 tumors), the use of shorter course of adjuvant chemotherapy should be tailored to the individual patient.

7.3. Irinotecan and Cetuximab ± Vemurafinib

Patients with metastatic CRC that carry the $BRAF^{V600}$ mutation tend to respond poorly to standard chemotherapy and/or the BRAF inhibitor vemurafenib. In vitro blockade of $BRAF^{V600}$ mutation by vemurafenib has been shown to up-regulate epidermal growth factor receptor (EGFR); a combination of the EGFR inhibitor cetuximab and irinotecan can block the EGFR-mediated signaling events. A randomized clinical study aimed to investigate a combination of irinotecan and cetuximab with or without vemurafenib in $BRAF^{V600}$-mutated metastatic CRC (SWOG S1406). In this study, 106 patients with $BRAF^{V600}$ mutated and RAS wild-type metastatic CRC were enrolled. The patients had received 1 or 2 prior chemotherapy, 39% of the patients received prior irinotecan, and none had prior anti-EGFR antibodies [28]. Addition of vemurafenib to irinotecan and cetuximab improved anti-tumor response and patient survival (Table 12). Results of this study suggest the combination of vemurafenib with cetuximab and irinotecan as a potential treatment option for patients with $BRAF^{V600}$ mutated and RAS wild-type metastatic CRC.

Table 12. Results of a clinical study to investigate the addition of vemurafenib to irinotecan and cetuximab in metastatic colorectal carcinoma with $BRAF^{V600}$ mutation and wild-type RAS.

Regimen	Vemurafenib + Irinotecan and Cetuximab	Irinotecan and Cetuximab
PFS (months)	4.4 (5.7 if no prior irinotecan)	2.0 (1.9 if no prior irinotecan)
RR (%)	16 # $P = 0.08$	4
DCR (%)	67%	22

DCR: disease control rate. PFS: progression-free survival. RR: response rate. # P indicates a trend for statistical significance.

7.4. Trifluridine/Tipiracil and Bevacizumab

Previous study has demonstrated a significant overall survival benefit of TAS-102, a combination of trifluridine and tipiracil, in patients with refractory metastatic CRC. A phase I/II, open-label, single-arm, multi-center clinical trial aimed to investigate TAS-102 in combination with bevacizumab in patients with metastatic CRC that had been refractory or intolerant to chemotherapy, anti-VEGF therapy, and anti-EGFR therapy, but had not received regorafenib. In this study, 25 patients were enrolled; 6 patients in phase 1 (dose-escalation) and 19 in phase II. The recommended phase II dose was determined for TAS-102 (35 mg/m^2 orally twice daily on days 1 to 5 and days 8 to 12 of every 28-day cycle) in combination with bevacizumab (5 mg/kg iv over 30 min every 2 weeks). Results of this study demonstrate a PFS of 42.9% (80% confidence interval 27.8 to 59.0) at 16 weeks, with myelosuppression as the most common grade 3 or 4 adverse event. The mutational statuses of RAS, TP53, APC, and PIK3CA were not associated with survival. These data suggest the combination of TAS-102 with bevacizumab as a new potential treatment option for patients with refractory metastatic CRC [29].

For patients with advanced or metastatic CRC, new therapeutic tools have become available, and new potential treatment options are underway. Since FDA's approval of nivolumab for treatment of patients with previously treated metastatic CRC with MSI-H or dMMR, molecular analysis for MSI and MMR should be routinely conducted. Any improvement of survival benefit by combination of nivolumab with other therapeutic agents is under active investigation. A 3-month course of adjuvant FOLFOX or CAPOX is expected to be the standard of care for low-risk CRC in patients who will likely benefit from reduced chemotherapy-induced toxicity, particularly peripheral neuropathy.

The combination of vemurafenib with cetuximab and irinotecan has the potential of becoming a treatment option for patients with metastatic CRC that carry $BRAF^{V600}$ mutation and wild-type RAS. The combination of trifluridine/tipiracil and bevacizumab appears an attractive option for patients with refractory metastatic CRC. A phase III clinical study to compare the efficacy and safety of this combination with the current standard treatment, and even addition of oxaliplatin or irinotecan to the combination may be considered in future investigation.

8. Conclusions and Future Perspectives

In this article, the presentations on the new development in systemic treatment of various malignant diseases in the digestive system at the Multi-Disciplinary Patient Care in Gastrointestinal Oncology Conference on 29 September 2017 are summarized. These include highlights of the recent clinical trials that investigated chemotherapy, targeted therapy, and immunotherapy in the malignant diseases of various digestive organs. Results of some of the clinical studies have led to U.S. FDA approval of nivolumab in HCC and CRC with dMMR or MSI-H, and pembrolizumab in GC/GEJC expressing PD-L1. The recent FDA's approval of pembrolizumab for treatment of solid tumors, including those in the digestive organs, that display dMMR also needs to be mentioned [30]. Peri-operative FLOT for resectable GC and GEJC, adjuvant capecitabine for resected (R0) BTC, and 3 months of adjuvant FOLFOX or CAPOX for low-risk CRC are expected to become new standard of care. Various targeted therapeutic agents, and new combinations of chemotherapy and targeted therapy demonstrate the potential of providing new treatment options for patients with cancers of the digestive system.

Author Contributions: Nelson S. Yee conceived the study, reviewed the literature, and wrote the paper.

Conflicts of Interest: The author declares no conflict of interest.

References

1. Yee, N.S.; Kazi, A.A.; Yee, R.K. Current systemic treatment and emerging therapeutic strategies in pancreatic adenocarcinoma. *Curr. Clin. Pharmacol.* **2015**, *10*, 256–266. [CrossRef] [PubMed]
2. Yee, N.S. Towards the goal of personalized therapy in pancreatic cancer by targeting the molecular phenotype. *Adv. Exp. Med. Biol.* **2013**, *779*, 91–143. [PubMed]
3. Hingorani, S.R.; Bullock, A.J.; Seery, T.E.; Zheng, L.; Sigal, D.; Ritch, P.S.; Braiteh, F.S.; Zalupski, M.; Bahary, N.; Harris, W.P.; et al. Randomized phase II study of PEGPH20 plus nab-paclitaxel/gemcitabine vs. nab-paclitaxel plus gemcitabine in patients with untreated, metastatic pancreatic ductal adenocarcinoma. *J. Clin. Oncol.* **2017**, *35*. [CrossRef]
4. Bekaii-Saab, T.S.; Starodub, A.; El-Rayes, B.F.; O'Neil, B.H.; Shahda, S.; Ciombor, K.K.; Noonan, A.M.; Hanna, W.T.; Sehdev, A.; Shaib, W.L.; et al. A phase Ib/II study of cancer stemness inhibitor napabucasin in combination with gemcitabine (gem) & nab-paclitaxel (nabPTX) in metastatic pancreatic adenocarcinoma (mPDAC) patients (pts). *Ann. Oncol.* **2017**, *28* (Suppl. S3). [CrossRef]
5. Krall, A.S.; Xu, S.; Graeber, T.G.; Braas, D.; Christofk, H.R. Asparagine promotes cancer cell proliferation through use as an amino acid exchange factor. *Nat. Commun.* **2016**, *7*, 11457. [CrossRef] [PubMed]
6. Hammel, P.; Bachet, J.B.; Portales, F.; Mineur, L.; Metges, J.P.; de la Fouchardiere, C.; Louvet, C.; El Hajbi, F.; Faroux, R.; Guimbaud, R.; et al. A phase 2b of eryaspase in combination with gemcitabine or FOLFOX as second-line therapy in patients with metastatic pancreatic adenocarcinoma. *Ann. Oncol.* **2017**, *28* (Suppl. S5), v209–v268. [CrossRef]
7. Fonkoua, L.K.; Yee, N.S. Immunotherapy in gastric carcinoma: Current status and emerging strategies. *Clin. Cancer Drugs* **2015**, *2*, 91–99. [CrossRef]
8. Al-Batran, S.E.; Homann, N.; Schmalenberg, H.; Kopp, H.G.; Haag, G.M.; Luley, K.B.; Schmiegel, W.H.; Folprecht, G.; Probst, S.; Prasnikar, N.; et al. Perioperative chemotherapy with docetaxel, oxaliplatin, and fluorouracil/leucovorin (FLOT) versus epirubicin, cisplatin, and fluorouracil or capecitabine (ECF/ECX) for resectable gastric or gastroesophageal junction (GEJ) adenocarcinoma (FLOT4-AIO): A multicenter, randomized phase 3 trial. *J. Clin. Oncol.* **2017**, *35*. [CrossRef]

9. Fuchs, C.S.; Doi, T.; Jang, R.W.; Muro, K.; Satoh, T.; Machado, M.; Sun, W.; Jalal, S.I.; Shah, M.A.; Metges, J.P.; et al. KEYNOTE-059 cohort 1: Efficacy and safety of pembrolizumab (pembro) monotherapy in patients with previously treated advanced gastric cancer. *J. Clin. Oncol.* **2017**, *35*. [CrossRef]
10. Kang, Y.K.; Satoh, T.; Ryu, M.H.; Chao, Y.; Kato, K.; Chung, H.C.; Chen, J.S.; Muro, K.; Kang, W.K.; Yoshikawa, T.; et al. Nivolumab (ONO-4538/BMS-936558) as salvage treatment after second or later-line chemother-apy for advanced gastric or gastro-esophageal junction cancer (AGC): A double-blinded, randomized, phase III trial. *J. Clin. Oncol.* **2017**, *35*. [CrossRef]
11. Janjigian, Y.Y.; Ott, P.A.; Calvo, E.; Kim, J.W.; Ascierto, P.A.; Sharma, P.; Peltola, K.J.; Jaeger, D.; Evans, T.J.; De Braud, F.G.; et al. Nivolumab ± ipilimumab in pts with advanced (adv)/metastatic chemotherapy-refractory (CTx-R) gastric (G), esophage-al (E), or gastroesophageal junction (GEJ) cancer: CheckMate 032 study. *J. Clin. Oncol.* **2017**, *35*. [CrossRef]
12. Doi, T.; Piha-Paul, S.A.; Jalal, S.I.; Saraf, S.; Lunceford, J.; Koshiji, M.; Bennouna, J. Safety and antitumor activity of the anti-programmed death-1 antibody pembrolizumab in patients with advanced esophageal carcinoma. *J. Clin. Oncol.* **2017**, *35*. [CrossRef] [PubMed]
13. Marks, E.I.; Yee, N.S. Molecular genetics and targeted therapy in hepatocellular carcinoma. *Curr. Cancer Drug Targets* **2016**, *16*, 53–70. [CrossRef] [PubMed]
14. Todd, S.C.; El-Khoueiry, A.B.; Yau, T.; Melero, I.; Sangro, B.; Kudo, M. Nivoluman in sorafenib-naïve and–experienced patients with advanced hepatocellular carcinoma: CheckMate040 Study. *J. Clin. Oncol.* **2017**, *35* (Suppl. 15), 4013.
15. Zhu, A.X.; Baron, A.D.; Malfertheiner, P.; Kudo, M.; Kawazoe, S.; Pezet, D.; Weissinger, F.; Brandi, G.; Barone, C.A.; Okusaka, T.; et al. Ramucirumab as second-line treatment in patients with advanced hepatocellular carcinoma analysis of REACH trial results by child-pugh score. *JAMA Oncol.* **2017**, *3*, 235–243. [CrossRef] [PubMed]
16. Cheng, A.L.; Finn, R.S.; Qin, S.; Han, K.H.; Ikeda, K.; Piscaglia, F.; Baron, A.D.; Park, J.W.; Han, G.; Jassem, J.; et al. Phase III trial of lenvatinib (LEN) vs. sorafenib (SOR) in first-line treatment of patients (pts) with unresectable hepatocellular carcinoma (uHCC). *J. Clin. Oncol.* **2017**, *35*. [CrossRef]
17. Wu, A.-L.; Coulter, S.; Liddle, C.; Wong, A.; Eastham-Anderson, J.; French, D.M.; Peterson, A.S.; Sonoda, J. FGF19 regulates cell proliferation, glucose and bile acid metabolism via FGFR4-dependent and independent pathways. *PLoS ONE* **2011**, *6*, e17868. [CrossRef] [PubMed]
18. Kang, Y.-K.; Macarulla, T.; Yau, T. Clinical activity of Blu-554, a potent, highly-selective FGFR4 inhibitor in advanced hepatocellular carcinoma (HCC) with FGFR4 pathway activation. Presented at 2017 ILCA Annual Conference, Seoul, Korea, 15–17 September 2017. Abstract 0-032.
19. Marks, E.I.; Yee, N.S. Molecular genetics and targeted therapeutics in biliary tract carcinoma. *World J. Gastroenterol.* **2016**, *22*, 1335–1347. [CrossRef] [PubMed]
20. Wyluda, E.; Yee, N.S. Systemic treatment of advanced biliary tract cancer: Emerging roles of targeted therapy and molecular profiling. *Clin. Cancer Drugs* **2015**, *2*, 80–86. [CrossRef]
21. Ghidini, M.; Tomasello, G.; Botticelli, A.; Barni, S.; Zabbialini, G.; Seghezzi, S.; Passalacqua, R.; Braconi, C.; Petrelli, F. Adjuvant chemotherapy for resected biliary tract cancers: A systemic review and meta-analysis. *HPB* **2017**, *19*, 741–748. [CrossRef] [PubMed]
22. Ben-Josef, E.; Guthrie, K.A.; El-Khoueiry, A.B.; Corless, C.L.; Zalupski, M.M.; Lowy, A.M.; Thomas, C.R., Jr.; Alberts, S.R.; Dawson, L.A.; Micetich, K.C.; et al. SWOG S0809: A phase II intergroup trial of adjuvant capecitabine and gemcitabine followed by radiotherapy and concurrent capecitabine in extrahepatic cholangiocarcinoma and gallbladder carcinoma. *J. Clin. Oncol.* **2015**, *33*, 2617–2622. [CrossRef] [PubMed]
23. Primrose, J.N.; Fox, R.; Palmer, D.H.; Prasad, R.; Mirza, D.; Anthoney, D.A.; Corrie, P.; Falk, S.; Wasan, H.S.; Ross, P.J.; et al. Adjuvant capecitabine for biliary tract cancer: The BILCAP randomized study. *J. Clin. Oncol.* **2017**, *35*. [CrossRef]
24. Shroff, R.T.; Borad, M.J.; Xiao, L.; Kaseb, A.O.; Varadhachary, G.R.; Wolff, R.A.; Raghav, K.P.; Iwasaki, M.; Masci, P.; Ramanathan, R.K.; et al. A phase II trial of gemcitabine (G), cisplatin (C), and nab-paclitaxel (N) in advanced biliary tract cancers (aBTCs). *J. Clin. Oncol.* **2017**, *35*. [CrossRef]
25. Overman, M.J.; McDermott, R.; Leach, J.L.; Lonardi, S.; Lenz, H.-J.; Morse, M.A.; Desai, J.; Hill, A.; Axelson, M.; Moss, R.A.; et al. Nivolumab in patients with metastatic DNA mismatch repair-deficient or microsatellite instability-high colorectal cancer (CheckMate 142): An open-label, multicenter, phase 2 study. *Lancet Oncol.* **2017**, *18*, 1182–1191. [CrossRef]

26. Shi, Q.; Sobrero, A.F.; Shields, A.F.; Yoshino, T.; Paul, J.; Taieb, J.; Sougklakos, I.; Kerr, R.; Labianca, R.; Meyerhardt, J.A.; et al. Prospective pooled analysis of six phase III trials investigating duration of adjuvant (adjuv) oxaliplatin-based therapy (3 vs. 6 months) for patients (pts) with stage III colon cancer (CC): The IDEA (International Duration Evaluation of Adjuvant chemotherapy) collaboration. *J. Clin. Oncol.* **2017**, *35*. [CrossRef]
27. Iveson, T.; Kerr, R.; Saunders, M.P.; Hollander, N.H.; Tabernero, J.; Haydon, A.M.; Glimelius, B.; Harkin, A.; Scudder, C.; Boyd, K.; et al. Final DFS results of the SCOT study: An international phase III randomized (1:1) non-inferiority trial comparing 3 versus 6 months of oxaliplatin based adjuvant chemotherapy for colorectal cancer. *J. Clin. Oncol.* **2017**, *35*. [CrossRef]
28. Kopetz, S.; McDonough, S.L.; Lenz, H.J.; Magliocco, A.M.; Atreya, C.E.; Diaz, L.A.; Allegra, C.J.; Raghav, K.P.; Morris, V.K.; Wang, S.E.; et al. Randomized trial of irinotecan and cetuximab with or without vemurafenib in BRAF-mutant metastatic colorectal cancer (SWOG S1406). *J. Clin. Oncol.* **2017**, *35*. [CrossRef]
29. Kuboki, Y.; Nishina, T.; Shinozaki, E.; Yamazaki, K.; Shitara, K.; Okamoto, W.; Kajiwara, T.; Matsumoto, T.; Tsushima, T.; Mochizuki, N.; et al. TAS-102 plus bevacizumab for patients with metastatic colorectal cancer refractory to standard therapies (C-TASK FORCE): An investigator-initiated, open-label, single-arm, multicenter, phase 1/2 study. *Lancet Oncol.* **2017**, *18*, 1172–1181. [CrossRef]
30. Le, D.T.; Durham, J.N.; Smith, K.N.; Wang, H.; Bartlett, B.R.; Aulakh, L.K.; Lu, S.; Kemberling, H.; Wilt, C.; Luber, B.S.; et al. Mismatch repair deficiency predicts response of solid tumors to PD-1 blockade. *Science* **2017**, *357*, 409–413. [CrossRef] [PubMed]

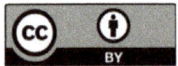

© 2018 by the author. Licensee MDPI, Basel, Switzerland. This article is an open access article distributed under the terms and conditions of the Creative Commons Attribution (CC BY) license (http://creativecommons.org/licenses/by/4.0/).

MDPI
St. Alban-Anlage 66
4052 Basel
Switzerland
Tel. +41 61 683 77 34
Fax +41 61 302 89 18
www.mdpi.com

Biomedicines Editorial Office
E-mail: biomedicines@mdpi.com
www.mdpi.com/journal/biomedicines

www.ingramcontent.com/pod-product-compliance
Lightning Source LLC
LaVergne TN
LVHW071956080526
838202LV00064B/6759